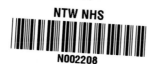

Manual of Botulinum Toxin Therapy
Second Edition

Manual of Botulinum Toxin Therapy

Second Edition

Daniel Truong
The Parkinson and Movement Disorder Institute, Orange Coast Memorial Medical Center, Fountain Valley, CA, USA

Mark Hallett
Department of Neurology, The George Washington University School of Medicine and Health Sciences, Washington, DC, USA

Christopher Zachary
Department of Dermatology, University of California, Irvine, Irvine, CA, USA

Dirk Dressler
Movement Disorders Section, Department of Neurology, Hannover Medical School, Hannover, Germany

Medical Illustration: Mayank Pathak

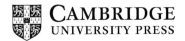
CAMBRIDGE
UNIVERSITY PRESS

CAMBRIDGE
UNIVERSITY PRESS

University Printing House, Cambridge CB2 8BS, United Kingdom

Cambridge University Press is part of the University of Cambridge.

It furthers the University's mission by disseminating knowledge in the pursuit of education, learning, and research at the highest international levels of excellence.

www.cambridge.org
Information on this title: www.cambridge.org/9781107025356

© Cambridge University Press 2013

First published 2013
1st edition 2009
Reprinted 2014

Printed in the United States of America by Sheridan Books Inc.

A catalog record for this publication is available from the British Library

Library of Congress Cataloging in Publication data
Manual of botulinum toxin therapy / [edited by] Daniel Truong . . . [et al.]. – 2nd ed.
 p. ; cm.
Includes bibliographical references and index.
ISBN 978-1-107-02535-6 (hardback)
I. Truong, Daniel, M. D.
[DNLM: 1. Botulinum Toxins – therapeutic use.   2. Neuromuscular Agents – therapeutic use.   3. Botulinum Toxins –
pharmacology.   4. Movement Disorders – drug therapy.   5. Neuromuscular Diseases – drug therapy. QV 140]
RL120.B66
615′.778–dc23

2013014807

ISBN 978-1-107-02535-6 Hardback

To my wife, Diane Truong and my children, Karl, Christian, and Gianni, whose love I cherish; to Norman Seiden, whose idealism I adore; and for Thomas Collins, for whose support I am grateful

Daniel Truong

To my wife and family and to the patients whose participation in research helps to move knowledge forward

Mark Hallett

To my wife Janellen, and to my children Laura, George, Cameron, Tague and Alexa, all of whom make my life so entertaining

Christopher Zachary

I am most grateful to my colleagues for their discussions, my patients for their encouragement and most of all to my wife, Doctor Fereshte Adib Saberi, for her professional and emotional support

Dirk Dressler

Contents

Contents

Contributors

Katharine E. Alter
Mount Washington Pediatric Hospital, Baltimore, MD, USA

Vito Annese
University Hospital, Careggi, Department of Medical and Surgical Sciences, Gastroenterology, SOD2, Florence, Italy

Alfredo Berardelli
Department of Neurology and Psychiatry, Sapienza University of Rome, Rome, Italy

Roongroj Bhidayasiri
Chulalongkorn Center of Excellence on Parkinson's Disease and Related Disorders, Faculty of Medicine, Chulalongkorn University Hospital, Bangkok, Thailand

Hans Bigalke
Institute of Toxicology, Hannover Medical School, Hannover, Germany

Allison Brashear
Department of Neurology, Wake Forest University Baptist Medical Center, Winston-Salem, NC, USA

Stefano Carda
Department of Clinical Neuroscience Service of Neuropsychology and Neurorehabilitation, Lausanne University Hospital, Lausanne, Switzerland

Francisco Cardoso
Departament of Clinical Medine, Universidade Federal de Minas Gerais Belo Horizonte, Minas Gerais, Brazil

Carlo Colosimo
Department of Neurology and Psychiatry, Sapienza University of Rome, Rome, Italy

Cynthia L. Comella
Department of Neurological Sciences, Rush University Medical Center, Chicago, IL, USA

Chandi Das
Neurology Department, Canberra Hospital, Garren Act Health, ACT, Australia

José De Andrés
Department of Surgical Specialties, Valencia School of Medicine and Anesthesia Department of Anesthesiology, Critical Care and Pain Management, Valencia University General Hospital, Valencia, Spain

Dirk Dressler
Movement Disorder Section, Department of Neurology, Hannover Medical School, Hannover, Germany

Frank J. Erbguth
Department of Neurology, Nuremberg Municipal Academic Hospital, Nuremberg, Germany

Gustavo Fabregat
Department of Surgical Specialties, Valencia School of Medicine and Department of Anesthesiology, Critical Care and Pain Management, Valencia University General Hospital, Valencia, Spain

Pietro Fiore
Department of Physical Medicine and Rehabilitation, "Policlinico Hospital" Bari and University of Foggia, Foggia, Italy

Loren M. Fishman
Department of Rehabilitation and Regenerative Medicine, Columbia College of Physicians and Surgeons, New York, USA

Karen Frei
The Parkinson and Movement Disorder Institute, Orange Coast Memorial Center, Fountain Valley, CA, USA

Jürgen Frevert
Institute of Toxicology, Hannover Medical School, Hannover, Germany

Holger G. Gassner
Department of Otolaryngology, University of Regensburg, Regensburg, Germany

Dee Anna Glaser
Department of Dermatology, Saint Louis University School of Medicine, St. Louis, MO, USA

H. Kerr Graham
University of Melbourne, Royal Children's Hospital, Parkville, Victoria, Australia

Daniele Gui
Department of Surgery, Università Cattolica del Sacro Cuore, Policlinico "A. Gemelli", Rome, Italy

Mark Hallett
Department of Neurology, The George Washington University School of Medicine and Health Sciences, Washington, DC, USA

Henning Hamm
Department of Dermatology, University of Würzburg, Würzburg, Germany

Chaur-Jong Hu
Department of Neurology, Shuang-Ho Hospital, Taipei Medical University, New Taipei City, Taiwan

Oleg Olegovich Ivanov
Department of Neurology for Stroke Patients, City Clinical Hospital Number 1, Novokuznetsk, Russia

Bahman Jabbari
Department of Neurology, Yale University School of Medicine, New Haven, CT, USA

Joseph Jankovic
Parkinson's Disease Center and Movement Disorder Clinic, Department of Neurology, Baylor College of Medicine, Houston, TX, USA

Barbara Illowsky Karp
Combined NeuroScience IRB, National Institute of Neurological Disorders and Stroke, National Institutes of Health, Bethesda, MD, USA

Rainer Laskawi
Department of Otolaryngology, Head and Neck Surgery, University of Göttingen, Göttingen, Germany

Shivam Om Mittal
Department of Neurology, Case Western Reserve University, Cleveland, OH, USA

Franco Molteni
Valduce Hospital, Villa Beretta, Rehabilitation Center, Costa Masnaga, Lecco, Italy

Markus K. Naumann
Department of Neurology, Augsburg Hospital, Augsburg, Germany

Michael W. Neumeister
Department of Plastic Surgery, Southern Illinois University School of Medicine, Carbondale, IL, USA

Arno Olthoff
Department of Phoniatrics and Pediatric Audiology, University of Göttingen, Göttingen, Germany

Mayank S. Pathak
The Parkinson and Movement Disorder Institute, Orange Coast Memorial Medical Center, Fountain Valley, CA, USA

Gerhard Reichel
Center for Movement Disorders, Clinic Paracelsus, Zwickau, Germany

Diana Richardson
Department of Neurology, Yale University School of Medicine, New Haven, CT, USA

Peter Roggenkamper
Department of Ophthalmology, University of Bonn, Bonn, Germany

Andrea Santamato
Department of Physical Medicine and Rehabilitation, "OORR" Hospital, University of Foggia, Foggia, Italy

Sarah B. Schmidhofer
Department of Psychiatry, Warren Alpert Medical School, Brown University, Providence, RI, USA.

Brigitte Schurch
Department of Clinical Neuroscience, Service of Neuropsychology and Neurorehabilitation, Lausanne University Hospital, Lausanne, Switzerland

Alan Scott
Strabismus Research Institute, San Francisco, CA, USA

Stephen D. Silberstein
Jefferson Headache Center, Thomas Jefferson University, Philadelphia, PA, USA

Jasvinder A. Singh
Department of Medicine, University of Alabama at Birmingham, Birmingham, AL, USA, and Mayo Clinic College of Medicine, Rochester, MN, USA

Joshua Spanogle
Department of Dermatology, University of California, Irvine, Irvine, CA, USA

Ann Tilton
Louisiana State University Health Sciences Center, New Orleans, LA, USA

Dorina Tiple
Dipartimento di Biologia Cellulare Neuroscienze, Istituto Superiore di Sanita, Roma, Italy

Daniel Truong
The Parkinson and Movement Disorder Institute, Orange Coast Memorial Medical Center, Fountain Valley, CA, USA

Kelli Webb
Department of Plastic Surgery, Southern Illinois University School of Medicine, Carbondale, IL, USA

Bettina Westhoff
Department of Orthopaedics, Heinrich-Heine-University Hospital, Duesseldorf, Germany

Szu-Kuan Yang
Department of Neurology, Shuang-Ho Hospital, Taipei Medical University, New Taipei City, Taiwan

Christopher Zachary
Department of Dermatology, University of California, Irvine, Irvine, CA, USA

Preface

The clinical use of botulinum neurotoxin comes into its third decade of existence with many new off-label indications for a host of different medical conditions. Originally used specifically for strabismus, blepharospasm and spasmodic torticollis, botulinum neurotoxin is now commonly employed in diverse disciplines by many specialists. Its unique properties requires local application for efficacy ... and while this is relatively simple in some locations such as the skin and superficial muscles of the face, it is much more complicated in others, at times requiring ultrasound guidance or endoscopic assistance. Not all neurotoxins are the same and, therefore, an in-depth understanding of their pharmacological actions, limitations and complications is required.

This book tries to answer many of the questions posed above with the contributions from a team of international experts. As in the first edition, the emphasis in this book is on technique, so it is richly endowed with illustrations concerning accurate access techniques to help physicians to become familiar and fully competent.

The readers will find instruction and discussion about widely accepted treatments, and others that are less known. While some treatments will gain wide acceptance, others may be passing fads, and we recommend that the readers evaluate them critically. We hope that the book will serve as teaching aid for the beginner, and a practical resource for the advanced user.

We are grateful to the contributors of this book and trust that physicians who employ botulinum neurotoxin in their practices will find it valuable.

We thank Michael Tsao, Mary Ann Chapman and Lisa Brauer for their assistance; Dr Hiep Truong for drawing some of the pictures. We also express our appreciation to our families and friends for their support and understanding during the preparation of this book.

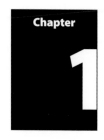

The pretherapeutic history of botulinum neurotoxin

Frank J. Erbguth

Unintended intoxication with botulinum neurotoxin (botulism) occurs only rarely, but its high fatality rate makes it a great concern for the general public and the medical community. In the USA, an average of 110 cases of botulism are reported each year. Of these, approximately 25% are food borne, 72% are infant botulism and the rest are wound botulism. Outbreaks of food-borne botulism involving two or more persons occur most years and are usually caused by eating contaminated home-canned foods.

Botulism in ancient times

Botulinum neurotoxin poisoning probably has afflicted humankind through the mists of time. As long as humans have preserved and stored food, some of the chosen conditions would be optimal for the presence and growth of the toxin-producing pathogen *Clostridium botulinum*: for example, the storage of ham in barrels of brine, poorly dried and stored herring, trout packed to ferment in willow baskets, sturgeon roe not yet salted and piled in heaps on old horsehides, lightly smoked fish or ham in poorly heated smoking chambers and insufficiently boiled blood sausages.

However, in ancient times there was no general knowledge about the causal relationship between the consumption of spoiled food and a subsequent fatal paralytic disease, nowadays recognized as botulism. Only some historical sources reflect a potential understanding of the life-threatening effects of consuming food intoxicated with botulinum neurotoxin. Louis Smith, for example, reported in his textbook on botulism a dietary edict announced in the tenth century by Emperor Leo VI of Byzantium (886–911), in which manufacturing of blood sausages was forbidden (Smith, 1977). This edict may have its origin in the recognition of some circumstances connected with

cases of food poisoning. Also, some ancient formulae suggested by shamans to Indian maharajas for the killing of personal enemies give hint of an intended lethal application of botulinum neurotoxin: a tasteless powder extracted from blood sausages dried under anaerobic conditions should be added to the enemies' food at an invited banquet. Because the consumer's death occurred after he or she had left the murderer's place, with a latency of some days, the host was probably not suspected (Erbguth, 2008).

Botulism outbreaks in Germany in the eighteenth and nineteenth centuries

Accurate descriptions of botulism emerge in the German literature from two centuries ago when the consumption of improperly preserved or stored meat and blood sausages gave rise to many deaths throughout the kingdom of Württemberg in southwestern Germany. This area near the city of Stuttgart developed as the regional focus of botulinum toxin investigations in the eighteenth and nineteenth centuries. In 1793, 13 people were involved in the first well-recorded outbreak of botulism in the small southwest German village of Wildbad; six died. Based on the observed mydriasis in all affected victims, the first official medical speculation was that the outbreak was caused by an atropine (*Atropa belladonna*) intoxication. However, in the controversial scientific discussion, the term "sausage poison" was introduced by the exponents of the opinion that the fatal disease in Wildbad was caused by the consumption of "Blunzen," a popular local food from cooked pork stomach filled with blood and spices.

The number of cases of suspected sausage poisoning in southwestern Germany increased rapidly at the end of the eighteenth century. Poverty followed the

Manual of Botulinum Toxin Therapy, 2nd edition, ed. Daniel Truong, Mark Hallett, Christopher Zachary and Dirk Dressler.
Published by Cambridge University Press. © Cambridge University Press 2013.

devastating Napoleonic Wars (1795–1813) and led to the neglect of sanitary measures in rural food production (Grüsser, 1986). In July 1802, the Royal Government of Württemberg in Stuttgart issued a public warning about the "harmful consumption of smoked blood-sausages." In August 1811, the medical section of the Department of Internal Affairs of the Kingdom of Württemberg, on Stuttgart again, addressed the problem of "sausage poisoning," considering it to be caused by hydrocyanic acid, known at that time as "prussic acid." However, the members of the nearby Medical Faculty of the University of Tübingen disputed that prussic acid could be the toxic agent in sausages, suspecting a biological poison. One of the important medical professors of the University of Tübingen, Johann Heinrich Ferdinand Autenrieth (1772–1835), asked the government to collect the reports of general practitioners and health officers on cases of food poisoning for systematic scientific analyses. After Autenrieth had studied these reports, he issued a list of symptoms of the so-called "sausage poisoning" and added a comment, in which he blamed the housewives for the poisoning because they did not dunk the sausages long enough in boiling water while trying to prevent the sausages from bursting (Grüsser, 1998). The list of symptoms was distributed by a public announcement and contained characteristic features of food-borne botulism such as gastrointestinal problems, double vision, mydriasis and muscle paralysis.

In 1815, a health officer in the village of Herrenberg, J. G. Steinbuch (1770–1818), sent the case reports of seven intoxicated patients who had eaten liver sausage and peas to Professor Autenrieth. Three of the patients had died and the autopsies had been carried out by Steinbuch himself (Steinbuch, 1817).

Justinus Kerner's observations and publications on botulinum toxin 1817–1822

Contemporaneously with Steinbuch, the 29-year-old physician and Romantic poet Justinus Kerner (1786–1862) (Fig. 1.1), then medical officer in a small village, also reported a lethal food poisoning. Autenrieth considered the two reports from Steinbuch and Kerner as accurate and important observations and decided to publish them both in 1817 in the *Tübinger Blätter für Naturwissenschaften und Arzneykunde* [*Tübinger*

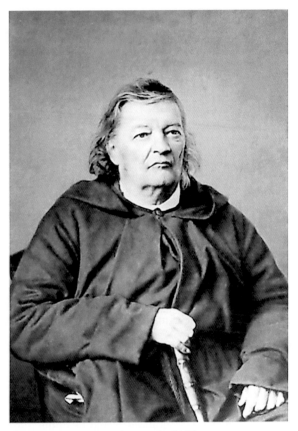

Fig. 1.1 Justinus Kerner; photograph of 1855.

Papers for Natural Sciences and Pharmacology] (Kerner, 1817; Steinbuch, 1817).

Kerner again disputed that an inorganic agent such as hydrocyanic acid could be the toxic agent in the sausages, suspecting a biological poison instead. After he had observed further cases, Kerner published a first monograph in 1820 on "sausage poisoning" in which he summarized the case histories of 76 patients and gave a complete clinical description of what we now recognize as botulism. The monograph was entitled "*Neue Beobachtungen über die in Württemberg so häufig vorfallenden tödlichen Vergiftungen durch den Genuss geräucherter Würste* [*New Observations on the Lethal Poisoning that occurs so frequently in Württemberg Owing to the Consumption of Smoked Sausages*] (Kerner, 1820). Kerner compared the various recipes and ingredients of all sausages that had produced intoxication and found that among the ingredients of blood, liver, meat, brain, fat, salt, pepper, coriander, pimento, ginger and bread the only common ones were fat and salt. Because salt was probably known to be "innocent," Kerner concluded that the toxic change in the sausage must take place in the fat and, therefore, called the suspected substance "sausage poison," "fat poison" or "fatty acid." Later Kerner speculated about the similarity of the "fat poison" to other known poisons, such as atropine, scopolamine, nicotine and snake venom, which led him to the conclusion that the fat poison was probably a biological poison (Erbguth, 2004).

In 1822, Kerner published 155 case reports including autopsy studies of patients with botulism and developed hypotheses on the "sausage poison" in a second monograph *Das Fettgift oder die Fettsäure und ihre Wirkungen auf den thierischen Organismus, ein Beytrag zur Untersuchung des in verdorbenen Würsten giftig wirkenden Stoffes* [The Fat Poison or the Fatty Acid and its Effects on the Animal Body System, a Contribution to the Examination of the Substance Responsible for the Toxicity of Bad Sausages] (Kerner, 1822) (Fig. 1.2). The monograph

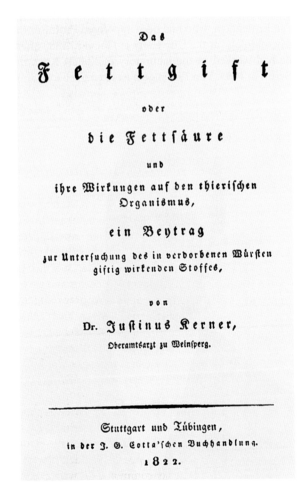

Fig. 1.2 Title of Justinus Kerner's second monograph on sausage poisoning, 1822.

contained an accurate description of all muscle symptoms and clinical details of the entire range of autonomic disturbances occurring in botulism, such as mydriasis, decrease of lacrimation and secretion from the salivary glands, and gastrointestinal and bladder paralysis. Kerner also experimented on various animals (birds, cats, rabbits, frogs, flies, locusts, snails) by feeding them with extracts from bad sausages and finally carried out high-risk experiments on himself. After he had tasted some drops of a sausage extract he reported: "...some drops of the acid brought onto the tongue cause great drying out of the palate and the pharynx" (Erbguth and Naumann, 1999).

Kerner deduced from the clinical symptoms and his experimental observations that the toxin acts by interrupting the motor and autonomic nervous signal transmission (Erbguth, 1996). He concluded: "The nerve conduction is brought by the toxin into a condition in which its influence on the chemical process of life is interrupted. The capacity of nerve conduction is interrupted by the toxin in the same way as in an electrical conductor by rust" (Kerner, 1820). Finally, Kerner tried in vain to produce an artificial "sausage poison."

In summary, Kerner's hypotheses concerning "sausage poison" were that (1) the toxin developed in bad sausages under anaerobic conditions, (2) the toxin acts on the motor nerves and the autonomic nervous system, and (3) the toxin is strong and lethal even in small doses (Erbguth and Naumann, 1999).

In Chapter 8 of the 1822 monograph, Kerner speculated about using the "toxic fatty acid" botulinum toxin for therapeutic purposes. He concluded that small doses would be beneficial in conditions with pathological hyperexcitability of the nervous system (Erbguth, 2004). Kerner wrote: "The fatty acid or zoonic acid administered in such doses, that its action could be restricted to the sphere of the sympathetic nervous system only, could be of benefit in the many diseases which originate from hyperexcitation of this system" and "by analogy it can be expected that in outbreaks of sweat, perhaps also in mucous hypersecretion, the fatty acid will be of therapeutic value." The term "sympathetic nervous system" as used during the Romantic period, encompassed nervous functions in general. "Sympathetic overactivity" then was thought to be the cause of many internal, neurological and psychiatric diseases. Kerner favored the "Veitstanz" (St. Vitus dance – probably identical with chorea minor) with its "overexcited nervous ganglia" to be a promising indication for the therapeutic use of the toxic fatty acid. Likewise, he considered other diseases with assumed nervous overactivity to be potential candidates for the toxin treatment: hypersecretion of body fluids, sweat or mucus; ulcers from malignant diseases; skin alterations after burning; delusions; rabies; plague; consumption from lung tuberculosis; and yellow-fever. However, Kerner conceded self-critically that all the possible indications mentioned were only hypothetical and wrote: "What is said here about the fatty acid as a therapeutic drug belongs to the realm of hypothesis and may be confirmed or disproved by observations in the future" (Erbguth, 1998).

Justinus Kerner also advanced the idea of a gastric tube, suggested by the Scottish physician Alexander Monro in 1811, and adapted it for the nutrition of patients with botulism; he wrote: "if dysphagia occurs, softly prepared food and fluids should be brought into the stomach by a flexible tube made from resin." He considered all characteristics of modern nasogastric tube application: the use of a guide wire with a cork at the tip and the lubrication of the tube with oil.

Botulism research after Kerner

After his publications on food-borne botulism, Kerner was well known to the German public and amongst his contemporaries as an expert on sausage poisoning, as well as for his melancholy poetry. Many of his poems were set to music by the great German Romantic composer Robert Schumann (1810–56), who had to quit his piano career because of the development of a pianist's focal finger dystonia. Kerner's poem *The Wanderer in the Sawmill* was the favourite poem of the twentieth century poet Franz Kafka (in full in Appendix 1.1). The nickname "Sausage Kerner" was commonly used and "sausage poisoning" was known as "Kerner's disease." Further publications in the nineteenth century by various authors (e.g. Müller, 1869) increased the number of reported cases of "sausage poisoning," describing the fact that the food poisoning occurred after the consumption not only of meat but also of fish. However, these reports added nothing substantial to Kerner's early observations. The term "botulism" (from the Latin *botulus*, sausage) appeared at first in Müller's reports and was subsequently used. Therefore, "botulism" refers to poisoning caused by sausages and not to the sausage-like shape of the causative bacillus discovered later (Torrens, 1998).

The discovery of *"Bacillus botulinus"* in Belgium

The next and most important scientific step was the identification of *Clostridium botulinum* in 1895–6 by the Belgian microbiologist Emile Pierre Marie van Ermengem of the University of Ghent (Fig. 1.3).

On December 14, 1895, an extraordinary outbreak of botulism occurred amongst the 4000 inhabitants of the small Belgian village of Ellezelles. The musicians of the local brass band "Fanfare Les Amis Réunis" played at the funeral of the 87-year-old Antoine Creteur and as it was the custom gathered to eat in the inn "Le Rustic" (Devriese, 1999). Thirty-four people were together and ate pickled and smoked ham. After the meal, the musicians noticed symptoms such as mydriasis, diplopia, dysphagia and dysarthria, followed by increasing muscle paralysis. Three of them died and ten nearly died. A detailed examination of the ham and an autopsy were ordered and conducted by van Ermengem, who had been appointed Professor of Microbiology at the University of Ghent in 1888 after he had worked in the laboratory of Robert Koch in Berlin in 1883. Van Ermengem isolated the bacterium

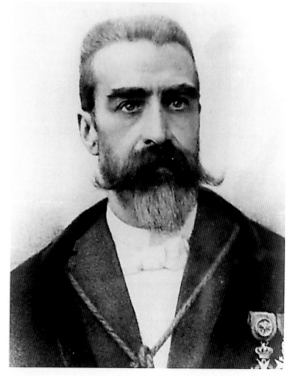

Fig. 1.3 Emile Pierre Marie van Ermengem 1851–1922.

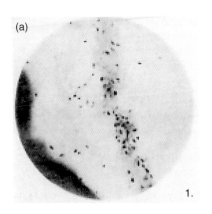
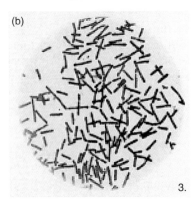

Fig. 1.4 Microscopy of the histological section of the suspect ham at the Ellezelles botulism outbreak. (a) Numerous spores among the muscle fibers (Ziehl ×1000). (b) Culture (gelatine and glucose) of mature rod-shaped forms of "Bacillus botulinus" from the ham on the eighth day (×1000). (From van Ermengem, 1897.)

in the ham and in the corpses of the victims (Fig. 1.4), grew it, used it for animal experiments, characterized its culture requirements, described its toxin, called it "Bacillus botulinus," and published his observations in the German microbiological journal *Zeitschrift für Hygiene und Infektionskrankheiten* [*Journal of Hygiene and Infectious Diseases*] in 1897 (an English translation was published in 1979) (van Ermengem, 1897). The pathogen was later renamed *Clostridium botulinum*. Van Ermengem was the first to correlate "sausage poisoning" with the newly discovered anaerobic microorganism and concluded that "it is highly probable that the poison in the ham was produced by an anaerobic growth of specific micro-organisms during the salting process." Van Ermengem's milestone investigation yielded all the major clinical facts about botulism and botulinum neurotoxin: (1) botulism is an intoxication, not an infection; (2) the toxin is produced in food by a bacterium; (3) the toxin is not produced if the salt concentration in the food is high; (4) after ingestion, the toxin is not inactivated by the normal digestive process; (5) the toxin is susceptible to inactivation by heat; and (6) not all species of animals are equally susceptible.

Botulinum neurotoxin research in the early twentieth century

In 1904, when an outbreak of botulism in the city of Darmstadt, Germany, was caused by canned white beans, the opinion that the only botulinogenic foods were meat or fish had to be revised. The bacteria isolated from the beans by Landmann (1904) and from the Ellezelles ham were compared by Leuchs (Leuchs, 1910) at the Royal Institute of Infectious Diseases in Berlin. He found that the strains differed and the toxins were serologically distinct. The two types of Bacillus botulinus did not receive their present letter designations of serological subtypes until Georgina Burke, who worked at Stanford University, designated them as types A and B (Burke, 1919). Over the next decades, increases in food canning and food-borne botulism went hand in hand (Cherington, 2004). The first documented outbreak of food-borne botulism in the USA was caused by commercially conserved pork and beans and dates from 1906 (Drachmann, 1971; Smith, 1977). Techniques for killing the spores during the canning process were subsequently developed. The correct pH (<4.0), the osmolarity needed to prevent clostridial growth and toxin production, and the requirements for toxin inactivation by heating were defined.

In 1922, type C was identified in the USA by Bengston and in Australia by Seddon; type D and type E were characterized some years later (type D in the USA in 1928 by Meyer and Gunnison; type E in the Ukraine 1936 by Bier) (Kriek and Odendaal, 1994; Geiges, 2002). Type F and type G toxins were identified in 1960 in Scandinavia by Moller and Scheibel and in 1970 in Argentina by Gimenex and Ciccarelli (Gunn, 1979; Geiges, 2002). In 1949, Burgen and his colleagues in London discovered that botulinum toxin blocked the release of acetylcholine at neuromuscular junctions (Burgen *et al.*, 1949). The essential insights into the molecular actions of botulinum toxin were gained by various scientists after 1970 (Dolly *et al.*, 1990; Schiavo *et al.*, 1992, 1993; Dong *et al.*, 2006; Mahrhold *et al.*, 2006), when its use as a therapeutic agent was pioneered by Edward J. Schantz and Alan B. Scott.

Until the last century, botulism was thought to be caused exclusively by food that was contaminated with preformed toxin. This view has changed since the 1950s, as spores of *C. botulinum* were discovered in contaminated wounds (wound botulism) in the 1950s and in the intestines of babies in 1976 (infant botulism) (Merson and Dowell, 1973; Pickett *et al.*, 1976; Arnon *et al.*, 1977). The number of cases of food-borne and infant botulism has changed little in recent years, but wound botulism has increased because of the use of black-tar heroin, especially in California.

Swords to ploughshares

Before the therapeutic potential of botulinum neurotoxin was discovered, around 1970, its potential use as a weapon was recognized during World War I (Lamb, 2001). The basis for its use as a toxin was investigations by Hermann Sommer and colleagues working at the Hooper Foundation, University of California, San Francisco in the 1920s: the researchers were the first to isolate pure botulinum neurotoxin type A as a stable acid precipitate (Snipe and Sommer, 1928; Schantz, 1994). With the outbreak of World War II, the USA Government began intensive research into biological weapons, including botulinum toxin, particularly in the laboratory at Camp Detrick (later named Fort Detrick) in Maryland. Development of concentration and crystallization techniques at Fort Detrick was pioneered by Carl Lamanna and James Duff in 1946. The methodology was subsequently used by Edward J. Schantz to produce the first batch of toxin, which was the basis for the later clinical product (Lamanna *et al.*, 1946). The entrance of botulinum toxin into the medical therapeutic armamentarium in Europe also came from military laboratories to hospitals: in the UK, botulinum toxin research was conducted in the Porton Down laboratories of the military section of the Centre for Applied Microbiology and Research (CAMR), which later provided British clinicians with a therapeutic formulation of the toxin (Hambleton *et al.*, 1981).

Appendix *The Wanderer in the Sawmill* (Justinus Kerner 1826)

Down yonder in the sawmill
I sat in good repose
and saw the wheels go spinning
and watched the water too.

I saw the shiny saw blade,
as if I had a dream,
which carved a lengthy furrow
into a fir tree trunk.

The fir tree as if living,
in saddest melody,
through all its trembling fibres
sang out these words for me:

At just the proper hour,
o wanderer! you come,
it's you for whom this wounding
invades my heart inside.

It's you, for whom soon will be,
when wanderings cut short,
these boards in earth's deep bosom,
a box for lengthy rest.

Four boards I then saw falling,
my heart was turned to stone,
one word I would have stammered,
the blade went round no more.

References

Arnon SS, Midura TF, Clay SA, Wood RM, Chin J (1977). Infant botulism: epidemiological, clinical and laboratory aspects. *JAMA*, **237**, 1946–51.

Burgen A, Dickens F, Zatman, L (1949). The action of botulinum toxin on the neuromuscular junction. *J Physiol*, **109**, 10–24.

Burke GS (1919). The occurrence of Bacillus botulinus in nature. *J Bacteriol*, **4**, 541–53.

Cherington, M (2004). Botulism: update and review. *Semin Neurol*, **24**, 155–63.

Devriese PP (1999). On the discovery of *Clostridium botulinum*. *J Hist Neurosci*, **8**, 43–50.

Dolly JO, Ashton AC, McInnes, C *et al.* (1990). Clues to the multi-phasic inhibitory action of botulinum neurotoxins on release of transmitters. *J Physiol*, **84**, 237–46.

Dong M, Yeh F, Tepp WH *et al.* (2006). SV2 is the protein receptor for botulinum neurotoxin A. *Science*, **312**, 592–6.

Drachmann DB (1971). Botulinum toxin as a tool for research on the nervous system. In Simpson LL (ed.) *Neuropoisons: Their Pathophysiology Actions*, Vol. 1. New York: Plenum Press, pp. 325–47.

Erbguth, F (1996). Historical note on the therapeutic use of botulinum toxin in neurological disorders. *J Neurol Neurosurg Psychiatry*, **60**, 151.

Erbguth, F (1998). Botulinum toxin, a historical note. *Lancet*, **351**, 1280.

Erbguth FJ (2004). Historical notes on botulism, *Clostridium botulinum*, botulinum toxin, and the idea of the therapeutic use of the toxin. *Mov Disord*, **19**(Suppl 8), S2–6.

Erbguth FJ (2008). From poison to remedy: the chequered history of botulinum toxin. *J Neural Transm*, **115**, 559–65.

Erbguth F, Naumann, M (1999). Historical aspects of botulinum toxin: Justinus Kerner (1786–1862) and the "sausage poison." *Neurology*, **53**, 1850–3.

Geiges ML (2002). The history of botulism. In Kreyden OP, Böne R, Burg G (eds.) *Current Problems in Dermatology*, Vol. 30: *Hyperhidrosis and Botulinum Toxin in Dermatology*. Basel: Karger, pp. 77–93.

Grüsser OJ (1986). Die ersten systematischen Beschreibungen und tierexperimentellen Untersuchungen des Botulismus. Zum 200. Geburtstag von Justinus Kerner am 18. September 1986. *Sudhoffs Arch*, **10**, 167–87.

Grüsser OJ (1998). Der "Wurstkerner". Justinus Kerners Beitrag zur Erforschung des Botulismus. In H. Schott (ed.) *Justinus Kerner als Azt und Seelenforscher*, 2nd edn. Weinsberg: Justinus Kerner Verein, pp. 232–56.

Gunn RA (1979). Botulism: from van Ermengem to the present. A comment. *Rev Infect Dis*, **1**, 720–1.

Hambleton P, Capel B, Bailey N, Tse CK, Dolly O (1981). Production, purification and toxoiding of *Clostridium botulinum* A toxin. In Lewis G (ed.) *Biomedical Aspects of Botulism*. New York: Academic Press, pp. 247–60.

Kerner J (1817). Vergiftung durch verdorbene Würste. *Tübinger Blätter für Naturwissenschaften und Arzneykunde*, **3**, 1–25.

Kerner J (1820). *Neue Beobachtungen über die in Württemberg so häufig vorfallenden tödlichen Vergiftungen durch den Genuss geräucherter Würste. [New Observations on the Lethal Poisoning that occurs so frequently in Württemberg Owing to the Consumption of Smoked Sausages.]* Tübingen: Osiander.

Kerner J (1822). *Das Fettgift oder die Fettsäure und ihre Wirkungen auf den thierischen Organismus, ein Beytrag zur Untersuchung des in verdorbenen Würsten giftig wirkenden Stoffes. [The Fat Poison or the Fatty Acid and its Effects on the Animal Body System, a Contribution to the Examination of the Substance Responsible for the Toxicity of Bad Sausages.].* Tübingen: Cotta.

Kriek NPJ, Odendaal MW (1994). Botulism. In Coetzer JAW, Thomson GR, Tustin RC (eds.) *Infectious Diseases of Livestock*. Cape Town: Oxford University Press, pp. 1354–71.

Lamanna C, Eklund HW, McElroy OE (1946). Botulinum toxin (type A); including a study of shaking with chloroform as a step in the isolation procedure. *J Bacteriol*, **52**, 1–13.

Lamb A (2001). Biological weapons: the facts not the fiction. *Clin Med*, **1**, 502–4.

Landmann G (1904). Über die Ursache der Darmstädter Bohnenvergiftung. *Hyg Rundschau*, **10**, 449–52.

Leuchs J (1910). Beiträge zur Kenntnis des Toxins und Antitoxins des Bacillus botulinus. *Z Hyg Infektionskrankh*, **65**, 55–84.

Mahrhold S, Rummel A, Bigalke H, Davletov B, Binz T (2006). The synaptic vesicle protein 2C mediates the uptake of botulinum neurotoxin A into phrenic nerves. *FEBS Lett*, **580**, 2011–14.

Merson MH, Dowell J (1973). Epidemiologic, clinical and laboratory aspects of wound botulism. *N Engl J Med*, **289**, 1105–10.

Müller H (1869). *Das Wurstgift*. Deutsche Klinik, pulserial publication, **35**, 321–3, 37, 341–3, 39, 357–9, 40, 365–7, 381–3, 49, 453–5.

Pickett J, Berg B, Chaplin E, Brunstetter-Shafer MA (1976). Syndrome of botulism in infancy: clinical and electrophysiologic study. *N Engl J Med*, **295**, 770–2.

Schantz EJ (1994). Historical perspective. In Jankovic J, Hallett M (eds.) *Therapy with Botulinum Toxin*. New York: Marcel Dekker, pp. xxiii–vi.

Schiavo G, Benfenati F, Poulain B *et al.* (1992). Tetanus and botulinum-B toxins block transmitter release by proteolytic cleavage of synaptobrevin. *Nature*, **359**, 832–5.

Schiavo G, Cantucci A, Das Gupta BR *et al.* (1993). Botulinum neurotoxin serotypes A and E cleave SNAP-25 at distinct COOH-terminal peptide bonds. *FEBS Lett*, **335**, 99–103.

Smith LD (1977). *Botulism. The Organism, its Toxins, the Disease*. Springfield, IL: Charles C Thomas.

Snipe PT, Sommer H (1928). Studies on botulinus toxin. 3. Acid preparation of botulinus toxin. *J Infect Dis*, **43**, 152–60.

Steinbuch JG (1817). Vergiftung durch verdorbene Würste. *Tübinger Blätter für Naturwissenschaften und Arzneykunde*, **3**, 26–52.

Torrens JK (1998). *Clostridium botulinum* was named because of association with "sausage poisoning." *BMJ*, **316**, 151.

van Ermengem EP (1897). Über einen neuen anaeroben Bacillus und seine Beziehung zum Botulismus. *Z Hyg Infektionskrankh*, **26**, 1–56 (English version: Van Ermengem EP (1979). A new anaerobic bacillus and its relation to botulism. *Rev Infect Dis*, **1**, 701–19).

Botulinum neurotoxin: history of clinical development

Daniel Truong and Mark Hallett

The clinical development of botulinum neurotoxin began in the late 1960s with the search for an alternative to surgical realignment of strabismus. At that time, surgery of the extraocular muscles was the primary treatment for strabismus, but it was unsatisfactory for some patients because of the variability in results, consequent high reoperation rates and its invasive nature. In an attempt to find an alternative, Alan B. Scott, an ophthalmologist from the Smith–Kettlewell Eye Research Institute in San Francisco, investigated the effects of different compounds injected locally into the extraocular muscles to chemically weaken them. The drugs tested initially proved unreliable, short acting or necrotizing (Scott *et al.*, 1973).

About this time, Scott became aware of Daniel Drachman, a renowned neuroscientist at Johns Hopkins University and his work, in which he had been injecting minute amounts of botulinum neurotoxin directly into the hind limbs of chickens to achieve local denervation (Drachman, 1964). Drachman introduced Scott to Edward Schantz (1908–2005), who was producing purified botulinum neurotoxins for experimental use and generously making them available to the academic community. Schantz himself credits Vernon Brooks with the idea that botulinum neurotoxin might be used for weakening muscle (Schantz, 1994). Brooks worked on the mechanism of action of botulinum toxin for his PhD under the mentorship of Arnold Burgen, who suggested the project to him (Brooks, 2001). Schantz had left the US Army Chemical Corps at Fort Detrick, Maryland, in 1972 to work at the Department of Microbiology and Toxicology, University of Wisconsin in Madison. Using acid precipitation purification techniques worked out at Fort Detrick by Lamanna and Duff, Schantz was able to make purified botulinum toxins.

In extensive animal experiments, low doses of botulinum neurotoxin produced the desired long-lasting, localized, dose-dependent muscle weakening, reportedly without any systemic toxicity and without any necrotizing side effects (Scott *et al.*, 1973). Based on these results, the US Food and Drug Administration (FDA) permitted Scott in 1977 to test botulinum neurotoxin in humans under an Investigational New Drug (IND) license for the treatment of strabismus. These tests proved successful and the results of 67 injections were published in 1980 (Scott, 1980). With this publication, botulinum neurotoxin was established as a novel therapeutic. Scott approached several drug companies to take the drug on and manufacture it. However, he had disclosed the drug in earlier publications and thus could not get it patented. Without this, none of the manufacturers would undertake it. Scott then moved the activity from Smith–Kettlewell, setting up his own company, Oculinum, in Berkeley California. Dennis Honeychurch, a pharmacist, joined him and devised many of the tests for safety, potency, stability, sterility and water retention in the freeze-dried product that were required before botulinum toxin could be registered as a drug by the FDA. In addition to establishing a laboratory for testing and record keeping, a sterile facility for filling and freeze-drying was required. This was found at Adria Labs in Albuquerque, where Scott and Honeychurch went several times a year to fill 8000–10 000 vials.

Some time in the 1960s, Robert Crone, a professor of ophthalmology in Amsterdam, whose interest was in strabismus, was able to get the Porton group to send him dried toxin from the UK, with the idea of use in strabismus. The package was damaged, and dried toxin leaked out – probably enough to kill all of Amsterdam (A. Scott, personal communication)! Crone decided not to pursue it further. By the early 1980s, Scott and

---

Manual of Botulinum Toxin Therapy, 2nd edition, ed. Daniel Truong, Mark Hallett, Christopher Zachary and Dirk Dressler.
Published by Cambridge University Press. © Cambridge University Press 2013.

colleagues had injected botulinum neurotoxin for the treatment of strabismus, blepharospasm, hemifacial spasm, cervical dystonia and thigh adductor spasm (Scott, 1994). Prior to FDA approval, the neurotoxin was made available to a group of investigators for research, including Calne, Dykstra, Fahn, Hallett, Jankovic, Roggenkamper, Tanner and Truong. Stanley Fahn's group at Columbia University reported in 1985 the first double-blind study testing Scott's toxin in improving the symptoms of blepharospasm (Fahn *et al.*, 1985). Also in 1985, Tsui and colleagues reported the successful use of botulinum neurotoxin for treatment of cervical dystonia in 12 patients based on earlier dosage data from Scott's injections (Tsui *et al.*, 1985). This was followed by the first double-blind, crossover study in which botulinum neurotoxin was significantly superior to placebo at reducing the symptoms of cervical dystonia, including pain (Tsui *et al.*, 1986). Therapeutic use of botulinum neurotoxin for the treatment of blepharospasm and hemifacial spasm proceeded along similar lines, with several groups reporting success for these indications by the mid 1980s and documenting the benefits of repeated injections after the effects waned (Frueh *et al.*, 1984; Mauriello, 1985; Scott *et al.*, 1985). Brin *et al.* (1987) reported on use of Scott's toxin to treat multiple dystonias (e.g. cranial, cervical, laryngeal, limb) and related hyperkinetic disorders. Reports of the successful use of botulinum neurotoxin in many conditions of focal muscle overactivity continued, including spasmodic dysphonia (Blitzer *et al.*, 1986; Truong *et al.*, 1991), oromandibular dystonia (Jankovic and Orman, 1987), dystonias of the hand (Cohen *et al.*, 1989) and limb spasticity (Das and Park, 1989). Soon, botulinum neurotoxin was accepted as safe and efficacious for blepharospasm, cervical dystonia and other focal dystonias, and was the treatment of choice for some indications (National Institutes of Health, 1991).

In December 1989, the FDA licensed the manufacturing facilities and batch 79–11 of botulinum neurotoxin type A, manufactured by Scott and Schantz in November 1979. The therapeutic preparation contained 100 mouse units of neurotoxin per vial. A mouse unit was defined as the LD_{50} for Swiss Webster mice. Scott named this drug Oculinum (**ocu** and **lin**ing-up) and it was recognized as an orphan drug for the treatment of strabismus, hemifacial spasm and blepharospasm. According to Scott (personal communication), he asked FDA to approve 88–4, a four times more potent batch for which he had ample data. However, the FDA required the use of 79–11 in the USA because it was used for generating most of the clinical data on which approval was based. Some European regulatory agencies accepted 88–4 with the initial filings. All current neurotoxins have greater specific potency than 79–11 and are equal to or better than 88–4. For about 2 years, Scott's Oculinum Inc. was the licensed manufacturer, with Allergan Inc. (Irvine, CA, USA) the sole distributor. Manufacturing rights and license were acquired by Allergan in late 1991; a different batch of Botox was distributed in 1998. This and subsequent batches of Botox contained less protein per unit, which may have made them less liable to elicit antibodies than the original 79–11.

The name Botox was perhaps first used by Stanley Fahn and Mitchell Brin, who did not think of it as a possible trade name. Around 1985, Scott trademarked the name B-botox for the type B neurotoxin that he studied. Finding type B was inferior to type A, he abandoned it and also the name. "Botox" is a name readily derived from laboratory lingo for toxins, probably newly invented several times prior to Allergan's use (A. Scott, personal communication). The non-proprietary name is now onabotulinumtoxinA.

In 2000, a product containing the botulinum neurotoxin B serotype, NeuroBloc/MyoBloc, was registered with the FDA by Elan Pharmaceuticals (South San Francisco, CA, USA) with the indication of cervical dystonia. MyoBloc is the trade name in the USA and NeuroBloc is the trade name used elsewhere. The name NeuroBloc was coined by Mitchell Brin and MyoBloc by Lloyd Glenn (Elan). The initial research on botulinum toxin B was carried out by Tsui, Truong and O'Brien. MyoBloc was eventually sold to Solstice Neurosciences Inc. (Malvern, PA, USA) and recently to US WorldMeds (Louisville, KY, USA). The non-proprietary name is rimabotulinumtoxinB. Botox was also approved for cervical dystonia in 2000.

In Europe, botulinum neurotoxin was first produced for therapeutic purposes at the Defence Science and Technology Laboratory in Porton Down, UK. When commercialized, manufacturing operations were renamed several times – to Centre of Applied Microbiology and Research (CAMR), Porton Products, Public Health Laboratory Service (PHLS) and Speywood Pharmaceuticals. In 1994, Speywood Pharmaceuticals was acquired by Ipsen (Paris, France). The UK botulinum neurotoxin product was first registered in 1991 as

Dysport (**dys**tonia **Port**on Products; non-proprietary name now abobotulinumtoxinA). It is manufactured for worldwide use by Ipsen (Slough, UK). It was approved in the USA for cervical dystonia and glabellar facial wrinkles in April 2009. It was first used to treat strabismus and blepharospasm in the UK not long after Scott's initial reports (Elston 1985; Elston *et al.*, 1985). The movement disorders group of C. David Marsden at the National Hospital of Neurology and Neurosurgery, London pioneered its use in neurology (Stell *et al.*, 1988). Soon afterwards, Dirk Dressler, a student of Marsden, introduced this product (Dysport) to continental European neurology (Dressler *et al.*, 1989). However, it was Roggenkamper who personally carried botulinum neurotoxin (Oculinum) that he received from Alan Scott to Germany and who initiated investigations in patients with blepharospasm (Roggenkamper, 1986). A flabbergasted German custom officer waved Roggenkamper with his hand-carried botulinum neurotoxin into Germany without even looking as he perceived Roggenkamper's declaration as a joke (Roggenkamper, personal communication). More details about the expansion of botulinum neurotoxin therapy in continental European are described by Homann *et al.* (2002).

Subsequently, another botulinum neurotoxin drug named Xeomin (incobotulinumtoxinA) was marketed by Merz Pharmaceuticals (Frankfurt/M, Germany). It is a botulinum neurotoxin type A preparation with high specific biological activity and, as a consequence, a reduced protein load (Dressler and Benecke, 2006). Structurally, it is free of the complexing botulinum neurotoxin proteins. It is currently approved in most European countries, USA, Canada, some middle and South American countries, as well as several Asian countries. Besides blepharospasm, cervical dystonia and glabellar lines, it is also approved for spasticity and some other indications depending on the country.

An additional source of therapeutic botulinum neurotoxin type A is the Lanzhou Institute of Biological Products (Lanzhou, Gansu Province, China), where the manufacturing expertise comes from Wang Yinchun, a former collaborator of Schantz. Wang used the protocol for acid precipitation of the crystalline toxin from the cultures worked out at the Army Chemical Laboratories at Fort Detrick (A. Scott, personal communication). Its product was registered as Hengli in China in 1993. In some other Asian and South American markets, it is distributed as CBTX-A, Redux or Prosigne. The international

marketing is provided by Hugh Source International Ltd (Kowloon, Hong Kong). Registration of this product in the USA and in Europe seems unlikely. Publications about this product are scarce.

In South Korea and some other Asian countries, Neuronox, a botulinum neurotoxin type A drug manufactured by Medy-Tox (Ochang, South Korea), is distributed. Other botulinum neurotoxin drugs are under development at Tokushima University, Tokushima City, Japan and at the Mentor Corporation (Santa Barbara, CA, USA).

Over the years that these other products were developed, the clinical applications for botulinum neurotoxin continued to expand. Botox, which has most indications, was further approved by the FDA for glabellar rhytides in 2002 and for primary axillary hyperhidrosis in 2004. In 2010, Botox was approved for chronic migraine and upper limb spasticity in adults, in 2011 for the treatment of neurogenic detrusor overactivity and in 2013 for overactive bladder. Off-label use by physicians is widespread and includes tremor, anal fissure, achalasia, various conditions of pain and others (Dressler, 2000; Moore and Naumann, 2003; Truong and Jost, 2006). Outside the USA, there are at least 20 indications in 83 countries. Numerous formal therapeutic trials for registration are in progress. The use of Botox for wrinkles has been very popular and is perhaps the indication best known by general public.

These expanded uses were paralleled by increased understanding of the mechanism of action of botulinum neurotoxins from basic research (Lalli *et al.*, 2003). The multistep mechanism of action postulated by Simpson (1979) was verified, and research on botulinum neurotoxin has itself contributed much to the understanding of vesicular neurotransmitter release. It has also been demonstrated that botulinum neurotoxin, which was once believed to exert its activity solely on cholinergic neurons, can, under certain conditions, inhibit the evoked release of several other neurotransmitters (Welch *et al.*, 2000; Durham *et al.*, 2004). These discoveries continue to intrigue basic scientists and clinicians alike, as the therapeutic uses and applications of botulinum neurotoxin appear destined to increase still further in the years to come.

Acknowledgment

Some historical information was provided by Mitchell F. Brin, MD (Allergan, Irvine, CA, USA).

References

Blitzer A, Brin MF, Fahn S, Lange D, Lovelace RE (1986). Botulinum toxin (BOTOX) for the treatment of "spastic dysphonia" as part of a trial of toxin injections for the treatment of other cranial dystonias. *Laryngoscope*, **96**, 1300–1.

Brin MF, Fahn S, Moskowitz C *et al.* (1987). Localized injections of botulinum toxin for the treatment of focal dystonia and hemifacial spasm. *Mov Disord*, **2**, 237–54.

Brooks V (2001). Vernon Brooks. In Squire LR (ed). *The History of Neuroscience in Autobiography,* Vol. 3. New York: Academic Press, pp. 76–116.

Cohen LG, Hallett M, Geller BD, Hochberg F (1989). Treatment of focal dystonias of the hand with botulinum toxin injections. *J Neurol Neurosurg Psychiatry*, **52**, 355–63.

Das TK, Park DM (1989). Effect of treatment with botulinum toxin on spasticity. *Postgrad Med J*, **65**, 208–10.

Drachman DB (1964). Atrophy of skeletal muscle in chick embryos treated with botulinum toxin. *Science.* **145**, 719–21.

Dressler D (2000). *Botulinum Toxin Therapy*. Stuttgart: Thieme-Verlag.

Dressler D, Benecke R (2006). Xeomin eine neue therapeutische Botulinum Toxin Typ A-Präparation. *Akt Neurol*, **33**, 138–41.

Dressler D, Benecke R, Conrad B (1989). Botulinum Toxin in der Therapie kraniozervikaler Dystonien. *Nervenarzt*, **60**, 386–93.

Durham PL, Cady R, Cady R (2004). Regulation of calcitonin gene-related peptide secretion from trigeminal nerve cells by botulinum toxin type A: implications for migraine therapy. *Headache*, **44**, 35–42.

Elston JS (1985). The use of botulinum toxin A in the treatment of strabismus. *Trans Ophthalmol Soc UK*, **104**, 208–10.

Elston JS, Lee JP, Powell CM, Hogg C, Clark P (1985). Treatment of strabismus in adults with botulinum toxin A. *Br J Ophthalmol*, **69**, 718–24.

Fahn S, List T, Moskowitz CB *et al.* (1985). Double-blind controlled study of botulinum toxin for blepharospasm. *Neurology*, **35**(Suppl 1), 271.

Frueh BR, Felt DP, Wojno TH, Musch DC (1984). Treatment of blepharospasm with botulinum toxin. A preliminary report. *Arch Ophthalmol*, **102**, 1464–8.

Homann CN, Wenzel K, Kriechbaum N *et al.* (2002). Botulinum Toxin: Die Dosis macht das Gift. Ein historischer Abriß. *Nervenheilkunde*, **73**, 519–24.

Jankovic J, Orman J (1987). Botulinum A toxin for cranial-cervical dystonia: a double-blind, placebo-controlled study. *Neurology*, **37**, 616–23.

Lalli G, Bohnert S, Deinhardt K, Verastegui C, Schiavo G (2003). The journey of tetanus and botulinum neurotoxins in neurons. *Trends Microbiol*, **11**, 431–437.

Mauriello JA Jr. (1985). Blepharospasm, Meige syndrome, and hemifacial spasm: treatment with botulinum toxin. *Neurology*, **35**, 1499–500.

Moore P, Naumann M (2003). *Handbook of Botulinum Toxin Treatment,* 2nd edn. Malden, MA: Blackwell Science.

National Institutes of Health (1991). National Institutes of Health Consensus Development Conference. Clinical use of botulinum toxin. National Institutes of Health Consensus Development Statement, November 12–14, 1990. *Arch Neurol*, **48**, 1294–8.

Roggenkamper P (1986). [Blepharospasm treatment with botulinum toxin (follow-up).] *Klin Monbl Augenheilkd*, **189**, 283–5.

Schantz EJ (1994). Historical perspective. In Jankovic J, Hallett M (eds). *Therapy with Botulinum Toxin*. New York: Marcel Dekker, pp. xxiii–xxvi.

Scott AB (1980). Botulinum toxin injection into extraocular muscles as an alternative to strabismus surgery. *Ophthalmology*, **87**, 1044–9.

Scott AB (1994). Foreword. In Jankovic J, Hallett M (eds.) *Therapy with Botulinum Toxin*. New York: Marcel Dekker, pp. vii–ix.

Scott AB, Rosenbaum A, Collins CC (1973). Pharmacologic weakening of extraocular muscles. *Invest Ophthalmol*, **12**, 924–7.

Scott AB, Kennedy RA, Stubbs HA (1985). Botulinum A toxin injection as a treatment for blepharospasm. *Arch Ophthalmol*, **103**, 347–50.

Simpson LL (1979). The action of botulinal toxin. *Rev Infect Dis*, **1**, 656–62.

Stell R, Thompson PD, Marsden CD (1988). Botulinum toxin in spasmodic torticollis. *J Neurol Neurosurg Psychiatry*, **51**, 920–3.

Truong DD, Jost WH (2006). Botulinum toxin: clinical use. *Parkinsonism Relat Disord*, **12**, 331–55.

Truong DD, Rontal M, Rolnick M, Aronson AE, Mistura K (1991). Double-blind controlled study of botulinum toxin in adductor spasmodic dysphonia. *Laryngoscope*, **101**, 630–4.

Tsui JK, Eisen A, Mak E *et al.* (1985). A pilot study on the use of botulinum toxin in spasmodic torticollis. *Can J Neurol Sci*, **12**, 314–16.

Tsui JK, Eisen A, Stoessl AJ, Calne S, Calne DB (1986). Double-blind study of botulinum toxin in spasmodic torticollis. *Lancet*, **ii**, 245–7.

Welch MJ, Purkiss JR, Foster KA (2000). Sensitivity of embryonic rat dorsal root ganglia neurons to *Clostridium botulinum* neurotoxins. *Toxicon*, **38**, 245–58.

Pharmacology of botulinum neurotoxins

Daniel Truong and Mark Hallett

Introduction

Botulinum neurotoxins (BoNTs) are proteins derived from the bacterium *Clostridium botulinum* that have been formulated as drug products for clinical use. These biologics are typically injected into muscles where they act locally to inhibit the release of acetylcholine at the neuromuscular junction. Botulinum neurotoxins can also act on cholinergic autonomic terminals following injection into smooth muscle, where they inhibit contractions, or nearby glands, where they inhibit glandular secretions. Additionally, they can inhibit release of inflammatory peptides at pain endings.

Synthesis and structure

C. botulinum produces BoNTs as protein complexes that contain non-toxin hemagglutinin and non-hemagglutinin proteins in addition to the neurotoxin itself. The type and number of non-toxin proteins are determined by the strain of the bacteria, and these proteins form complexes with the neurotoxin that range in molecular weight from approximately 300 kDa to approximately 900 kDa (Sakaguchi *et al.*, 1984). Seven different BoNTs serotypes are produced by different clostridial strains, A, B, C_1, D, E, F and G. Only types A and B are commercially available; types C and F have been tried in humans on an experimental basis only.

The BoNT is synthesized as a single protein chain with a molecular weight of approximately 150 kDa and has little biological activity. Proteases cleave this single chain into a light chain of approximately 50 kDa and a heavy chain of approximately 100 kDa, linked together by a disulfide bond. It is this two-chain molecule that exhibits biological activity.

Mechanism of action

When injected into the body, BoNTs exert their biological activity through a multistep mechanism that was first described in the late 1970s and early 1980s (Simpson, 1981) and has been elaborated over the years. The heavy chain portion of the neurotoxin protein contains the domain that binds to gangliosides on neuronal membranes. This first binding step enables a second step in which the BoNT binds to a synaptic vesicle protein that is exposed during vesicular neurotransmitter release (Dong *et al.*, 2006). The BoNT is then internalized into the cytoplasm of the neuron within the vesicle.

Once the endosome is inside the cytosol, the BoNT molecule undergoes a conformational change in response to acidification in the endosome and chemical gradient changes across its membrane (Montal, 2009). The heavy chain then forms a channel in the endosomal membrane that enables the light chain to enter the cytosol. Botulinum neurotoxin light chains are zinc endopeptidases that interact with one or more of the proteins that form the vesicular neurotransmitter release complex. These SNARE proteins (soluble *N*-ethylmalemide sensitive factor attachment receptor) include synaptosomal associated protein-25 (SNAP-25), synaptobrevin and syntaxin.

Each BoNT serotype acts at a specific site on one or more of the SNARE proteins. Serotypes A, C_1 and E target SNAP-25, whereas serotypes B, D, F and G target synaptobrevin (also known as vesicle-associated membrane protein-2 [VAMP-2]). Serotype C_1 also targets syntaxin. Without these proteins, the SNARE complex does not form properly and vesicular neurotransmitter release is inhibited. This manifests clinically as reduced muscular contractions or decreased glandular secretion.

Manual of Botulinum Toxin Therapy, 2nd edition, ed. Daniel Truong, Mark Hallett, Christopher Zachary and Dirk Dressler. Published by Cambridge University Press. © Cambridge University Press 2013.

The effects of BoNTs are not permanent but reverse over time in response to neuronal sprouting forming transient new synapses and an eventual recovery of neurotransmitter release in the original terminals (de Paiva *et al.*, 1999). The clinical duration of action of BoNTs is approximately 3 to 4 months when injected into striated muscle and may be several months longer when injected into smooth muscle for the treatment of overactive bladder or into a sudomotor region for the treatment of hyperhidrosis. Duration of action also varies with the BoNT serotype (Foran *et al.*, 2003).

Clinical pharmacology

Botulinum neurotoxin products

Several different BoNT products are approved for clinical use, with the specific indications varying based on country or region and each supported by its own set of data. As is typical for biologics, doses for all BoNT products are expressed as units of biological activity. However, no international standard exists for botulinum neurotoxins and units are not interchangeable among products. In the USA, each of these products has a unique non-proprietary name. Although there are seven different BoNT serotypes, types A and B have been the most consistently studied and all of the commercially available products are based on one of these two serotypes. The most widely used BoNT products are shown in Table 3.1.

Onset and duration of action

Clinical effects of BoNTs develop gradually and are typically evident within a week of injection (Moore and Naumann, 2003). As noted previously, duration of action is approximately 3 to 4 months when administered into skeletal muscle and patients typically request reinjection around this time. Longer durations may be seen following injection into autonomic terminal regions, as in the case of overactive bladder and axillary hyperhidrosis.

Once the effects wear off, BoNTs may be reinjected and many patients with neurological conditions receive repeated BoNT treatment for years or decades. The response is typically maintained over many years (Lungu *et al.*, 2011), although the injected muscles may need to be altered in response to changes in the pattern of muscle activity over time (Gelb *et al.*, 1991).

Immunogenicity

As with most protein therapies, there is the potential for antibody formation with BoNT therapy. The extremely small amounts of BoNT protein needed to produce a biological effect likely help to minimize immunogenicity, but patients occasionally develop antibodies over time. Neutralizing antibodies can interfere with the clinical effects of BoNT (Brin *et al.*, 2008) and patients may need to switch to a different serotype or different therapy altogether. Neutralizing antibody development may be influenced by the dose/amount of BoNT complex, frequency of injections,

Table 3.1 Summary of different commercial botulinum neurotoxin products

	Botox	Dysport	Xeomin	NeuroBloc/MyoBloc
Non-proprietary name (USA)	OnabotulinumtoxinA	AbobotulinumtoxinA	IncobotulinumtoxinA	RimabotulinumtoxinB
Serotype	A	A	A	B
Product format	Vacuum-dried powder	Lyophilized powder	Lyophilized powder	Buffered solution
SNARE protein target	SNAP-25	SNAP-25	SNAP-25	Synaptobrevin (VAMP-2)
Neurotoxin protein complex size	~900 kDa	Not formally reported	~150 kDa neurotoxin without associated proteins	~700 kDa
Excipients	HSA, sodium chloride	HSA, lactose	HSA, sucrose	HSA, sodium chloride, sodium succinate

HSA, human serum albumin; SNAP-25, synaptosomal associated protein-25; VAMP-2, vesicle-associated membrane protein-2.

and choice of BoNT product, as well as by individual factors that have not been well characterized.

Before concluding that a patient's non-response is caused by neutralizing antibodies, however, it may be prudent to consider other factors. Administrative errors, muscle selection, product storage or reconstitution errors, expectation effects or emotional/social factors related to the underlying physical illness may all influence clinical response (Moore and Naumann, 2003). Given these possibilities, some experts recommend that another injection cycle be tried at the same dose in patients who experience a reduced response, provided that side effects were not intolerable (Moore and Naumann, 2003). While there are serological tests available for antibodies, the best way to check is functionally with small injections into sites where the effect should be obvious. These sites include the unilateral brow, the extensor digitorum brevis muscle in the foot and the abductor digiti minimi in the hand.

Adverse events

In general, BoNT injections are well tolerated and show acceptable safety across a wide range of conditions and disorders (Naumann and Jankovic, 2004; Brin et al., 2009). The most frequent adverse events are local weaknesses in nearby muscles, and these tend to be mild or moderate in severity (Naumann and Jankovic, 2004). However, severe adverse events do occasionally occur with BoNTs and, therefore, it is always advisable to follow injection guidelines for each individual product and not to exceed the upper recommended doses for the product.

Because BoNTs have local actions within the injected regions, they do not typically interact with systemic medications. This is an advantage for all patients but particularly for those who are taking multiple medications to treat multisymptom conditions such as poststroke neurological damage.

All BoNT serotype A drugs have similar adverse effect profiles. The adverse effect profile of the BoNT serotype B drug (rimabotulinumtoxinB) is slightly different. The type B drug frequently produces autonomic adverse effects, including dryness of mouth (Dressler and Benecke, 2003); however, the frequency of motor adverse effects is similar after types A and B. Type B may have an advantage over type A in the treatment of autonomic disorders such as sialorrhea.

Future developments

The development of BoNT products is proceeding along several lines. First, manufacturers of current products are conducting clinical trials to expand the conditions for which they are indicated or approved in various regions of the world. The commonality among all of these conditions is that a focal reduction in cholinergic tone is beneficial. The exception to this rule may be the use of BoNTs for various conditions of pain, which is supported by preclinical evidence that BoNT serotype A inhibits the release of pain-related neurochemicals such as substance P and calcitonin gene-related peptide (Purkiss et al., 2000; Durham et al., 2004).

A second development is the increase in the number of different BoNT products. In addition to the products outlined in Table 3.1, which are all available in many countries worldwide, a number of other products are only available in certain regions, such as China. The lucrative facial esthetic market has also spurred the availability of counterfeit toxins, which are not approved in any country but are available via the Internet. It is important to note that these products have not undergone the necessary safety and biological activity testing required of approved products and, therefore, may be dangerous. Indeed, a 2006 report described four patients who received a highly concentrated, unlicensed BoNT preparation for cosmetic purposes (Chertow et al., 2006). These patients experienced serious side effects, illustrating the importance of using only licensed products at recommended doses.

A third path of BoNT development is the modification of the toxin molecule. For example, some scientists are attempting to engineer proteins that retain the endopeptidase activity of the toxin but possess an altered binding domain, such that the BoNT shows specificity for a different type of cell (Chen, 2012). The altered binding domain may also be coupled with a modified light chain designed to cleave non-neuronal SNARE proteins such as SNAP-23, which plays a role in the secretion of airway mucus in asthma (Chen, 2012). It is clear from these studies that much remains to be learned and gleaned from this interesting neurotoxin.

References

Brin MF, Comella CL, Jankovic J, Lai F, Naumann M (2008). Long-term treatment with botulinum toxin type A in cervical dystonia has low immunogenicity by mouse protection assay. *Mov Disord*, **23**, 1353–60.

Brin MF, Boodhoo TI, Pogoda JM *et al.* (2009). Safety and tolerability of onabotulinumtoxinA in the treatment of facial lines: a meta-analysis of individual patient data from global clinical registration studies in 1678 participants. *J Am Acad Dermatol*, **61**, 961–70.

Chen S (2012). Clinical uses of botulinum neurotoxins: current indications, limitations and future developments. *Toxins*, **4**, 913–39.

Chertow DS, Tan ET, Maslanka SE *et al.* (2006). Botulism in 4 adults following cosmetic injections with an unlicensed, highly concentrated botulinum preparation. *JAMA*, **296**, 2476–9.

de Paiva A, Meunier FA, Molgo J, Aoki KR, Dolly JO (1999). Functional repair of motor endplates after botulinum neurotoxin type A poisoning: biphasic switch of synaptic activity between nerve sprouts and their parent terminals. *Proc Natl Acad Sci USA*, **96**, 3200–5.

Dong M, Yeh F, Tepp WH *et al.* (2006). SV2 is the protein receptor for botulinum neurotoxin A. *Science*, **312**, 592–6.

Dressler D, Benecke R (2003). Autonomic side effects of botulinum toxin type B treatment of cervical dystonia and hyperhidrosis. *Eur Neurol*, **49**, 34–8.

Durham PL, Cady R, Cady R (2004). Regulation of calcitonin gene-related peptide secretion from trigeminal nerve cells by botulinum toxin type A: implications for migraine therapy. *Headache*, **44**, 35–42; discussion 42–3.

Foran PG, Mohammed N, Lisk GO *et al.* (2003). Evaluation of the therapeutic usefulness of botulinum neurotoxin B, C1, E, and F compared with the long lasting type A. Basis for distinct durations of inhibition of exocytosis in central neurons. *J Biol Chem*, **278**, 1363–71.

Gelb DJ, Yoshimura DM, Olney RK, Lowenstein DH, Aminoff MJ (1991). Change in pattern of muscle activity following botulinum toxin injections for torticollis. *Ann Neurol*, **29**, 370–6.

Lungu C, Karp BI, Alter K, Zolbrod R, Hallett M (2011). Long-term follow-up of botulinum toxin therapy for focal hand dystonia: outcome at 10 years or more. *Mov Disord*, **26**, 750–3.

Montal M (2009). Translocation of botulinum neurotoxin light chain protease by the heavy chain protein-conducting channel. *Toxicon*, **54**, 565–9.

Moore P, Naumann M (2003). General and clinical aspects of treatment with botulinum toxin. In Moore P, Naumann M (eds.) *Handbook of Botulinum Toxin Treatment*, 2nd edn. Malden, MA: Blackwell Science, pp. 28–75.

Naumann M, Jankovic J (2004). Safety of botulinum toxin type A: a systematic review and meta-analysis. *Curr Med Res Opin*, **20**, 981–90.

Purkiss J, Welch M, Doward S, Foster K (2000). Capsaicin-stimulated release of substance P from cultured dorsal root ganglion neurons: involvement of two distinct mechanisms. *Biochem Pharmacol*, **59**, 1403–6.

Sakaguchi G, Kozaki S, Ohishi, I (1984). Structure and function of botulinum toxins. In Aiouf JE (ed.) *Bacterial Protein Toxins*. London: Academic Press, pp. 435–43.

Simpson LL (1981). The origin, structure, and pharmacological activity of botulinum toxin. *Pharmacol Rev*, **33**, 155–88.

Chapter 4

Immunological properties of botulinum neurotoxins

Hans Bigalke, Dirk Dressler and Jürgen Frevert

Introduction

Botulinum neurotoxins (BoNTs) are used to treat a large number of muscle hyperactivity disorders including dystonia, spasticity, tremor and autonomic disorders (e.g. hyperhidrosis and hypersalivation), as well as facial wrinkles. Commercially available products differ with respect to serotype, formulation and purity. Not all products are approved in all countries. Serotype A-containing products are Botox (onabotulinumtoxinA), Dysport (abobotulinumtoxinA) and Xeomin (incobotulinumtoxinA), whereas NeuroBloc/ MyoBloc (rimabotulinumtoxinB) contains serotype B. The active ingredient in all products is BoNT, a two-chain protein with a molecular weight of 150 kDa. BoNT type A (BoNT-A) inhibits release of the neurotransmitter acetylcholine by cleaving synaptosomal associated protein-25, a SNARE protein, while BoNT type B (BoNT-B) cleaves synaptobrevin (vesicle-associated membrane protein-2).

Since BoNTs are foreign proteins, the human immune system may respond to them with the production of specific anti-BoNT antibodies. The probability of developing such antibodies increases with the BoNT doses applied (Göschel et al., 1997; Lange et al., 2009). Whether other drug-related factors might contribute to immune responses is discussed below. Patient-related factors may also be involved in triggering antibody formation to BoNT. Recently, a patient was reported who was treated with abobotulinumtoxinA for several years with good results until he developed anti-BoNT-induced therapy failure after he received BoNT following a wasp sting (Paus et al., 2006). Since components of wasp poison are effective immunostimulants, a preactivation of lymphocytes may have triggered antibody formation against BoNT-A. In the following, a method is

presented for the quantification of anti-BoNT in sera; the immune cell reactions to antigens are described and drug-related immune responses are discussed.

Detection and quantification of neutralizing antibodies to botulinum neurotoxins

A method to detect anti-BoNT antibodies must test the function of each domain of the neurotoxin – binding, translocation and catalytic activity of the enzyme – either in one assay or a set of assays, because antibodies can be directed against each domain. If a single assay is to be developed, this can only be achieved by using intact cellular systems. The easiest method is to inject the neurotoxin into animals (e.g. mice) and determine their survival rate. This assay, the so-called mouse bioassay, is presently considered the gold standard because the median lethal dose (LD_{50}) can be determined very accurately. The LD_{50} increases when anti-BoNT antibodies are present. With the help of a calibration curve based upon standard anti-BoNT antibody concentrations, titers in patients' sera can be calculated. The test has, however, many disadvantages. The test is costly, requires several days before it can be evaluated and, most important, exposes the test animals to prolonged agony including respiratory failure.

Since the endpoint of the test is the paralysis of the respiratory muscle, a truncated version of the test is represented by an isolated nerve–muscle, the phrenic–hemidiaphragm preparation (mouse diaphragm assay). When BoNT is applied to an organ bath in which a muscle has been placed, the contraction amplitude of the nerve-stimulated muscle continuously declines until it disappears completely

---

Manual of Botulinum Toxin Therapy, 2nd edition, ed. Daniel Truong, Mark Hallett, Christopher Zachary and Dirk Dressler.
Published by Cambridge University Press. © Cambridge University Press 2013.

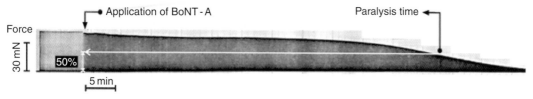

Fig. 4.1 Development of paralysis. A mouse hemidiaphragm was continuously stimulated via the phrenic nerve at a frequency of 1 Hz. After equilibration, the muscle was exposed to 1 ng/ml botulinum neurotoxin type A (BoNT-A). The arrows indicate when the neurotoxin was applied and when the amplitude was reduced by 50% of its initial value, respectively. Paralysis time is defined as the time elapsed until the contraction amplitude has been halved.

(Fig. 4.1). The contractions of the diaphragm can be recorded isometrically, using a commercially available force transducer, while commercially available software allows the analysis of the contraction amplitude over time. The time period between application of BoNT to the organ bath and the point when the contraction amplitude is reduced to half of its original height (paralysis time or $t_{1/2}$) is used to characterize the efficacy and potency of the BoNT. This paralysis time is closely correlated to the toxicity as measured in the LD_{50} (Fig. 4.2) (for details see Wohlfarth *et al.*, 1997). With the help of the mouse diaphragm assay, it is possible to detect anti-BoNT antibodies quantitatively. Using a calibration curve with increasing concentrations of either standard anti-BoNT-A or standard anti-BoNT-B, antibody titers in sera can be measured (Fig. 4.3) (Göschel *et al.*, 1997; Dressler *et al.*, 2005).

Reactions of the organism to botulinum neurotoxin

As BoNT is a foreign protein, it should be recognized by B-cells, which would bind BoNT with the help of specific, preformed antigen receptors. Subsequently, the BoNT is internalized and proteolysed to small peptides of 9–20 amino acid residues. These peptides are presented to the outside of the B-cells associated with proteins of the major histocompatibility complex (MHC). These antigen-presenting B-cells are bound by T-helper cells in the presence of costimulatory molecules. As a result, the T-cells release cytokines; these, together with the MHC-bound peptides, stimulate the B-cells to differentiate into plasma cells. Plasma cells then produce and release specific BoNT-binding immunoglobulins, anti-BoNT. These antibodies protect the host either by neutralizing BoNT, which then loses its toxic properties, or simply by binding the BoNT. These complexes of BoNT and anti-BoNT antibodies may retain toxicity but because

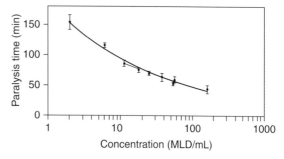

Fig. 4.2 Concentration–response curves for a standard batch of botulinum neurotoxin type A. One curve was constructed using samples containing pure neurotoxin in a median lethal dose (MLD) concentration range of 2 to 162 MLD/ml, the other from the same batch but in the range 11–56 MLD/ml. The curve with the lower range was fitted by linear regression.

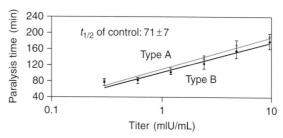

Fig. 4.3 Calibration curves for botulinum neurotoxin types A and B. Antibody titers are plotted against paralysis times in the ex vivo model (*n* = 3 ±SD). The standard antibody was taken from Botulism Antitoxin from Behring, Marburg, Germany (750 U/ml). Paralysis time in the antibody-free control was 71 minutes. With increasing titers, the paralysis time was prolonged. Use of paralysis time allows antibody titers in patients' sera to be calculated when these sera are supplemented with the same neurotoxin concentration as used for the calibration curves.

of the linked antibody the complexes can be easily recognized and phagocytosed by accessory cells (clearing antibodies; Shankar *et al.*, 2007). Recently, positive T-cell responses to BoNT-A have been shown in 95 patients who were treated with the neurotoxin, but there was no difference in the T-cell response between the BoNT-A-responsive patients and the non-responsive patients (Oshima *et al.*, 2011).

Some exogenic factors can facilitate the immune response. It is well known that certain lectins, such as wheat germ agglutinin, phytohemagglutinin, concanavalin A, the B-unit of cholera toxin, or ricin, and others (e.g. components of wasp venom) may stimulate immune cells. These lectins may act as immune adjuvants enhancing antibody concentration. Another factor stimulating immune responses is the amount of antigen exposed to the immune system. In exposure to BoNT-A, the probability of stimulating the immune system increases with the dose of BoNT applied (Göschel et al., 1997; Lange et al., 2009).

Product specificity of immune responses

The therapeutic use of proteins is always associated with immune reactions. Even drugs based on proteins of human origin such as insulin, human growth hormone and erythropoietin may induce antibody formation (Kromminga and Schellekens, 2005). The factors that trigger immunogenicity are impurities, aggregation, formulation and degradation (e.g. oxidation). In addition to these product-specific factors, host-specific factors (e.g. host immune competence) can also determine the immunological response (Kromminga and Schellekens, 2005).

As BoNT is a foreign protein, it will be immunogenic. Prevention of antibody formation can only be avoided by administration of BoNT in extremely small quantities and with long intervals. Nevertheless, in a small number of patients, BoNT does elicit antibody formation, which can inactivate it. The formation of anti-BoNT antibodies in sufficient quantities effectively terminates BoNT therapy (Herrmann et al., 2004).

In the following, factors influencing the immunogenic potential of different BoNT drugs are discussed. Although onabotulinumtoxinA, abobotulinumtoxinA and incobotulinumtoxinA are based on the same active substance, the 150 kDa BoNT-A protein, they contain a different set of additional neurotoxin-associated proteins (except incobotulinumtoxinA). Moreover, they are formulated differently. These differences can influence the immune response to the BoNT drugs.

It has long been known that the neurotoxin-associated proteins (particularly the hemagglutinins) elicit antibodies in 40–60% of patients treated with the complex-containing products (Göschel et al., 1997; Critchfield, 2002), whereas the proportion of patients with anti-BoNT antibodies remains small. Antibodies

against the neurotoxin-associated proteins do not interfere with the neurotoxins, whereas anti-BoNT antibodies will neutralize BoNT and thus cause therapy failure (Göschel et al., 1997).

Whereas the non-toxic non-hemagglutinating protein is responsible for binding the neurotoxin into the complex (Shenyan et al., 2012), some of the other neurotoxin-associated proteins are hemagglutinins thought to facilitate the absorption of BoNT from the gut (Fujinaga et al., 2009). They act, however, as lectins with high specificity to galactose-containing glycoproteins or glycolipids. Other lectins are known to act as immune adjuvants. For example, the cell-binding subunit of ricin that resembles one of the C. botulinum hemagglutinin (HA-1) stimulates antibody production against a virus antigen (Choi et al., 2006).

Concomitant administration of an adjuvant strongly facilitates the immune response against a single antigen (Critchfield, 2002). In an immunization experiment, Lee et al. (2006) showed that hemagglutinins act as adjuvants, enhancing the antibody titer against BoNT-B. They also demonstrated a hemagglutinin-induced increase of the production of interleukin-6 (a B-cell-activating cytokine). However, Lee et al. (2005) used a formalin-inactivated toxin (toxoid) in a dose 100 000 times greater than therapeutic doses. In addition, they injected at weekly intervals, which does not reflect therapeutic recommendations, as already discussed by Atassi (2006). Therefore, it is difficult to estimate the immunological role of the neurotoxin-associated proteins when therapeutic doses are applied, even though hemagglutinins possess an immune adjuvant activity.

The amount of BoNT that is actually exposed to the immune system is also influenced by the specific potency of the BoNT used in the therapeutic preparation (Göschel et al., 1997; Dressler and Hallett, 2006). In onabotulinumtoxinA, approximately 40% of the original BoNT potency is lost during the manufacturing process, thus producing toxoid that cannot be used for therapeutic purposes but which still acts as an antigen (Hunt, 2007).

The specific potency (activity related to the amount of clostridial protein) of abobotulinumtoxinA (1 U = 25 pg) is higher than that of onabotulinumtoxinA (1 U = 50 pg), which can be partly explained by the difference in size of the complex. Whereas onabotulinumtoxinA consists of the 900 kDa complex, abobotulinumtoxinA contains the 300 kDa complex in addition to the

600 kDa complex (Hambleton, 1992). There is no information about the specific activity of the active substance before formulation; therefore, it is not known if there is any denatured neurotoxin in the final product. Despite the fact that abobotulinumtoxinA has to be administered in three times higher doses than onabotulinumtoxinA numerically, the actual dose applied is probably lower because, owing to a low concentration of albumin in this product, some of the toxin binds irreversibly to glass and plastic surfaces. This bound toxin will not reach the patient's tissue; consequently, the dose applied is probably as low as a respective dose of onabotulinumtoxinA.

The active substance of abobotulinumtoxinA shows some impurities not related to the complexing proteins (Pickett *et al.*, 2005). It is notable that a flagellin is present, a protein which is known for its immunostimulatory properties (Honko *et al.*, 2006). It reacts with the Toll-like receptor-5 and induces the maturation of dendritic cells that activate T-cells. It was shown that the addition of flagellin to tetanus toxoid in a vaccination experiment enhanced the antibody titer against tetanus toxin (Lee *et al.*, 2006). However, as discussed above for onabotulinumtoxinA, the doses of adjuvant proteins applied experimentically were much higher than the doses given therapeutically; also in this case, difficulties arise about the assessment of the role flagellin plays in patients treated with abobotulinumtoxinA.

In contrast to onabotulinumtoxinA and abobotulinumtoxinA, incobotulinumtoxinA only contains the purified neurotoxin and no other clostridial proteins; it, therefore, shows the highest specific activity (1 U = 4.4 pg) (Frevert, 2010).

The immunogenic potential of BoNT-B versus BoNT-A has not been well investigated. In people vaccinated with the pentavalent botulinum toxoid vaccine, the antibody titer against BoNT-A is markedly higher than the titer against BoNT-B (Siegel, 1989), but the vaccine contains toxins inactivated by treatment with formalin, which could influence their antigenic potential. It has to be considered that BoNT-B is not fully activated. The unnicked, non-activated proportion of BoNT-B (about 25%) is inactive and could act as a toxoid (Aoki, 2002). The specific activity of rimabotulinumtoxinB is remarkably higher (1 U = 11 pg) than the specific activity of BoNT-A-containing products, but this is only true when mice are involved (Callaway, 2004). A single mutation in the gene for the human BoNT-B receptor, synaptotagmin-II, results in a drastic decrease in the the the receptor's affinity for the toxin, of approximately 100-fold (Strotmeier *et al.*, 2012). Therefore, this type has to be applied in much higher doses to achieve a therapeutic effect. If one considers that this substantially higher dose of rimabotulinumtoxinB has to be injected, the specific potency in humans is much lower (estimated 40-fold; Dressler, 2006). This substantially increases the risk of developing antibodies. Therefore, more than 40% of de novo patients treated with rimabotulinumtoxinB for cervical dystonia developed complete antibody-induced therapy failure after only a few treatments (Dressler and Bigalke, 2004). Table 4.1 summarizes the average protein load contained in doses of BoNT products used for the treatment of cervical dystonia.

The relatively high amount of BoNT-B administered with rimabotulinumtoxinB explains why

Table 4.1 Doses of botulinum neurotoxin for the treatment of cervical dystonia

	OnabotulinumtoxinA	AbobotulinumtoxinA	IncobotulinumtoxinA	RimabotulinumtoxinB
Average dose (units)	200	600	200	8000
Amount of administered clostridial protein (ng)	10	5.2	1	88
Calculated amount of neurotoxin (ng)	1.5	1.7[a]	0.9[b]	22[c]

According to [a]Panjwani *et al.* (2008), [b]Frevert (2010) and [b]Callaway (2004) based on the calculated proportion of neurotoxin in onabotulinumtoxinA of approximately 20% (150 kDa/900 kDa), in abobotulinumtoxinA of 33% (150 kDa/(300 kDa + 600 kDa)/2, and in rimabotulinumtoxinB of 25% (150 kDa/600 kDa).

patients develop antibodies and become non-responders to BoNT-B after a few injections (Dressler and Hallett, 2006), whereas the percentage of patients who have developed antibodies against onabotulinumtoxinA and abobotulinumtoxinA is much lower, approximately 1–3% (Kessler et al., 1999). A more recently published trial, however, reported a low incidence of antibody formation also for BoNT-B-treated patients (Chinnapongse et al., 2012). IncobotulinumtoxinA, which has been available since 2005, has not produced a documented case of antibody-induced therapy failure (Dressler, 2012).

Avoidance of antibody formation is of major importance. If therapy failure occurs, appropriate antibody tests should be used. In 50% of patients, therapy failure is caused by antibody formation (Lange et al., 2009). In the remaining patients, non-responsiveness is frequently caused by inappropriate injection schemes.

References

Aoki KR (2002). Immunological and other properties of therapeutic botulinum toxin serotypes. In Brin MF, Jankovic J, Hallett M (eds.) *Scientific and Therapeutic Aspects of Botulinum Toxin*. Philadelphia, PA: Lippincott, Williams & Wilkins, pp. 103–13.

Atassi MZ (2006). On the enhancement of anti-neurotoxin antibody production by subcomponents HA1 and HA3b of *Clostridium botulinum* type B 16S toxin-haemagglutinin. *Microbiology*, **152**, 1891–5.

Callaway JE (2004). Botulinum toxin type B (Myobloc˚): pharmacology and biochemistry. *Clin Dermatol*, **22**, 23–8.

Chinnapongse RB, Lew MF, Ferreira JJ et al. (2012). Immunogenicity and long-term efficacy of botulinum toxin type B in the treatment of cervical dystonia: report of 4 prospective, multicenter trials. *Clin Neuropharmacol*, **35**, 215–23.

Choi NW, Estes MK, Langridge WH (2006). Ricin toxin B subunit enhancement of rotavirus NSP4 immunogenicity in mice. *Viral Immunol*, **19**, 54–63.

Critchfield J (2002). Considering the immune response to botulinum toxin. *Clin J Pain*, **18**(Suppl), S133–41.

Dressler D (2006). Pharmacological aspects of therapeutic botulinum toxin preparations. *Nervenarzt*, **77**, 912–21.

Dressler D (2012). Five-year experience with incobotulinumtoxinA (Xeomin). The first botulinum toxin drug free of complexing proteins. *Eur J Neurol*, **19**, 385–9.

Dressler D, Bigalke H (2004). Antibody-induced failure of botulinum toxin type B therapy in de novo patients. *Eur Neurol*, **52**, 132–5.

Dressler D, Hallett M (2006). Immunological aspects of Botox˚, Dysport˚ and Myobloc˚/NeuroBloc˚. *Eur J Neurol*, **13**(Suppl 1), 11–15.

Dressler D, Lange M, Bigalke H (2005). The mouse diaphragm assay for detection of antibodies against botulinum toxin type B. *Mov Disord*, **20**, 1617–19.

Frevert J (2010). Content of botulinum neurotoxin in Botox˚/Vistabel˚, Dysport˚/Azzalure˚, and Xeomin˚/Bocouture˚. *Drugs R D*, **10**, 67–73.

Fujinaga Y, Matsumura T, Jin Y, Takegahara Y, Sugawara Y (2009). A novel function of botulinum toxin-associated proteins: HA proteins disrupt intestinal epithelial barrier to increase toxin absorption. *Toxicon*, **54**, 583–6.

Göschel H, Wohlfarth K, Frevert J, Dengler R, Bigalke H (1997). Botulinum A toxin therapy: neutralizing and nonneutralizing antibodies: therapeutic consequences. *Exp Neurol*, **147**, 96–102.

Hambleton P (1992). *Clostridium botulinum* toxins: a general review of involvement in disease, structure, mode of action and preparation for clinical use. *J Neurol*, **239**, 16–20.

Herrmann J, Geth K, Mall V et al. (2004). Clinical impact of antibody formation to botulinum toxin in children. *Ann Neurol*, **55**, 732–5.

Honko AN, Sriranganathan N, Lees CJ, Mizel SB (2006). Flagellin is an effective adjuvant for immunization against lethal respiratory challenge with Yersinia pestis. *Infect Immun*, **74**, 1113–20.

Hunt TJ (2007). Botulinum toxin composition. *US Patent Application 2007/0025019*.

Kessler KR, Skutta M, Benecke R (1999). Long-term treatment of cervical dystonia with botulinum toxin A: efficacy, safety, and antibody frequency. German Dystonia Study Group. *J Neurol*, **246**, 265–74.

Kromminga A, Schellekens H (2005). Antibodies against erythropoietin and other protein-based therapeutics: an overview. *Ann N Y Acad Sci*, **1050**, 257–65.

Lange O, Bigalke H, Dengler R et al. (2009). Neutralizing antibodies and secondary therapy failure after treatment with botulinum toxin type A: much ado about nothing? *Clin Neuropharmacol*, **32**, 213–18.

Lee JC, Yokota K, Arimitsu H et al. (2005). Production of anti-neurotoxin antibody is enhanced by two subcomponents, HA1 and HA3b, of *Clostridium botulinum* type B 16S toxin-haemagglutinin. *Microbiology*, **151**, 3739–47.

Lee SE, Kim SY, Jeong BC et al. (2006). A bacterial flagellin, *Vibrio vulnificus* FlaB, has a strong mucosal adjuvant activity to induce protective immunity. *Infect Immun*, **74**, 694–702.

Oshima M, Deitiker PR, Jankovic J et al. (2011). Human T-cell responses to botulinum neurotoxin. Proliferative responses in vitro of lymphocytes from botulinum neurotoxin A-treated movement disorder patients. *J Neuroimmunol*, **237**, 66–72.

Panjwani N, O'Keeffe R, Pickett A (2008). Biochemical, functional and potency characteristics of type A botulinum toxin in clinical use. *Botulinum J*, **1**, 153–66.

Paus S, Bigalke H, Klockgether T (2006). Neutralizing antibodies against botulinum toxin A after a wasp sting. *Arch Neurol*, **63**, 1808–9.

Pickett, A, Shipley S, Panjwani N, O'Keeffe R, Sing BR (2005). Characterisation and consistency of botulinum A toxin-hemagglutinin complex used for clinical therapy. In *Proceedings of the International Conference on Basic and Therapeutic Aspects of Botulinum and Tetanus Toxins*, Denver, 23–25 June 2005.

Shankar G, Pendley C, Stein KE (2007). A risk-based bioanalytical strategy for the assessment of antibody immune responses against biological drugs. *Nat Biotechnol*, **25**, 555–61.

Shenyan G, Rumpel S, Zhou J et al. (2012). Botulinum neurotoxin is shielded by NTNHA in an interlocked complex. *Science*, **335**, 977–81.

Siegel LS (1989). Evaluation of neutralizing antibodies to type A, B, E, and F botulinum toxins in sera from human recipients of botulinum pentavalent (ABCDE) toxoid. *J Clin Microbiol*, **27**, 1906–8.

Strotmeier J, Willjes G, Binz T, Rummel A (2012). Human synaptotagmin-II is not a high affinity receptor for botulinum neurotoxin B and G: increased therapeutic dosage and immunogenicity. *FEBS Lett*, **586**, 310–13.

Wohlfarth K, Goschel H, Frevert J, Dengler R, Bigalke H (1997). Botulinum A toxins: units versus units. *Naunyn-Schmiedeberg Arch Pharmacol*, **355**, 335–40.

Treatment of cervical dystonia

Daniel Truong, Karen Frei and Cynthia L. Comella

Introduction

Cervical dystonia (CD), originally known as spasmodic torticollis and first described by Foltz in 1959, is a neurological syndrome characterized by abnormal head and neck posture caused by tonic involuntary contractions in a set of cervical muscles. However, CD and spasmodic torticollis are not interchangeable: CD is the preferred term when referring to idiopathic focal dystonia of the neck. Spasmodic torticollis is now considered to be one of four types of CD. Cervical dystonia is classified into four types based on the principal direction of head posture:

- torticollis: abnormal rotation of the head to the right or to the left in the transverse plane
- laterocollis: the head tilts toward the right or left shoulder
- antecollis: the head pulls forward with neck flexion
- retrocollis: the head pulls back with the neck hyperextended.

Cervical dystonia is slightly more common in females, with a male to female ratio of 1:1.2 (Kessler *et al.*, 1999). Onset is usually insidious, although in some patients the onset has been reported as sudden. Cervical dystonia may develop in patients of all age groups, but the peak age of onset is 41 years (Kessler *et al.*, 1999). Idiopathic CD usually progresses in severity over the first 5 years until it reaches a plateau, after which it remains fairly constant and becomes a lifelong condition. Although remission can occur, it is rare and the dystonia usually returns after a period of time. The cervical component may also exist as part of a more extensive form of dystonia, in which the dystonia can spread to involve adjacent structures such as the face or the arm(s). When dystonia involves several contiguous body parts, it is considered segmental dystonia. When it involves several parts of the body that are not contiguous, such as the neck and foot, it is called multifocal, and when it involves the majority of the body, it is referred to as generalized dystonia.

Characteristic traits of CD include transient relief from symptoms with a sensory trick or "geste antagoniste". A common form of a sensory trick in CD is placing the hand lightly on the cheek. This allows the head to return to a more normal posture. Resting the head against the headrest while driving or against a pillow while watching TV are examples of sensory tricks. Patients may obtain temporary relief from symptoms of CD in the morning hours following sleep; this is referred to as the "honeymoon" effect (Truong *et al.*, 1991). Stress can exacerbate the symptoms. Neck pain is common and has been reported in 70–80% of affected patients (Van Zandijcke, 1995). Cervical dystonia is often a major source of disability. Degenerative disc disease seems to be accelerated in CD, which can aggravate the pain associated with this disorder.

Multichannel electromyography (EMG) may help to elicit the involved muscle patterns producing the particular posture. Evidence of prolonged bursts of electrical activity detected with EMG that correlate with the involved musculature is helpful in diagnosing CD. Testing agonist–antagonist pairs of muscles allows the comparison of overall activity, which can also assist in distinguishing the most active muscles involved in producing the CD posture.

In the first part of the last century, CD was thought to be of psychogenic origin, although today an organic basis for the syndrome is well accepted. There are cases of heritable forms of CD, such as the *DYT7* locus, but the majority of heritable dystonia types are variable in presentation and may include different

Manual of Botulinum Toxin Therapy, 2nd edition, ed. Daniel Truong, Mark Hallett, Christopher Zachary and Dirk Dressler. Published by Cambridge University Press. © Cambridge University Press 2013.

forms of dystonia, such as blepharospasm, limb dystonia and CD. Heritable forms of dystonia generally have autosomal dominant transmission and incomplete penetrance. With the incomplete penetrance of these disorders, not all family members with the mutation will have dystonia. Moreover, affected family members may present with different signs/symptoms in different body regions – not all affected family members will have CD. Cervical dystonia is often a component of various secondary dystonias that manifest in a number of neurodegenerative diseases. Secondary causes of CD include neuroleptic medication exposure or trauma. A form of CD known as posttraumatic CD may occur following a relatively mild trauma. This form usually begins within days of an incident, lacks the sensory trick response and tends to be more resistant to treatment with botulinum neurotoxin (BoNT) (Truong et al., 1991; Frei et al., 2004).

The clinical spectrum of abnormal head and neck posture is extremely variable. The reason for this is the wide variety of the dystonic muscle patterns within the 54 muscles involved in head and neck posture. Furthermore, muscles can be involved on one side or on both sides. Dystonic muscles can show a dominant tonic activity, myoclonic activity or tremulous activity, often in complex mixtures. The extent of secondary changes in the muscles and connective and bony tissues may present differently from patient to patient and in their contribution to abnormal postures.

Intramuscular injections of BoNT are considered the first line of treatment in CD. Both serotype A (BoNT-A) (old and new onabotulinumtoxinA, abobotulinumtoxinA, incobotulinumtoxinA) and serotype B (BoNT-B) (rimabotulinumtoxinB) have been used. Medications such as the anticholinergic trihexyphenidyl (Artane) and benztropine (Cogentin) have some beneficial effects and can be used in more severe cases alongside BoNT injections. Other medications that have mild or limited usefulness include benzodiazepines, such as diazepam (Valium) or lorazepam (Ativan) and tricyclic antidepressants, such as amitriptyline (Elavil) and nortriptyline (Pamelor).

Surgical treatment with selective peripheral denervation has been reported in open studies to be helpful in some patients with severe CD that does not respond to either oral medications or chemodenervation. Surgical myectomy has also been used; however, the dystonia tends to involve other muscles or continues to involve remnants of the resected muscles, thus producing less favorable results. Deep brain stimulation, with electrodes placed in the globus pallidus interna, has been successfully used for treatment of generalized dystonia. Increasingly, deep brain stimulation has been employed in the treatment of CD and further improvements may be possible with advanced development of electrode placement and/or programming.

Botulinum neurotoxin in cervical dystonia

BoNT injections into the affected muscles remain the most effective treatment for CD. In 1985, Tsui and colleagues (Tsui et al., 1985) published the results of BoNT-A injections into the neck muscles of 12 patients with CD, and followed a year later with a double-blind, placebo-controlled trial in 21 patients (Tsui et al., 1986). Since then, several controlled trials have confirmed that BoNT-A injections improve CD (Blackie and Lees 1990; Greene et al., 1990; Lorentz et al., 1991; Moore and Blumhardt, 1991; Truong et al., 2010; Comella et al., 2011), with only one exception (Gelb et al., 1989). In a double-blind study by Naumann and colleagues (2002), 133 patients were injected with BoNT-A (onabotulinumtoxinA), produced from original and current bulk toxin sources, using a crossover design. The percentage improvement measured by the Toronto Western Spasmodic Torticollis Rating Scale (TWSTRS) amounted to about 35% after injections of both toxin sources.

Three double-blind, placebo-controlled studies using BoNT-B (rimabotulinumtoxinB) for treatment of CD have been performed. One study tested BoNT-B in unselected patients with CD (Lew et al., 1997). Another study examined BoNT-B in patients who were responsive to BoNT-B injections and compared placebo with either 5000 U or 10 000 U BoNT-B (Brashear et al., 1999). A further study tested BoNT-B in patients who were BoNT-A resistant, comparing placebo with 10 000 U BoNT-B (Brin et al., 1999). In all studies, total scores on the TWSTRS significantly improved from baseline 2 weeks after BoNT-B, with the greater improvement observed in the group receiving 10 000 U BoNT-B.

Table 5.1 provides a summary of the effects of BoNT-A and BoNT-B treatment in CD as published in a number of open and double-blind investigations (Tsui et al., 1986; Gelb et al., 1989; Stell et al., 1989; Blackie and Lees 1990; Greene et al., 1990, Jankovic and Schwartz, 1990; Jankovic and Brin 1991; Hambleton et al., 1992; Benecke 1993; Hatheway and

Table 5.1 Treatment effects of botulinum neurotoxin injections in cervical dystonia

Study	No. patients	Dose (units)	Assessment scale	Improvement (%)
OnabotulinumtoxinA (type A)				
Tsui et al. (1986)[a]	19	100	Tsui	30
Gelb et al. (1989)[a]	20	280	Tsui	20
Gelb et al. (1991)[a]	28	280	Tsui	20
Greene et al. (1990)[a]	34	240	GIR (0–3)	33
Comella et al. (1992)[b]	52	374	TWSTRS	>10
Naumann et al. 2002[b]	133	155	TWSTRS	>10
IncobotulinumtoxinA (type A)				
Benecke et al. (2005)[b]	231	140	TWSTRS	40
Comella et al. (2011)[a]	233	120–240	TWSTRS	25
AbobotulinumtoxinA (type A)				
Blackie and Lees (1990)[a]	19	960	Tsui	22
Stell et al. (1989)[b]	10	1200	Tsui	47
Poewe et al. (1992)[b]	37	632	Tsui	>50
Wissel and Poewe (1992)[b]	180	594	Tsui	>50
Kessler et al. (1999)[b]	616	778	Tsui	>60
Truong et al. (2010)	116	500	TWSTRS	32
Truong et al. (2005)	80	500	TWSTRS	22
RimabotulinumtoxinB (type B)				
Lew et al. (1997)[a]	122	2500	TWSTRS	25.5
		5000		27.6
		10 000		34.5
Brin et al. (1999)[a]	77	10 000	TWSTRS	21
Brashear et al. (1999)[a]	109	5000–10 000	TWSTRS	17.8–24.9

GIR, Global Improvement Rating (comparative study of two type A preparations only including responders, pain reduction 52%); TWSTRS, Toronto Western Spasmodic Torticollis Rating Scale.
[a] Double-blind study.
[b] Open study.

Dang 1994; Benecke 1999; Kessler et al., 1999; Naumann et al., 2002; Benecke at al., 2005). Studies are listed that evaluated responder rates and/or percentage improvements only.

Use of BoNT therapy is indicated in all forms of CD. Worsening of CD while being treated with BoNT could reflect resistance to BoNT or an actual increase in severity – often, the wrong muscles have been injected. Treatment with BoNT should be initiated as early as possible, since secondary changes to the muscles involved (contractures) and of connective tissues, bony tissues and cervical discs may occur with long-standing CD.

Treatment with BoNT results in the improvement of neck posture, muscle hypertrophy and pain. The effect begins 3 to 12 days after an injection and is sustained for approximately 3 months. Injections at 3-month intervals (or longer) are thought to reduce the risk of antibodies arising to BoNT. Less experienced physicians should perform EMG recordings from sternocleidomastoid, splenius capitis, trapezius (upper portion) and levator scapulae muscles to confirm their clinical impression on the basis of head posture and muscle palpation – particularly prior to the first BoNT treatment session. Needle EMG is needed for deeper muscles, but sometimes can even be useful for superficial muscles when they are close together. It may also be useful to employ EMG when response to BoNT treatment becomes unsatisfactory, in order to determine whether injected muscles are denervated and to assist in identifying overactive muscles that may not have been injected. There may also be a change in the dystonic posturing of the head and EMG can also assist in modifying injection pattern when this occurs.

The number of injection sites within a muscle ranges from one site in smaller muscles to eight sites in larger muscles. There is little evidence to assist in determining the optimum number of injection sites. Although a study by Borodic and colleagues (1992) suggests that multiple injection sites may provide an improved result, this has not been adequately evaluated. Multiple injections with smaller doses might well also limit diffusion and reduce side effects. This might be particularly relevant in the neck, where dysphagia might result if there is excessive spread. Patients should be re-examined prior to each treatment. Muscle hypertrophy and involved muscle patterns may change over time, necessitating the alteration of injection sites over the course of repeated treatments. It is important to document the injected muscles as well as the dosage given. Upon follow-up, this can help when adjusting injection patterns and dosage.

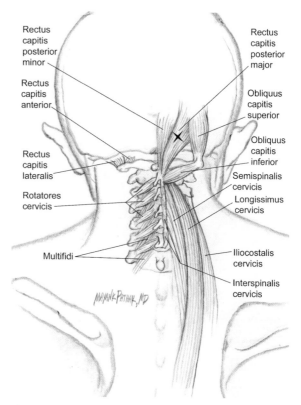

Fig. 5.1 The major neck muscles, which play some role in retrocollis but are usually not injected.

Neck muscles and their functions

Figures 5.1 to 5.4 show the location of the muscles, which are described below.

Iliocostalis cervicis. The iliocostalis cervicis arises from the angles of the third, fourth, fifth and sixth ribs, and is inserted into the posterior tubercles of the transverse processes of C4–C6. The iliocostalis flexes the head laterally. When both iliocostalis cervicis are activated bilaterally they extend the neck dorsally (Fig. 5.1).

Interspinalis cervicis. These muscles lie between the spinosus processes of the cervical vertebrae. They assist in dorsal extension (Fig. 5.1).

Intertransversarii cervicis. These muscles are arranged in pairs, passing between the anterior and the posterior tubercles, respectively, to the transverse processes of two contiguous vertebræ. The anterior primary division of the cervical nerve separates the intertransversarii anteriores cervicis muscle from the posterior intertransversarii. They assist in the lateral and the dorsal flexion of the neck (Fig. 5.2).

Levator scapulae. The levator scapulae arises from the transverse processes of C1–C4 and inserts into the medial border of the scapula. This muscle elevates the medial border of the scapula while rotating the lateral angle downward. Together with the rhomboid and trapezius muscles, it pulls the scapula upward and medially, as well as tilts the neck ipsilaterally (Fig. 5.3).

Longissimus cervicis. The longissimus cervicis is located laterally to the semispinalis. It is the longest subdivision of the sacrospinalis and extends forward into the transverse processes of the posterior cervical vertebrae. Arising from long, thin tendons at the transverse processes of the upper four or five thoracic vertebræ, it is inserted into the posterior tubercles of the transverse processes of the C2–C6. It tilts the head ipsilaterally. When the longissimus cervicis muscles are activated bilaterally, they extend the neck dorsally (Fig. 5.1).

25

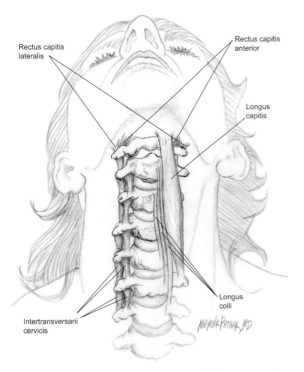

Rectus capitis
lateralis

Rectus capitis
anterior

Longus
capitis

Longus
colli

Intertransversarii
cervicis

MAYANK PATHAK, MD

Fig. 5.2 The juxta-vertebral muscles of the neck. The longus colli muscle is sometimes injected in anterocollis.

Longus capitis. The longus capitis arises by four tendinous slips from the anterior tubercles of the transverse processes of C3–C6 and ascends, converging toward its fellow of the opposite side, to be inserted into the inferior surface of the basilar part of the occipital bone (Fig. 5.2).

Longus colli. The longus colli originates from the lower anterior vertebral bodies and transverse processes and inserts into the anterior vertebral bodies and transverse processes several segments above, flexing the head (Fig. 5.2).

Multifidi. The mutifidus muscle fills up the groove on each side of the spinous processes of the vertebrae. It arises, in the cervical region, from the articular processes of the lower four vertebrae and inserts into the spinous process of one of the vertebræ above. It rotates the neck contralaterally. When both multifidus are activated they extend the neck (Fig. 5.1).

Obliquus capitis inferior. This muscle arises from the spinous process of the axis and inserts into the inferior and dorsal part of the transverse process of the atlas. It rotates the head and the first cervical vertebra ipsilaterally (Fig. 5.1).

Obliquus capitis superior. The oblique capitis superior originates in the atlas mass, inserting into the lateral half of the inferior nuchal line of the occipital bone. At the atlanto-occipital joint, it extends and flexes the head ipsilaterally (Fig. 5.1).

Rectus capitis anterior. The rectus capitis anterior is a small muscle originating in the anterior base of the transverse process of the atlas and inserting into the occipital bone anterior to the foramen magnum, flexing the head. Furthermore, the rectus capitis anterior stabilizes the atlanto-occipital joint (Fig. 5.2).

Rectus capitis lateralis. The rectus capitis lateralis originates in the transverse process of the atlas and inserts into the jugular process of the occipital bone. It tilts the head laterally (Fig. 5.2).

Rectus capitis posterior major. This muscle arises from the spinous process of the axis, ascending into the lateral part of the inferior nuchal line of the occipital bone. As the two muscles of the two rectus capitis posterior major pass upward and laterally, they create a triangular space occupied by the recti capitis posteriores minores. The rectus capitis posterior major extends the head and rotates it to the same side (Fig. 5.1).

Rectus capitis posterior minor. This is a muscle of triangular form arising from the posterior arch of the atlas and inserting into the medial part of the occipital bone at, and below, the nuchal line. It extends the head (Fig. 5.1).

Rotatores cervicis. The rotatores cervicis arises from the transverse spinosus process and inserts into the above vertebrae, extending the neck and assisting in contralateral rotation (Fig. 5.1).

Scalene anterior. The scalene muscles are lateral vertebral muscles that begin at the first and second ribs and pass up into the sides of the neck. There are three of these muscles. The anterior scalene originates in the anterior tubercles of the transverse processes of C3–C6 and inserts into the first rib. It elevates the ribs for respiration and weakly rotates the head to the opposite side. When both anterior scalene muscles are contracted they flex the head forward (Fig. 5.3).

Scalene medius. The middle scalene arises from the transverse processes of all cervical vertebrae and inserts into the first rib (behind the anterior scalene). It bends the neck to the same side and

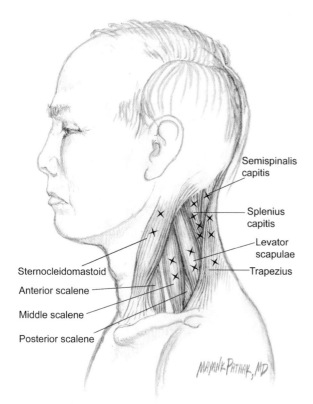

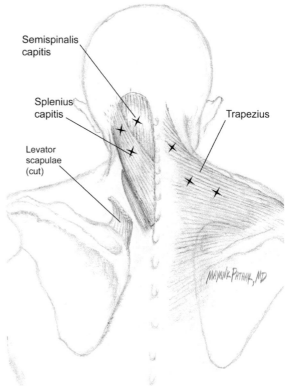

Fig. 5.3 Muscles of importance for genesis and treatment of torticollis. The sternocleidomastoid is injected contralaterally whereas the other muscles are injected on the ipsilateral side.

Fig. 5.4 Superficial muscles of the neck.

also can flex the neck as it lies anterior to the axis (Fig. 5.3).

Scalene posterior. This muscle arises from the posterior tubercles of the transverse processes of C5 and C6 cervical vertebrae and inserts into the second and/or third rib. The action of the posterior scalene is to elevate the second rib and tilt the neck to the same side (Fig. 5.3).

Semispinalis capitis. The semispinalis capitis originates in the transverse processes of the T6 and C7, as well as the articular processes of C4–C6. It inserts between the superior and inferior nuchal lines of the occipital bone. The semispinalis capitis is often a cause of neck pain. Even through its main action is extension, restriction in this muscle can cause pain on rotation at the end of the range. It also rotates the head to the opposite side (Fig. 5.3).

Semispinalis cervicis. This muscle arises from the transverse processes of the upper five or six thoracic vertebræ. It inserts into the spinous processes of C2–C5. The semispinalis tilts the head to the same side and rotates the head to the contralateral side. Working together, the two semispinalis cervicis extend the head backward. The semispinalis capitis and cervicis and longissimus capitis are commonly overused because of their role in supporting the head when leaning forward. They are often involved in headache pain (Fig. 5.1).

Splenius capitis. The splenius capitis originates in the spinal process of the body of C7 and the bodies of T1 to T3. It inserts into the mastoid process. This muscle turns and tilts the head ipsilaterally. Together, the two splenius capitis muscles extend the head backward (Fig. 5.4).

Splenius cervicis. This muscle arises from the spinosus processes of T3–T6. It is inserted, by tendinous fasciculi, into the posterior tubercles of the transverse processes of C1 to C3. This muscle turns the head ipsilaterally. When both splenius cervicis are activated, they extend the head backwards.

Table 5.2 Muscles anatomically involved and muscles commonly injected in torticollis[a]

Muscle name	Ipsilateral	Contralateral	Treated muscles
Splenius capitis and cervicis	X		X
Levator scapulae	X		X
Longissimus capitis and cervicis	X		X
Multifidi		X	
Rotatores cervicis		X	
Sternocleidomastoid		X	X
Trapezius (horizontal part)		X	X
Semispinalis capitis and cervicis		X	X

[a] The cervicis turns the head contralaterally; the semispinalis has weak effect on turning the head contralaterally and only in the upper part (C1–C3).

Table 5.3 Muscles anatomically involved and muscles commonly injected in laterocollis

Muscle name	Ipsilateral	Contralateral	Treated muscles
Sternocleidomastoid	X		X
Trapezius	X		X
Scalene medius and posterior	X		X
Splenius capitis and cervicis	X		X
Longissimus cervicis and capitis	X		X
Multifidi	X		
Intertransversarii cervicis	X		

Table 5.4 Muscles anatomically involved and muscles commonly injected in antecollis

Muscle name	Ipsilateral	Contralateral	Treated muscles
Sternocleidomastoid	X	X	X
Scalene anterior and medius	X	X	X
Longus colli	X	X	X
Longus capitis	X	X	
Infrahyoidal muscle	X	X	
Rectus capitis anterior	X	X	

Sternocleidomastoid. This muscle originates on the mastoid processes and inserts in two areas, one on the sternum and the other on the clavicle, hence the name sternocleidomastoid. It turns the head to the opposite side and the chin upward to the opposite side. It also tilts the head to the same side (Fig. 5.3).

Trapezius. The trapezius originates from the occipital protuberante, the ligamentum nuchae and the processes spinosus and inserts into the lateral third of the clavicle. The trapezius turns the head and neck contralaterally. It also elevates the shoulder (Fig. 5.4).

Table 5.5 Muscles anatomically involved and muscles commonly injected in retrocollis

Muscle name	Ipsilateral	Contralateral	Treated muscles
Levator scapulae	X	X	X
Splenius capitis and cervicis	X	X	X
Longissimus capitis and cervicis	X	X	X
Semispinalis capitis and cervicis	X	X	X
Iliocostalis cervicis	X	X	
Spinalis capitis and cervicis	X	X	
Rectus capitis posterior major and minor	X	X	
Rotatores cervicis	X	X	
Interspinalis cervicis	X	X	
Intertransversarii cervicis	X	X	

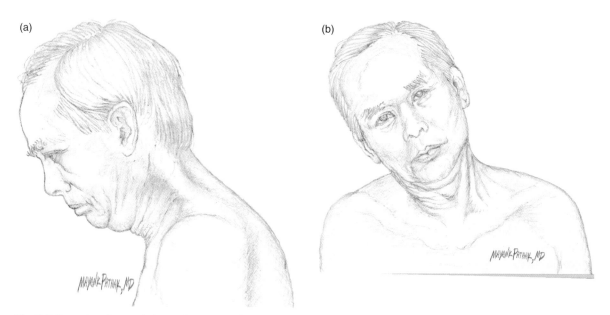

(a) (b)

Fig. 5.5 Illustration of postural abnormalities in pure forms of cervical dystonia: (a) antecollis; (b) laterocollis; (c) retrocollis; (d) torticollis.

Muscles involved in different subtypes of cervical dystonia

Based on the presentation of the head position (Fig. 5.5), different muscles are involved. The anatomical location, however, limits the muscles that can be treated. Tables 5.2 to 5.5 list the muscles that are anatomically involved and that are actually injected in torticollis (Table 5.2), laterocollis (Table 5.3), antecollis (Table 5.4) and retrocollis (Table 5.5).

Practical considerations for treatment of cervical dystonia with botulinum neurotoxin

The following questions must be answered before BoNT therapy of CD is considered:
1. Is the abnormal posture of the head and of the shoulder induced by dystonia or by another abnormality that only imitates CD?
2. Is the cervical dystonia the primary cause of disability?

(c)

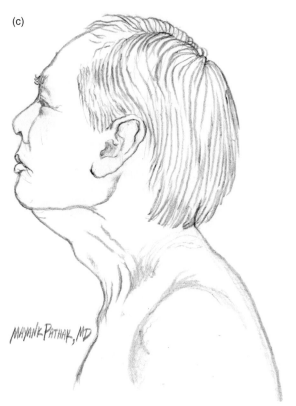

(d)

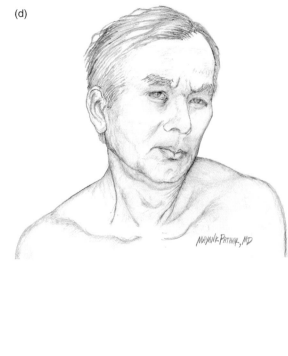

Fig. 5.5 (cont.)

3. Does the patient have myasthenia gravis or other neuromuscular junction disorders?
4. Are there already secondary changes of muscles or connective and bony tissues?

Physical examination of the patient with cervical dystonia

A high level of patient cooperation during the physical examination is necessary. Patients must be requested to release any compensatory voluntary muscle activities in non-dystonic muscles, avoid the use of sensory tricks (geste antagoniste) and report accurately on pain severity. They should be asked to perform slow head movements in all common directions: evaluation of head posture is performed with the patient standing, walking slowly and lying down. In a seated position, the patient should be asked to demonstrate his/her favorite sensory trick (e.g. touching the chin with the right hand). Finally, patients should be asked to hold their heads in a neutral position, with the assistance of

antagonistic compensatory muscle activity for as long as possible.

Videotaping is always recommended as a means of documenting the examination. As videotape is more complicated to use in routine clinical practice, we often help the patient to take a few photographs of themselves with their smart phone to use for comparison later. The most helpful picture is the one with the patient fully relaxed to register the degree of the neck deviation. Common CD rating scales include the TWSTRS and the Tsui Scale. Such rating scales are recommended not only for clinical trials but also for routine evaluation of CD and of BoNT treatment. They provide an objective detection of improvement of CD after BoNT injections, or lack of improvement in those patients who have developed antibodies.

Botulinum neurotoxin injection procedure

Physicians should obtain written, informed consent from the patient. Possible adverse effects and procedure complications should be clearly explained to the patient and the discussion documented in the patient's chart.

Muscle selection for treatment with BoNT is the next important step in developing an injection plan. Although there are 54 muscles that influence head and neck posture, as well as shoulder position, only a limited number of muscles are important to consider for injections. These muscles are the larger neck muscles that may be the most important factors in the abnormal postures.

The correct selection of doses for each individual muscle is the next step in the decision-making process, and perhaps the most difficult and most important part of BoNT treatment of CD. These decisions determine the success of treatment in an individual patient. Some general comments regarding BoNT dosing are:

- total and individual muscle doses may be higher in younger patients
- women with small necks usually require smaller doses
- men with larger necks or an athletic physique may require higher doses
- for bilateral injections in the sternocleidomastoid and infrahyoid muscles, the dose per muscle is half of the regular dose
- for bilateral injection into the splenius capitis and semispinalis capitis muscles, the individual dose per muscle should be reduced to 60 % of the regular dose to prevent neck weakness.

The requirement for decreased doses when giving bilateral injections results from increased severity and the prevalence of side effects. Swallowing problems happen more frequently with bilateral injections to the sternocleidomastoid and the infrahyoidal muscles. Neck muscle weakness, which may cause problems with holding the head upright, is more frequent if the splenius capitis and semispinalis capitis muscles are injected bilaterally.

Dose finding with the first injection treatment is more difficult than with subsequent treatments because the individual sensitivity of the muscles to BoNT and the probability of developing side effects are not known. For the average patient (suffering from pure torticollis, laterocollis or a combination of these abnormal head postures), the recommended total dose depends on the severity of CD. In general, a lower dose is used initially in the patient with newly diagnosed CD. Recommended total doses for the four products on the US market are given in Table 5.6. The total dose is divided into various portions, which are injected into individual dystonic muscles. Table 5.7 summarizes established dose ranges for the most important head and neck muscles. There is really no acceptable ratio between the four BoNT products, although some clinicians have used the following approximate relationship between the four commmercial products (Botox:Xeomin:Dysport:MyoBloc/NeuroBloc as 1:1:3:50). The US Food and Drug Administration also does not recommend a dosing ratio. So far, there is no evidence to support the superiority of any one brand of BoNT-A (Botox, Xeomin and Dysport).

In a recent study (Benecke et al., 2005), a new BoNT-A free of complexing proteins (incobotulinumtoxinA) was compared with onabotulinumtoxinA in patients with CD by means of a double-blind, non-inferiority trial. This study showed that incobotulinumtoxinA is not inferior to onabotulinumtoxinA and has a similar safety profile.

Side effects of BoNT include hypersensitivity reactions, injection site infections, injection site bleeding or bruising, dry mouth, dysphagia, upper respiratory infection, neck pain and headache. With bilateral posterior neck injections, neck weakness may occur, usually manifested by a feeling of instability when leaning forward or backward and often associated with pain. Dysphagia is associated with injections into the sternocleidomastoid muscle and is thought to be caused by the spread of the BoNT locally. Transient muscle

Table 5.6 Recommendations for total doses (units) in pure torticollis, laterocollis or combined form based on cervical dystonia severity measured by the Tsui Score

Score	OnabotulinumtoxinA	IncobotulinumtoxinA	AbobotulinumtoxinA	RimabotulinumtoxinB
12–15	200–300	200–300	700–1000	10 000
9–12	150–200	150–200	500–700	7500–10 000
6–9	100–150	100–150	300–500	5000–7500
3–6	80–120	80–120	320–400	4000–6000

Table 5.7 Recommended doses for individual muscles involved in cervical dystonia[a]

Muscle	Onabotulinum-toxinA (U)	Incobotulinum-toxinA (U)	Abobotulinum-toxinA (U)	Rimabotulinum-toxinB (U)
Sternocleidomastoid	20–50	20–50	100–200	1000–2500
Infrahyoid muscles	10–15	10–15	40–60	750–1000
Scalenus anterior	10–20	10–20	40–80	1000–1500
Scalenus medius	10–20	10–20	40–80	1000–1500
Scalenus posterior	10–50	10–50	40–80	1000–2500
Levator scapulae	10–50	10–50	40–100	1250–2500
Trapezius (upper portion)	50–75	50–75	80–200	2500–4000
Splenius capitis	50–100	50–100	200–300	2500–5000
Semispinalis capitis	15–30	15–30	60–120	1000–1500

[a] In bilateral injections of some muscles dose reduction is necessary (see text).

weakness may occur in muscles located adjacent to the injection site as a result of this diffusion.

To reduce the risk of developing resistance, a 3-month interval between injections is recommended. Prior to repeat injection, the patient should be asked to report on the effectiveness of the last injection, its time course, and the type, severity and duration of side effects. A clinical rating should be repeated and the actual scores compared with those prior to and 4 weeks after the last injection. Some patients will return prior to a waning effect of the BoNT. In these cases, it can be difficult to localize the muscles for reinjection because they are still denervated. If possible, these patients should be discouraged from receiving a repeat injection at that time and be rescheduled for injection 2–4 weeks later when symptoms begin to appear. If the patient fulfills the criteria for reinjection, total dose, dose per individual muscle and selection of muscles to be injected must be reconsidered.

Making a change to the individual injection plan depends on the effectiveness and the side effects of the previous injection(s). The total dose should be decreased if severe side effects occur. If dysphagia occurs, the dose for the sternocleidomastoid muscle(s) should be decreased. If neck pain and/ or neck weakness are prominent side effects, the dose for the splenius capitis muscle(s) and other posterior cervical muscles, including the upper trapezius, semispinalis and longissimus, should be reduced. The total dose should be increased when the peak effect (improvement) is less than 50–60%, or when the duration of the plateau phase is shorter than 4 weeks – provided that side effects of clinical relevance do not occur. A change in the injection plan may need to be considered particularly where high-dose therapy and/or considerable side effects, in conjunction with only low or moderate effectiveness, occur. Selection of the muscles to be injected may have to be reconsidered, preferably with assistance of EMG.

The official recommendation from the manufacturers is to reconstitute 100 U onabotulinumtoxinA or 500 U abobotulinumtoxinA in 1 ml or 2.5 ml unpreserved NaCl solution, respectively. IncobotulinumtoxinA 100 U is usually dissolved in 2.0 ml NaCl solution. RimabotulinumtoxinB does not require reconstitution and is already in a solution of 5000 U/ml. Systematic studies dealing with any differences in effectiveness at various concentrations of onabotulinumtoxinA and abobotulinumtoxinA are not available for treatment of CD; however, it is the experience of the authors that use of solutions of 400 U/ml abobotulinumtoxinA and 100 U/ml onabotulinumtoxinA may decrease the prevalence of side effects (Davis *et al.*, 1991; Bertrand 1993; Kessler *et al.*, 1999). This observation may reflect less pronounced diffusion of the BoNT injected at lower volumes, particularly for injections into the sternocleidomastoid muscle.

Notes regarding muscle injections

Prior to sternocleidomastoid muscle injections, the patient should be asked to tonically activate the muscle by rotating their head against the hand of the physician or their own hand, placed at the opposite chin side. In this condition, the sternocleidomastoid muscle will become maximally prominent; furthermore, the safety of injection sites can be improved when the sternocleidomastoid muscle is held firmly with the physician's fingers while reaching behind the muscle. This maneuver is particularly important in patients with obese necks. It is also recommended to concentrate the treatment on two injection sites in the upper third of the sternocleidomastoid in order to reduce the incidence of dysphagia (Truong *et al.*, 1989).

Injections into the lateral neck muscles are best performed when the head is in a straight, neutral position. Injections into the trapezius muscles can be made more easily when patients are asked to elevate their shoulders. During injections into the hyoid muscles, the head is extended backwards. Injections are normally carried out with a 2–5 ml syringe and a 27-gauge hypodermic needle.

In summary, BoNT injections are effective treatment for abnormal posture, muscle hypertrophy and pain associated with CD. In order to obtain optimal results, the use of EMG and a good knowledge of cervical anatomy are helpful in designing individualized injection patterns, which, in turn, help patients with CD to better manage the disorder.

Acknowledgments

The authors express their appreciation for the critiques and recommendations from Professor Sherry Downie, Departments of Anatomy and Structural Biology and Physical Medicine and Rehabilitation, Albert Einstein College of Medicine and the assistance of Professor Mark Lew, Department of Neurology, Keck/USC School of Medicine.

References

Benecke R (1993). Botulinum-Toxin A in der Behandlung der zervikalen Dystonien. In Richter HP, Braun V (eds.) *Schiefhals. Behandlungskonzepte des Torticollis Spasmodicus*. Berlin: Springer, pp. 63–78.

Benecke R (1999). Zervikale Dystonie. In Laskawi R, Roggenkaemper, P (eds.) *Botulinum-Toxin-Therapie im Kopf-Hals-Bereich*. Munich: Urban & Vogel, pp. 171–212.

Benecke R, Jost WH, Kanovsky MD *et al.* (2005). A new botulinum toxin type A free of complexing proteins for treatment of cervical dystonia. *Neurology*, **64**, 1949–51.

Bertrand CM (1993). Selective peripheral denervation for spasmodic torticollis: surgical technique, results, and observations in 260 cases. *Surg Neurol*, **40**, 96–103.

Blackie JD, Lees AJ (1990). Botulinum toxin treatment in spasmodic torticollis. *J Neurol Neurosurg Psychiatry*, **53**, 640–3.

Borodic GE, Pearce LB, Smith K, Joseph M (1992). Botulinum A toxin for spasmodic torticollis: multiple vs single injection points per muscle. *Head Neck*, **14**, 33–7.

Brashear A, Lew MF, Dykstra DD *et al.* (1999). Safety and efficacy of NeuroBloc (botulinum toxin type B) in type A-responsive cervical dystonia. *Neurology*, **53**, 1439–46.

Brin MF, Lew MF, Adler MD *et al.* (1999). Safety and efficacy of NeuroBloc (botulinum toxin type B) in type A-resistant cervical dystonia. *Neurology*, **53**, 1431–8.

Comella CL, Buchmann AS, Tanner CM, Brown-Toms NC, Goetz CG (1992). Botulinum toxin injection for spasmodic torticollis: increased magnitude of benefit with electromyographic assistance. *Neurology*, **42**, 878–82.

Comella CL, Jankovic J, Truong DD, Hanschmann A, Grafe S (2011). Efficacy and safety of incobotulinumtoxinA (NT 201, XEOMIN(R), botulinum neurotoxin type A, without accessory proteins) in patients with cervical dystonia. *J Neurol Sci*, **308**, 103–9.

Davis DH, Ahlskog JE, Litchy WJ, Root LM (1991). Selective peripheral denervation for torticollis: preliminary results. *Mayo Clin Proc*, **66**, 365–71.

Foltz EL, Knopp LM, Ward AA (1959). Experimental spasmodic torticollis. *J Neurosurg*, **16**, 55–72.

Frei K, Pathak M, Jenkens S, Truong DD (2004). The natural history of posttraumatic cervical dystonia. *Mov Disord*, **12**, 1492–8.

Gelb DJ, Lowenstein DH, Aminoff MJ (1989). Controlled trial of botulinum toxin injections in the treatment of spasmodic torticollis. *Neurology*, **39**, 80–4.

Gelb DJ, Yoshimura DM, Olney RK, Lowenstein DH, Aminoff MJ (1991). Change in pattern of muscle activity following botulinum toxin injections for torticollis. *Ann Neurol*, **29**, 370–6.

Greene P, Kang U, Fahn S *et al.* (1990). Double-blind, placebo-controlled trial of botulinum toxin injections for the treatment of spasmodic torticollis. *Neurology*, **40**, 1213–18.

Hambleton P, Cohen HE, Palmer VJ, Melling J (1992). Antitoxins and botulinum toxin treatment. *BMJ*, **304**, 959–60.

Hatheway CL, Dang C (1994). Immunogenicity of the neurotoxins of *Clostridium botulinum*. In Jankovic J, Hallett M (eds.) *Therapy with Botulinum Toxin*. New York: Dekker, p. 107.

Jankovic J, Brin MF (1991). Therapeutic uses of botulinum toxin. *N Engl J Med*, **324**, 1186–94.

Jankovic J, Schwartz PA (1990). Botulinum toxin injections for cervical dystonia. *Neurology*, **40**, 277–80.

Kessler KR, Skutta M, Benecke R (1999). Long-term treatment of cervical dystonia with botulinum toxin A: efficacy, safety, and antibody frequency. *J Neurol*, **246**, 265–74.

Lew MF, Adornato BT, Duane DD *et al.* (1997). Botulinum toxin type B. A double blind, placebo-controlled, safety and efficacy study in cervical dystonia. *Neurology*, **49**, 701–7.

Lorentz IT, Subramaniam SS, Yiannikas C (1991). Treatment of idiopathic spasmodic torticollis with botulinum toxin A: a double-blind study on twenty-three patients. *Mov Disord*, **6**, 145–50.

Moore AP, Blumhardt LD (1991). A double blind trial of botulinum toxin "A" in torticollis, with one year follow up. *J Neurol Neurosurg Psychiatry*, **54**, 813–16.

Naumann M, Yakovleff A, Durif F (2002). A randomized, double-masked, crossover comparison of the efficacy and safety of botulinum toxin type A produced from the original bulk toxin and current bold toxin source for the treatment of cervical dystonia. *J Neurol*, **249**, 57–63.

Poewe W, Schelosky L, Kleedorfer B *et al.* (1992). Treatment of spasmodic torticollis with local injections of botulinum toxin. One-year follow-up in thirty-seven patients. *J Neurol*, **239**, 21–5.

Stell R, Bronstein AM, Marsden CD (1989). Vestibulo-ocular abnormalities in spasmodic torticollis before and after botulinum toxin injections. *J Neurol Neurosurg Psychiatry*, **52**, 57–62.

Truong D, Lewitt P, Cullis P (1989). Effects of different injection techniques in the treatment of torticollis with botulinum toxin. *Neurology*, **39**(Suppl), 294.

Truong D, Dubinski R, Hermanowicz N *et al.* (1991). Posttraumatic torticollis. *Arch Neurol*, **48**, 221–3.

Truong D, Duane DD, Jankovic J *et al.* (2005). Efficacy and safety of botulinum type A toxin (Dysport) in cervical dystonia: results of the first US randomized, double-blind, placebo-controlled study. *Mov Disord* **20**, 783–91.

Truong D, Brodsky M, Lew M *et al.* for the Global Dysport Cervical Dystonia Study Group (2010). Long-term efficacy and safety of botulinum toxin type A (Dysport) in cervical dystonia. *Parkinsonism Relat Disord*, **16**, 316–23.

Tsui JK, Eisen A, Mak E *et al.* (1985). A pilot study on the use of botulinum toxin in spasmodic torticollis. *Can J Neurol Sci*, **12**, 314–16.

Tsui JK, Eisen A, Stoesl AJ, Calne S, Calne DB (1986). Double-blind study of botulinum toxin in spasmodic torticollis. *Lancet*, **ii**, 245–7.

Wissel J, Poewe W (1992). Dystonia: a clinical, neuropathological and therapeutic review. *J Neural Transm Suppl*, **38**, 91–104.

Van Zandijcke M (1995). Cervical dystonia (spasmodic torticollis). Some aspects of the natural history. *Acta Neurol Belg*, **95**, 210–15.

Examination and treatment of complex cervical dystonia

Gerhard Reichel

Introduction

Botulinum neurotoxin (BoNT) serotype A (BoNT-A) is the treatment of choice for cervical dystonia (CD). Treatment outcome can vary with the presentation of CD and is significantly dependent on the correct assessment of the muscle involved.

There are "simple" (movement disorders in one plane) and "complex" (movement disorder in two or more levels) forms of CD. The most common presentation is the rotation and tilting of the head. The difficulty lies in the treatment of complex CD. In large studies, rates of patient satisfaction with the BoNT therapy range from 50 to 60% (Comella *et al.*, 2000; Haussermann *et al.*, 2004; Truong *et al.*, 2010). The most common cause of unsatisfactory treatment is the selection of the wrong muscle. The selection of the treated muscles is most effective if the actual clinical picture of complex CD in a patient is considered as an individual situation.

In a large study with imaging (MRI, CT) in patients with CD, it was noted that the previous phenomenological classification of CD in four groups (torticollis, laterocollis, antecollis and retrocollis) is inadequate. There are clinical cases of CD in which only muscles that act on the head are involved, and others involving only muscles that act on the cervical spine (Reichel, 2009, 2012). Therefore, a more extensive complex cervical movement disorder clinical analysis beyond the four traditional groups is required. The objective is a precise delineation of an optimal individualized treatment strategy in the selection of muscle involved. As the selection of the treated muscles and finding the individual BoNT dose can be difficult, different diagnostic methods are used. They include ultrasound, CT neck soft tissue imaging (particularly the deep muscles of the neck), electromyography (EMG) of neck muscles and standardized photographs of patients with measurements of angles (head, neck, thorax). The

presence of a lateral shift or forward sagittal shift (very rarely backward) suggests a combination of two clinical pictures: lateral shift occurs when a laterocollis is combined with a laterocaput to the opposite side (Fig. 6.1a). A sagittal shift forward occurs when an antecollis is combined with a retrocaput. A sagittal shift to the rear is also possible (combination of retrocollis and antecaput) but occurs very rarely isolated, most likely with generalized dystonia.

The more differentiated is the examination of the patient, the better the likely success of therapy. Cervical dystonia may occur in principle in three axes (rotation, lateral flexion and sagittal flexion). The head or the neck can be affected alone in each of these planes of movement. Therefore, eight clinical forms can be distinguished: torticollis, laterocollis, antecollis, retrocollis, torticaput, laterocaput, antecaput and retrocaput (Fig. 6.2). In each plane of motion, the variations in the ratio 1:1:3 for each condition, such as for head turning, would be 1 torticollis pure to 1 pure torticaput to 3 both variants (Reichel, 2012).

Moreover, almost all types can occur at different levels together in combination: most common are the combination of lateral tilting and rotation.

Clinical studies and additional examinations

Observation of the patient in a sitting position from the front

The patient should assume a relaxed position on a swivel chair. The patient is asked to lean the upper body to the back of the chair with the eyes closed. The face is turned toward the examiner. The position of the head is observed in relaxation. The patient is asked to conduct the following movements:

Manual of Botulinum Toxin Therapy, 2nd edition, ed. Daniel Truong, Mark Hallett, Christopher Zachary and Dirk Dressler. Published by Cambridge University Press. © Cambridge University Press 2013.

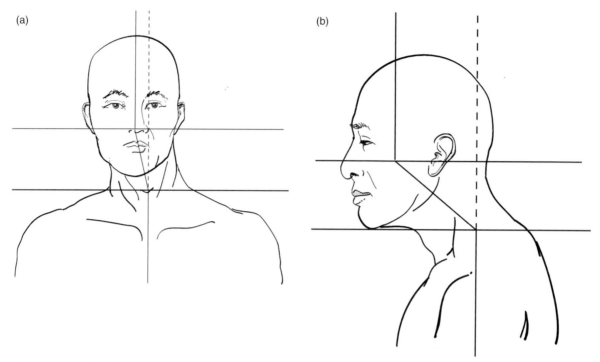

Fig. 6.1 Lateral shift or forward sagittal shift. (a) Lateral shift to the right: laterocollis to the right. The head is tilted on the neck line to the left: laterocaput to the left. (b) Sagittal shift forward: antecollis. The head is tilted in the neck line backward: retrocaput.

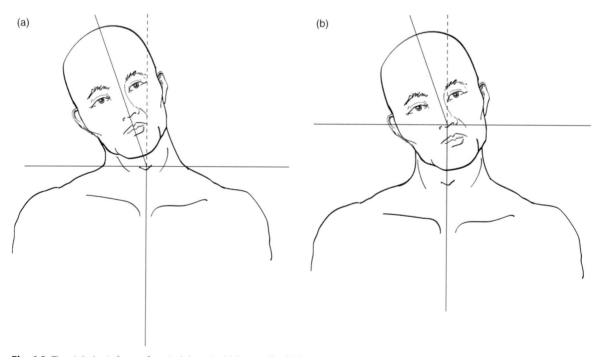

Fig. 6.2 The eight basic forms of cervical dystonia: (a) laterocollis; (b) laterocaput; (c) torticollis; (d) torticaput; (e) antecollis; (f) antecaput; (g) retrocollis; (h) retrocaput.

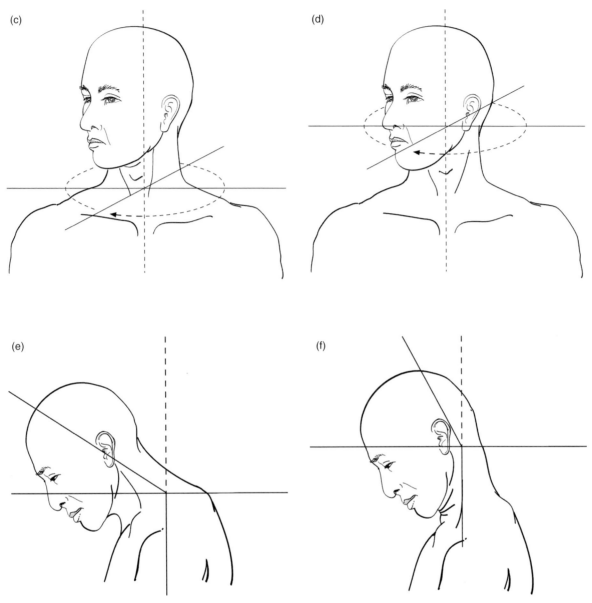

Fig. 6.2 (cont.)

- rotation of the head to the left and right and take a subjective center position
- tilting of the head to the left and right and then taking a subjective center position.

Observation of the patient in a sitting position from the side

The patient is again asked to take the relaxed sitting position and rotate so that he or she can be seen from the side. Throughout the investigation, the patient leans the upper body against the back of the chair and has eyes closed. The head position is observed in relaxation. Upon request, the patient moves through the following motions:

- tilting the head forward then returning to a subjective neutral head position
- tilting the head backward then returning to a subjective neutral head position.

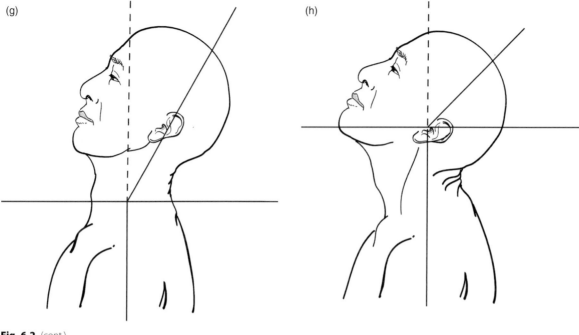

(g)

(h)

Fig. 6.2 (cont.)

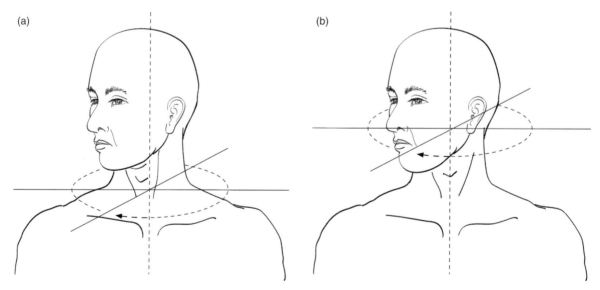

(a)

(b)

Fig. 6.3 Scheme of dystonic head rotation. (a) Rotation below C2 is torticollis. (b) Rotation in the lower head joint (between C1 and C2) is torticaput.

Investigation of the rotation: torticollis and torticaput

To distinguish between a torticollis and torticaput (Fig. 6.3), one must differentiate whether the area the rotation is in the range C3–C7 (torticollis), or in the lower head joint between C1 and C2 (torticaput). A mark (skin marker) is placed at the larynx above the superior thyroid notch and above the jugular notch at the manubrium sterni. If the mark on the throat shifts laterally from the mark on the manubrium at the turn of the head, this indicates the presentation of torticollis (Fig. 6.4a). In torticaput, the two marks stay perpendicular to each other on head rotation (Fig. 6.4b).

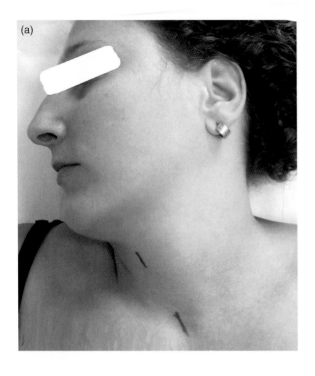

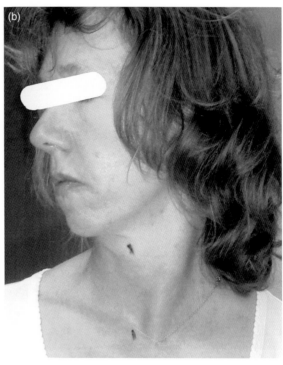

Fig. 6.4 Patients with head rotation. (a) The thyroid notch is clearly on the side of the jugular notch in torticollis. (b) The thyroid notch is located vertically above the jugular notch in torticaput.

When the analysis is uncertain, CT of the neck may help to clarify the situation, with a CT slice at the C3 level. The relationship between the position of C3 and the chin may help to clarify torticollis from torticaput.

In torticollis, C3 and the chin align in one direction, which indicates the rotation occurs below C3 (Fig. 6.5a). In torticaput, there is a rotation of the chin against C3, which indicates that the rotation occurs above C3, that is, at the lower head joint (Fig. 6.5b). For this differentiation, pictures from the CT bone window may be adequate.

In torticaput, the obliquus capitis inferior is often involved (Reichel, 2011). On CT, a short thick muscle on the side of the rotation at the level of the lower head–spine junction can be seen, with an elongated thinner muscle on the opposite side (Fig. 6.6a). In the CT reconstruction, the asymmetry of the obliquus capitis inferior muscles on either side can be seen in the coronal section (Fig. 6.6b).

Investigation of lateral flexion: laterocollis and laterocaput

During lateral bending, tilting at the head (laterocaput) or the cervical spine (laterocollis) can be differentiated (Fig. 6.7a).

When the tilting occurs at head level, the muscles involved are muscles that act at the bottom of the skull or head joints. In the lateral flexion of the neck, the muscles involved are muscles that arise and insert at the cervical spine.

Combination of laterocollis on one side and laterocaput to the opposite side results in the clinical picture of a lateral shift (Fig. 6.1a).

The patient often tries to normalize the position of the head or neck by raising the ipsilateral shoulder and with this keep the head straight with the use of a scoliosis in the cervical–thoracic region of the spine. If the patient is asked to have their eyes closed during the examination, the shoulder elevation may normalize. If a second person balances the shoulders, the shoulder elevation would show up as compensation for the laterocollis or laterocaput (Fig. 6.7b).

Investigation of sagittal flexion: retrocollis and retrocaput, antecollis and antecaput

Viewing the patient from the side will allow differentiation between retrocollis, retrocaput, antecollis and antecaput. The angle between the head and neck or cervical spine and thoracic spine can be determined in this position (Figs. 6.8 and 6.9).

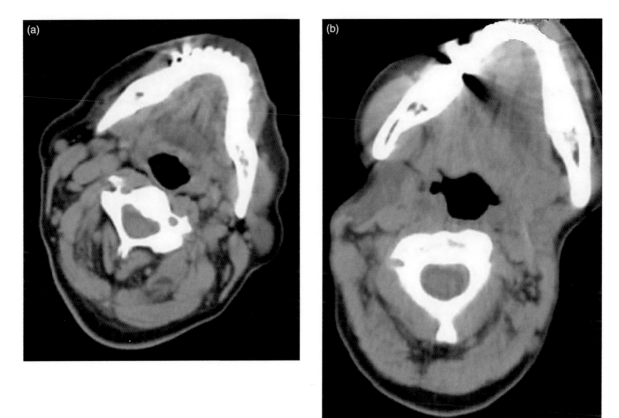

Fig. 6.5 The neck at the level of C3 in CT scans. (a) In torticollis, C3 and the chin point in one direction; (b) in torticaput, the chin is rotated compared with C3.

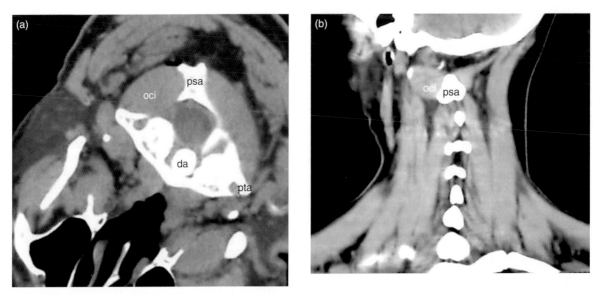

Fig. 6.6 The obliquus capitis inferior muscle. (a) The patient lies on her stomach for this view. In axial section, the dystonic obliquus capitis inferior (oci) is shown as thick and shortened. Note that the normal obliquus capitis inferior muscle of the opposite side is long and slender. (b) In the reconstruction (coronal section), the asymmetry of the obliquus capitis inferior muscle is evident. da, dens of the axis; psa, spinal process of the axis; pta, transverse process of the atlas.

(a)

(b)

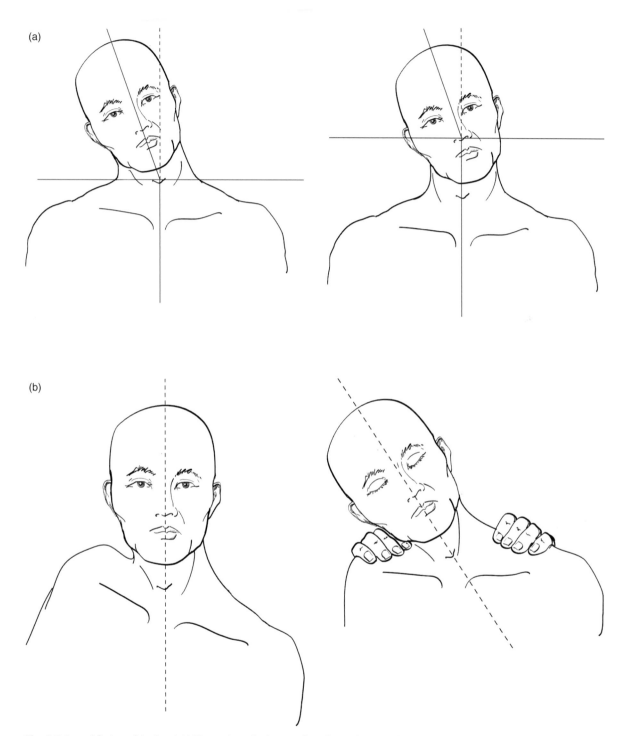

Fig. 6.7 Lateral flexion of the head. (a) The neck can be bent to the side in relation to the chest with the head straight on the neck (left). The head can be bent to the side in relation to the neck but the neck is not bent (right). (b) With open eyes, the patient compensates for the tilt of the head (laterocollis or laterocaput) by bending the spine, resulting in a higher shoulder (left). With eyes closed and after passive correction of the high shoulder stand, the tilting of the neck becomes obvious (here laterocollis) (right).

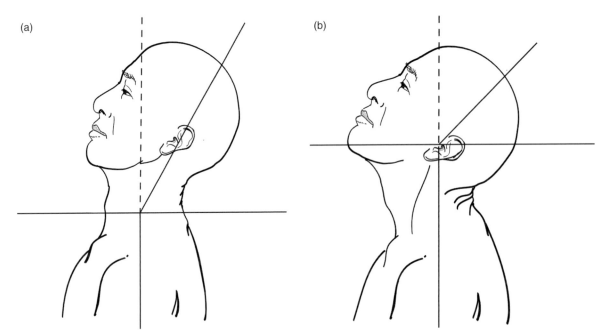

Fig. 6.8 Backward tilting of the neck/head. (a) The neck is extended against the chest toward the back and the head is straight on the neck. Extension backward is at the level of the clavicle in retrocollis. (b) The head is bent over the neck to the back and the neck is straight on the chest. Extension backward is at the level of the external auditory meatus in retrocaput. (Note the nuchal skin fold.)

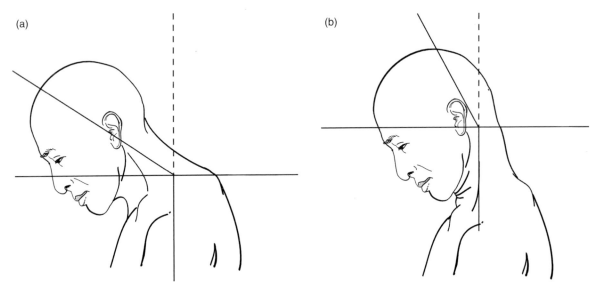

Fig. 6.9 Forward flexion of the head/neck. (a) The neck is flexed against the chest forward. The head is straight on the neck. The rotation forward is at the level of the clavicle and the external auditory meatus is anterior of the clavicle in antecollis. (b) The head is bent over the neck forward and the neck is straight on the chest. The axis of the rotation forward is at the level of the external auditory meatus in antecaput. (Note the double chin.)

The head rotates in antecollis and retrocollis in the lower cervical spine. In antecaput and retrocaput, the axis of the rotation occurs at the level of the external acoustic meatus.

The sagittal shift forward is the combination of antecollis and retrocaput. The investigation of the sagittal shift forward is also carried out by viewing the patient from the side. This allows the determination of the angle between the head and neck or cervical spine and thoracic spine (Fig. 6.1b).

Treatment of complex cervical dystonia with botulinum neurotoxin

After the clinical analysis has allowed phenomenological classification of the specific CD occurring, comparison of the muscle functions in the eight possible variants will narrow the circle of the muscle in question (Table 6.1).

The dystonic muscles can be identified on the relaxed patient with palpation, electromyography and ultrasound. For the first treatment we recommend injecting a maximum of three muscles. They should be the most clearly affected muscles. The following features are noteworthy:

Table 6.1 Muscles involved in the different head posture variants (from MRI measurements)

Form	Muscle	Origin	Insertion
Laterocollis	Levator scapulae	Processus transversus C1 – C4	Angulus superior scapulae
	Scalenus anterior	Processus transversus C4 – C6	Rib 1
	Scalenus medius	Processus transversus C2 – C7	Rib 1
	Semispinalis cervicis	Processus transversus T1 – T6	Processus spinosus C2 – C5
	Longissimus cervicis	Processus transversus T1 – T6	Processus transversus C2 – C5
Laterocaput	Sternocleidomastoideus	Sternum, clavicle	Processus mastoideus + linea nuchae superior
	Splenius capitis	Processus spinosus C4 – C7	Processus mastoideus
	Splenius cervicis	Processus spinosus T4 – T6	Processus transversus C1 + C2
	Trapezius pars descendens	Linea nuchae	Lateral third of clavicle
	Semispinalis capitis	Processus transversus C3 – C7, T1 – T6	Between lineae nuchae superior and inferior
	Longissimus capitis	Processus transversus T1 – T4, processus articularis C5 – C7	Processus mastoideus
	Levator scapulae	Processus transversus C1 – C4	Angulus superior scapulae
Torticollis	Longissimus cervicis	Processus transversus T1 – T6	Processus transversus C2 – C5
	Semispinalis cervicis	Processus transversus T1 – T6	Processus spinosus C2
Torticaput	Sternocleidomastoideus	Sternum, clavicle	Processus mastoideus + linea nuchae superior
	Trapezius pars descendens	Linea nuchae	Lateral third of clavicle
	Semispinalis capitis	Processus transversus C3 – C7, T1 – T6	Between lineae nuchae superior and inferior
	Splenius capitis	Processus spinosus C4 – C7	Processus mastoideus
	Splenius cervicis	Processus spinosus T4 – T6	Processus transversus C1 + C2
	Longissimus capitis	Processus transversus T1 – T4, processus articularis C5 – C7	Processus mastoideus
	Obliquus capitis inferior	Processus spinosus C2	Processus transversus C1
Antecollis bilateral	Scalenus anterior	Processus transversus C4 – C6	Rib 1
	Scalenus medius	Processus transversus C2 – C7	Rib 1
	Levator scapulae	Processus transversus C1 – C4	Angulus superior scapulae
	Longus colli pars recta	Bodies of C5 – C7, T1 – T3	Bodies of C2 – C4
	Longus collis pars obliqua inferior	Bodies of T1 – T3	Tubercula anteriora processus transversorum C5 and C6
Antecaput bilateral	Longus capitis	Tubercula anteriora processus transversorum C3 – C6	Pars basilaris ossis occipitalis
	Longus colli pars obliqua superior	Processus transversus C2 – C5	Tuberculum anterius C1
	Levator scapulae	Processus transversus C1 – C4	Angulus superior scapulae
Retrocollis bilateral	Longissimus cervicis	Processus transversus T1 – T6	Processus transversus C2 – C5
	Semispinalis cervicis	Processus transversus T1 – T6	Processus spinosus C2 – C5
Retrocaput bilateral	Sternocleidomastoideus	Sternum, clavicle	Processus mastoideus + linea nuchae superior
	Trapezius pars descendens	Linea nuchae	Lateral third of clavicle
	Semispinalis capitis	Processus transversus C4 – C7	Between lineae nuchae superior and inferior
	Splenius capitis	Processus spinosus C4 – C7	Processus mastoideus
	Splenius cervicis	Processus spinosus T4 – T6	Processus transversus C1 + C2
	Obliquus capitis inferior	Processus spinosus C2	Processus transversus C1

- the splenius cervicis is a muscle predominantly affecting the movements of the head and not the cervical spine despite its name, because it inserts on the lower head joint
- the levator scapula is the only muscle that acts on both the head and the cervical spine movements; it originates at the processus transversalis of C1 – C4
- the obliquus capitis is the most commonly affected in dystonia from all the deep neck muscles and leads to a torticaput; it originates on the spinous process of axis and inserts on the processus transversus atlantis.

For better identification of the muscle for the injection of BoNT we recommend the following methods:

Electromyography. The EMG guarantees that the BoNT is injected into the muscle tissue. The most frequent causes of lack of efficacy in the treatment with BoNT are missing the intended muscle – injection next to the muscle or piercing through the muscle. Use of EMG, however, cannot help to identify the specific muscle. The corresponding atlases are helpful (Jost *et al.*, 2008).

Ultrasound. The use of ultrasound allows precise mapping of the injection needle to the muscles. In the small deep neck muscles (obliquus capitis inferior, longus colli, etc.), the usefulness of the ultrasound examination is limited.

Computed tomography. This will help for deep muscles, when the ultrasound cannot identify reliably, particularly, when the obliquus capitis inferior is involved.

Injection of the small muscles of the neck under CT guidance

Patients are asked to lie on their stomachs with their heads in a relaxed position. The position of the obliquus capitis inferior can then be determined with CT (Fig. 6.10a). The lateral distance of the muscle to the midline (marked with an X-ray marker) and the depth from the surface to the muscle is measured on the CT image. After local anesthesia and disinfection of the skin, the cannula is inserted vertically with the penetration depth marked with a Steri-Strip (Fig. 6.10b). This is followed by a CT assessment of the needle position (Fig. 6.10c). If the needle tip is in the muscle, 25 mU onabotulinumtoxinA/incobotulinumtoxinA or 75 mU abobotulinumtoxinA is injected.

At the end of the procedure, a control CT can be performed if needed. The BoNT-injected muscle has a dark discoloration (Fig. 6.10d).

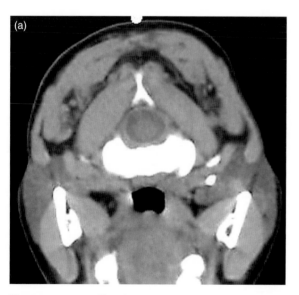

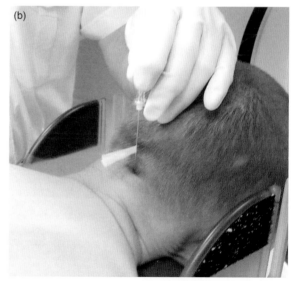

Fig. 6.10 Injection of botulinum neurotoxin into the obliquus capitis inferior under CT guidance. (a) Presentation of the soft tissue of the neck at the level of the obliquus capitis inferior as seen by CT. The dystonic muscle is slightly thicker and shorter than the normal opposite muscle. (b) Introduction of the injection needle with the Steri-Strip. (c) The neck soft tissue as seen by CT with the hypodermic needle in the obliquus capitis inferior. (d) After injection with botulinum neurotoxin in the inferior obliquus capitis.

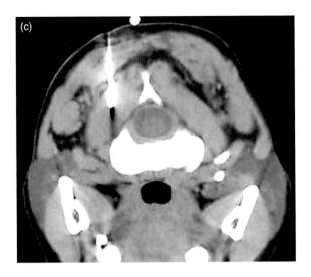

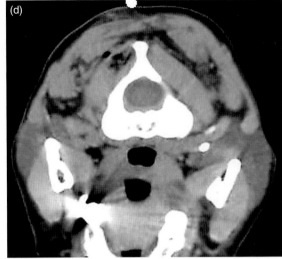

Fig. 6.10 (cont.)

In our experience, the rate of successful treatment for patients with torticaput increased by about 20% if treatment included the obliquus capitis inferior.

Summary

The treatment of complex CD requires a careful analysis of dystonic movement disorder in the eight subgroups. The basis for treatment decisions is the clinical examination and the assessment of the dystonic disorder in a relaxed patient who keeps his or her eyes closed.

Ultrasonography, EMG and CT are helpful in identification of the affected muscle. In the treatment of deep neck muscles, injection under CT guidance is helpful if ultrasound-assisted needle injections are unreliable.

Acknowledgment

The author expresses his appreciation for the extensive editing and rewriting of the article by Dr. Daniel Truong.

References

Comella CL, Jankovic J, Brin MF (2000). Use of botulinum toxin type A in the treatment of cervical dystonia. *Neurology*, **55**(Suppl 5), S15–21.

Haussermann P, Marczoch S, Klinger C *et al.* (2004). Long-term follow-up of cervical dystonia patients treated with botulinum toxin A. *Mov Disord*, **19**, 303–8.

Jost W (2008). *Pictorial Atlas of Botulinum Toxin Injection: Dosage, Localization, Application.* London: Quintessence.

Reichel G (2009). Zur Phänomenologie der zervikalen und kranialen Dystonien: Vorschlag einer neuen Behandlungsstrategie mit Botulinumtoxin. [The phenomenology of cervical dystonia: proposed new treatment strategy with botulinum toxin.] *Fortschr Neurol Psychiatry*, **77**, 1–6.

Reichel G (2011). Cervical dystonia: a new phenomenological classification for botulinum toxin therapy. *BaGa* **1**, 5–12.

Reichel G (2012). *Therapy Guide Spasticity: Dystonia*, 2nd edn. Bremen: UniMed.

Truong D, Brodsky M, Lew M *et al.* (2010). Global Dysport Cervical Dystonia Study Group. Long-term efficacy and safety of botulinum toxin type A (Dysport) in cervical dystonia. *Parkinsonism Relat Disord*, **16**, 316–23.

Ultrasound guidance for botulinum neurotoxin therapy: cervical dystonia

Katharine E. Alter

Introduction

The primary focus of this chapter is to provide a review of the technical requirements and techniques for performing brightness mode (B-mode) ultrasound (US) to guide botulinum neurotoxin (BoNT) injections for cervical dystonia (CD). A brief review of the advantages and disadvantages of various guidance techniques and the supporting literature is also presented.

Cervical dystonia

Idiopathic CD is the most common form of focal dystonia worldwide (Defazio *et al.*, 2004; Jankovic, 2004). It is characterized by sustained muscle contraction leading to abnormal postures and twisting movements of the head and neck. Patients with CD report functional limitations and pain associated with the muscle pulling or twisted postures. The combination of pain and posturing affect many activities of daily living and quality of life and limit participation in work, family life and avocational interests. A full review of the diagnosis, patterns of muscle involvement and range of therapies for CD is covered elsewhere in this text.

In brief, treatment options for patients with CD include manual or physical therapy, oral medications and BoNT therapy (Brans *et al.*, 1996; Brashear *et al.*, 1999; Useros-Olmo and Collado-Vázquez, 2010). Surgical procedures have been described but are rarely recommended. Because of its favorable side effect profile (compared with other treatments) clinicians frequently prescribe and patients often prefer BoNT therapy over oral medications. This is because BoNT therapy provides a long duration of symptomatic relief of the pain or postures associated with CD with minimal side effects (Comella *et al.*, 1992, 2011; Costa *et al.*, 2005; Simpson *et al.*, 2008, 2009; Truong *et al.*, 2010).

Traditional targeting techniques: anatomical reference guides, palpation, electromyography, electrical stimulation

For CD, or any other indication for BoNT therapy, accurately identifying and targeting problematic muscles (or other structures) is key to the success of the procedure and to reducing potential adverse events such as dysphagia or weakness in adjacent muscles (Speelman and Brans, 1995; Molloy *et al.*, 2002; Elovic *et al.*, 2009).

Commonly used targeting methods for chemodenervation procedures include manual needle placement based on palpation and/or anatomical reference guides, passive/active range of motion, electromyography (EMG) and electrical stimulation or combinations of these techniques. Each of these techniques has advantages and disadvantages, but currently there is no incontrovertible proof that one technique is superior to another. Additional studies are required to determine which technique provides the highest accuracy and whether increased accuracy leads to higher treatment efficacy and reduced adverse events associated with BoNT therapy (Lim *et al.*, 2011).

While the use of palpation and anatomical reference guides may seem simple, these techniques are subject to numerous limitations including:

- anatomical variations or rearrangements caused by spasticity/contractures

Manual of Botulinum Toxin Therapy, 2nd edition, ed. Daniel Truong, Mark Hallett, Christopher Zachary and Dirk Dressler. Published by Cambridge University Press. © Cambridge University Press 2013.

- variation in target depth because of variation in patient size, adipose tissue, muscle atrophy
- difficulty in palpating deep muscles or muscles in regions with complex overlapping architecture
- limitations in patient positioning to replicate anatomical reference guides.

The accuracy of BoNT injections guided by EMG is also affected by the limitations inherent to anatomical reference guides. In addition, the accuracy of EMG guidance is reduced by the presence of muscle co-contraction or poor selective motor control, which leads to widespread EMG activity or signals from the target and adjacent muscles. In the presence of co-contraction or impaired selective motor control, a clinician may falsely attribute EMG signal/muscle activity to the target when the needle is in another muscle.

While electrical stimulation may be a more accurate localization tool for BoNT injections than passive EMG, it is rarely if ever used in cervical muscles, likely because of the pain/discomfort associated with electrical stimulation.

Ultrasound and other imaging guidance techniques

A variety of imaging modalities are used for procedural guidance for BoNT/chemodenervation procedures include B-mode US, CT guidance, fluoroscopy and endoscopy (Jordan *et al.*, 2007; Botwin *et al.*, 2008; Danielson and Odderson, 2008; Glass *et al.*, 2009; Lee *et al.*, 2009; Torriani *et al.*, 2010; Hong *et al.*, 2012). Of these techniques, B-mode US has emerged as an accurate, clinician/patient friendly tool to guide BoNT therapy.

In US-guided BoNT procedures, B-mode and Doppler imaging are used to visualize the needle, injectate, target and other structures of interest (other muscles, vessels, nerves, organs). The distinct advantage of B-mode US is the provision of real-time continuous guidance for the needle and target throughout the procedure. Compared with other image guidance techniques, US also has a lower risk profile(no ionizing radiation), the equipment is portable, and procedures guided in this way are less costly than using fluoroscopy or CT. The technical requirements and techniques for US-guided BoNT procedures is covered in the technical section of this chapter.

Ultrasound versus other guidance techniques: what is the evidence?

In the last several years an increasing number of studies have compared US guidance with other guidance techniques. The majority of these studies evaluated the accuracy of US compared with another guidance technique(s) for upper or lower limb muscles. In the majority of these studies, US has been found to be more accurate (Henzel *et al.*, 2010; Boon *et al.*, 2011; Peck *et al.*, 2011; Schnitzler *et al.*, 2012).

While the literature specific to US-guided BoNT procedures for cervical muscles is limited, the current literature supports US as an accurate technique for cervical muscle localization (Lee *et al.*, 2009). One recent study also reported a reduced incidence of dysphagia for US-guided procedures compared with EMG-guided procedures for CD (Hong *et al.*, 2012). Given the complexity of cervical muscle anatomy, it is doubtful that the accuracy of cervical muscle targeting with blind insertion, landmark base localization or EMG would be higher than that reported in limb muscles. Therefore, the literature review includes studies related to US guidance for both cervical and limb muscles.

Ultrasound guidance compared with computed tomography or fluoroscopy for cervical dystonia

In a 2009 study, Lee *et al.* reported their initial experience with imaging guided US and CT for BoNT injections in patients with CD. Deep cervical muscle targeting was assessed in eight patients: in five US guidance was used, in two CT guidance, and in one both US and CT guidance. Muscles injected under imaging guidance included the oblique capitis inferioris and superioris (US guidance), longus colli (CT guidance), scalene (CT) and levator scapulae (CT). Both CT- and US-guided injection techniques were found to be accurate and all of the patients had marked improvement in symptoms after injection with either guidance system. Lee *et al.*, (2009) reported that, while both CT and US guidance techniques were accurate, US guidance was preferred because of its convenience.

A clear advantage of US guidance over CT or fluoroscopy is the lack of ionizing radiation. Given that BoNT injections for CD are frequently performed at 12-week intervals, the repeated use of CT or fluoroscopy guidance would, over time, lead to unacceptably high ionizing radiation exposure.

Hong *et al.* (2012) reported their experience with US-guided BoNT injections in treating five patients with CD who had a history of dysphagia with prior BoNT procedures. In these patients, US guidance was used for targeting, with the primary focus on US guidance for the sternocleidomastoid muscle. The authors reported a reduced incidence of dysphagia from 34% with EMG guidance to 0% with US-guided injections of the sternocleidomastoid and levator scapulae muscles (Hong *et al.*, 2012).

Several articles have documented the use of US, CT or fluoroscopy alone or with EMG to guide cervical muscle BoNT injections in the scalene muscles for thoracic outlet syndrome or cervicogenic pain syndromes (Jordan *et al.*, 2007; Botwin *et al.*, 2008; Danielson and Odderson, 2008; Torriani *et al.*, 2010). Jordan *et al.* (2007) compared combined EMG:fluoroscopy with EMG:US. The authors reported no difference in the success or complication rates between the two guidance methods. They concluded that US guidance combined with EMG was preferable because of the absence of ionizing radiation, convenience and lower cost of this procedure.

Ultrasound guidance compared with anatomical reference guides/palpation of limb muscles

A number of recent articles have evaluated the accuracy of manual, landmark-based targeting or EMG plus anatomical reference guides for needle insertion or limb muscle injections (Yang *et al.*, 2009; Henzel *et al.*, 2010; Boon *et al.*, 2011; Schnitzler *et al.*, 2012). In all of these articles, the accuracy of muscle targeting was substantially higher with US than with the other techniques.

Boon *et al.* (2011) compared the accuracy of blind placement and US-guided placement of fine wire in 14 lower limb muscles of fresh frozen cadavers. Blind placement was performed using standard EMG reference techniques by one experienced clinician (>10 years EMG experience) and a resident with 6 months of EMG training. The overall accuracy of blind placement was 39% in the 14 studied muscles compared with over 96% for the US-guided procedures. Accuracy with blind placement ranged from 0% in several muscles (rectus femoris, extensor hallucis longus, semitendinosus) to 100% (tibialis anterior). The accuracy of placement using US was 100% in all muscles except the semitendinosus (50%). Of note was that experience did not improve the accuracy of manual/blind wire insertion. Although the accuracy of the experienced clinician was slightly higher, only the accuracy of trajectory of the needle insertion reached statistical significance. This refutes the widely held belief that experience increases a clinician's accuracy when manually placing a needle into a muscle.

Yang *et al.* (2009) reported the accuracy of manual needle placement for BoNT injections in the gastrocnemius (checked by US). They found the accuracy of needle placement in the lateral gastrocnemius was unacceptably low at 64% (Yang *et al.*, 2009).

Schnitzler *et al.* (2012) evaluated the accuracy of manual targeting in the gastrocnemius in 30 cadaver gastrocnemius muscles. The accuracy of the injection (ink) was checked by anatomical dissection by a clinician and an anatomist. Overall, placement was only accurate in 43% of injections. As in the Boon *et al.* (2011) study, the results/accuracy was unrelated to clinician experience.

Henzel *et al.* (2010) evaluated two anatomical guidance techniques (Delagai, Bickerton) for upper limb muscles (flexor carpi ulnaris, flexor digitorum superficialis, flexor polices longus, pronator teres) comparing them with US muscle/fascicle localization. The investigators reported significant differences in muscle/muscle fascicle location when using US guidance compared with the reference guides for several flexor muscles both in proximal–distal and medial–lateral localization.

Ultrasound compared with electrical stimulation

In a randomized study, Picelli *et al.* (2012) compared the efficacy of BoNT injections into the gastrocnemius muscle of adults with spasticity after stroke using US, electrical stimulation or manual placement. A greater reduction in the Modified Ashworth Score and improvement in range of motion was reported in patients in whom injections were guided by US. No difference in the groups was noted in the Tardieu Scale.

Kwon *et al.* (2010) compared the efficacy of BoNT injections guided by electrical stimulation and US in treating spasticity in the gastrocnemius. A statistically significant improvement in gait (Physician Rating Scale) was noted in the US-guided group. No differences were noted in the Modified Ashworth Score or the Tardieu Scale.

Ultrasound-guided botulinum neurotoxin injections for cervical dystonia

Technical requirements and techniques

Equipment required to perform US-guided chemodenervation procedures includes a US machine, linear transducers of various frequencies and/or sizes, a coupling agent to reduce skin impedance (US gel or saline) and procedural supplies (transducer covers, needles, gloves, etc.) (Alter 2010; Davidson and Jayaraman, 2011; Alter *et al.*, 2012).

Ultrasound machines

Ultrasound machines include large cart-based systems and compact portable laptop style units. Proprietary differences between manufacturers influence transducer technology and thereby the image resolution provided by an individual machine. Clinicians are advised to evaluate several machines during live demonstrations, preferably head to head for diagnostic scanning and procedural guidance prior to purchasing equipment. This will ensure that the machine meets the needs of procedures to be performed by all of the clinicians who will be using the equipment.

The primary mode of US for chemodenervation procedures is B-mode, although Doppler imaging is a useful tool during chemodenervation procedures to visualize vascular structures, particularly when imaging head and neck structures. The majority of machines come with factory-installed musculoskeletal and/or glandular imaging presets. These presets speed system navigation, reduce the time for scanning or procedure set up and optimizes imaging of the structures of interest.

Transducers

When performing US-guided procedures, the importance of selecting the correct transducer cannot be overemphasized. Transducers come in various sizes and configurations. Linear transducers are best suited for US-guided BoNT procedures, including those for cervical muscles. The frequency of a transducer determines the depth of sound wave penetration as well as image resolution (through sampling frequency). Higher-frequency transducers always provide better image resolution but this is at the expense of depth of penetration. When performing diagnostic or procedural sonography, clinicians must select a transducer that allows imaging of the entire region of interest. For the vast majority of head and neck injections, a linear transducer with a frequency range between 5 and 12 MHz is sufficient. Higher frequencies may be useful when scanning superficial muscles or structures. A small footprint transducer such as a hockey stick is valuable for irregular surfaces, small spaces or smaller patients. A full discussion of US physics and equipment is beyond the scope of this chapter and the reader is referred to several reviews on this topic (Alter 2010; Alter *et al.*, 2012).

Ultrasound basics for tissues

With US imaging, structures are described based on their echotexture. During US imaging, structures appear hypoechoic or dark when few US waves are reflected back to the transducer. Structures will appear bright or hyperechoic when most, or many, of the US waves reflect off the tissue being imaged and, therefore, return back to the transducer. Muscle has a mixed echotexture appearance, with the contractile elements (fibers) appearing hypoechoic and the intramuscular connective tissue or surrounding fascia appearing relatively hyperechoic. Tendons are hyperechoic, highly anisotropic and fibrillar in appearance. Nerves are less hyperechoic or fibrillar than tendon. Vessels are anechoic (black). Bone is mirror-like and highly reflective of US. Therefore, the cortex of bone will appear hyperechoic and since no US penetrates the cortex posterior acoustic shadowing will be observed (Smith and Finnoff, 2009a; Alter 2010; Alter *et al.*, 2012).

Imaging techniques

The width of the US beam is narrower than the width/ footprint of the transducer. To completely image a structure or target requires the operator to "scan" or move the transducer up/down, back/forth to fully image the area of interest. A complete US scan of the area of interest is required prior to performing a procedure. This "scout" scan provides the clinician with useful information about structures of interest, the depth/location of the target, the best path to the target, structures to be avoided (nerves, vessels) and the

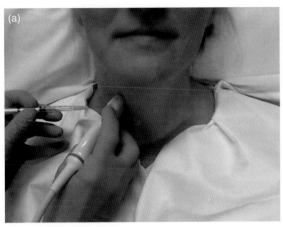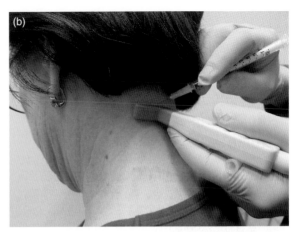

Fig. 7.1 Out-of-plane approach. (a) Longitudinal scan; (b) Transverse scan.

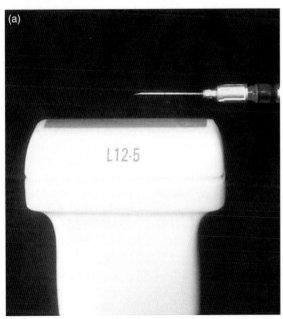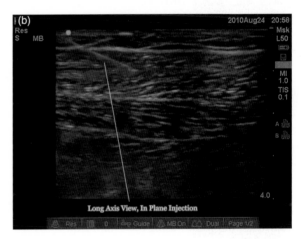

Fig. 7.2 Ultrasound-guided procedure for the in-plane approach. (a) Needle inserted along the length of the transducer; (b) In-plane view of needle path (white line).

presence of anatomical variations or masses (Smith and Finnoff, 2009a,b; Alter 2010; Alter *et al.*, 2012).

When scanning with US, muscles/structures can be imaged either in longitudinal or transverse plane (Fig. 7.1). It is recommended to scan in both planes to determine which provides the best view of the target and surrounding structures.

When used for procedural guidance, B-mode provides real-time imaging of a structure and the location of the needle throughout the procedure, but only if the

needle is kept within the beam produced by the transducer. Because the US beam created by the transducer is narrow, the sonographer must take care to keep the needle continuously within this beam otherwise visualization of the needle will be lost and the needle could be in an untargeted structure.

Needle insertion during US-guided procedures can be performed using either an "in-plane" or an "out-of-plane" approach. When using an in-plane approach (Fig. 7.2), the needle is inserted along the length of the

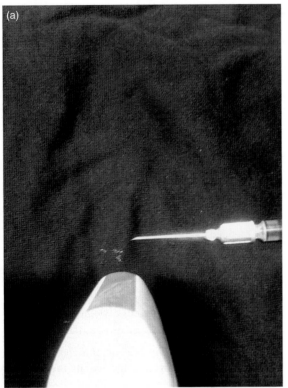

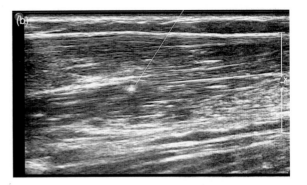

Fig. 7.3 Ultrasound-guided procedure for the out-of-plane approach. (a) Injection technique across the short access of the transducer; (b) Needle viewed as hyperechoic dot.

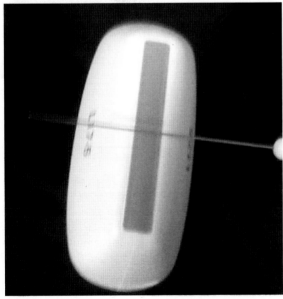

Fig. 7.4 Out-of-plane approach with needle tip incorrectly positioned out of the ultrasound beam and, therefore, potentially in an untargeted structure.

transducer. With this technique, the entire needle, including the tip will be visualized. In the out-of-plane approach, the needle is inserted through the short access of the transducer (Fig. 7.3a). When using an out-of-plane technique, the needle is viewed in short axis and, therefore, appears as a hyperechoic dot. When using the out-of-plane technique, both the tip and the shaft of the needle will appear as a hyperechoic dot (Fig. 7.3b). When using the out-of-plane technique, a "walk-down" technique is used to ensure that the *tip* of the needle is in the target structure (Fig. 7.4) (Smith and Finnoff, 2009b; Alter 2010; Alter *et al.*, 2012). When using a walk-down technique, the clinician jiggles or vibrates the needle during insertion, observing for movement as the needle penetrates the tissue passing from superficial layers to the target. The two techniques each have advantages and disadvantages and clinicians are advised to be skilled in both in-plane and out-of-plane approaches. While the in-plane technique is theoretically preferred (the entire needle is visualized), this technique can be technically challenging and difficult to perform when targeting superficial muscles. When performed carefully using a walk-down technique, the out-of-plane approach is easy and accurately performed in most muscles (Alter *et al.*, 2012).

In addition to providing direct assessment about the depth/location of the target and the needle, US also provides information about the volume of injectate and resulting distention of the muscle as the injection is performed. This added information can guide the clinician during the procedure to avoid injection of excess volume at one injection site.

Commonly targeted muscles

Anterior neck muscles

Sternocleidomastoid. The superficially located sternocleidomastoid can be imaged either in longitudinal or in transverse plane (Fig. 7.5). The transverse plane often provides a better assessment of the fascial planes between muscles, as well as the location of adjacent vascular structures (Fig. 7.6). Therefore, a scout scan should include scanning in both planes. The clinician can then choose a scanning plane which provides the best view of the sternocleidomastoid, carotid and jugular vessels. The sternocleidomastoid can be approached with either an in-plane or out-of-plane needle insertion. Injections are most often performed in the upper one-third or proximal portion of the muscle to reduce the risk of dysphagia (Truong *et al.*, 1989).

Longus colli and capitus. These muscles are located deep in the anterior cervical region. Without image guidance, these muscles are extremely challenging to target. Combined EMG guidance with US, fluoroscopy or CT is generally recommended. With US guidance, Doppler imaging should be employed as this will provide visualization of the carotid and internal and external jugular veins (Fig. 7.7). Longitudinal and transverse scans should be performed to determine which view provides the optimal view of the target as well as the structures to be avoided.

Scalene complex. The scalene muscles (anterior, middle, posterior) are located in the anterior

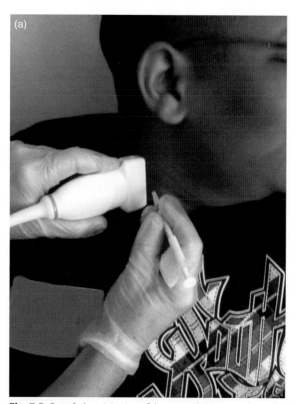

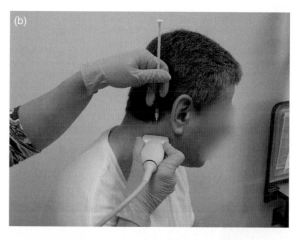

Fig. 7.5 Out-of-plane injection of the sternocleidomastoid muscle. (a) Longitudinal view; (b) transverse view.

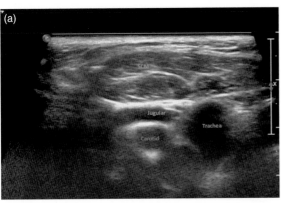

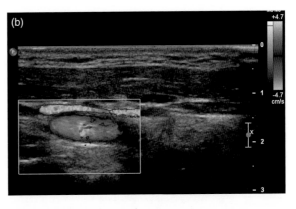

Fig. 7.6 Sternocleidomastoid muscle by ultrasound. (a) Transverse B-mode; (b) longitudinal color Doppler image.

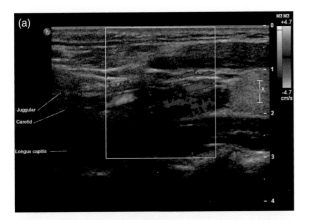

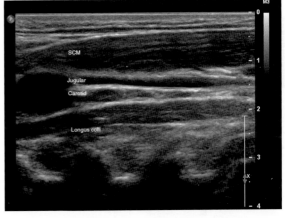

Fig. 7.7 Longus colli and capitis by ultrasound. (a) Longitudinal Doppler; (b) longitudinal B-mode; (c) transverse B-mode.

triangle of the neck, lateral, posterior and deep to the adjacent sternocleidomastoid. When performing US-guided scalene injections, a transverse view of the muscle usually provides the best view of the fascial planes between the sternocleidomastoid, scalene muscles, vessels and nerves (Fig. 7.8). In the transverse view, the roots/trunks of the brachial plexus are easily distinguished as they descend through the neck, running between the anterior and middle

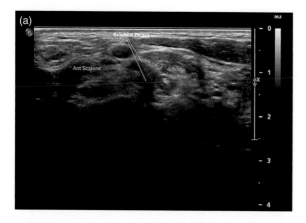

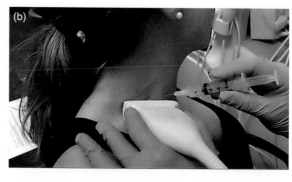

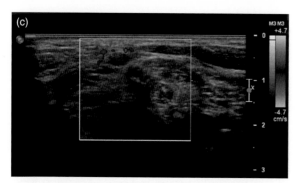

Fig. 7.8 Scalene muscles. (a) The brachial plexus can be distinguished from the scalene muscles by transverse B-mode ultrasound. (b) Clinical image showing the transverse scan for out-of-plane injection of the scalene muscles. (c) The brachial plexus and scalene muscles in transverse Doppler image.

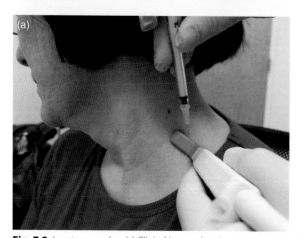

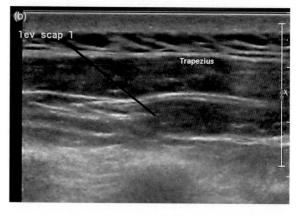

Fig. 7.9 Levator scapulae. (a) Clinical image showing anterior approach for a longitudinal scan; (b) corresponding B-mode image; (c) clinical image showing posterior approach.

scalene. Doppler imaging will confirm that these circular hypoechoic structures have no flow and are nerves, not vessels (Fig. 7.8c).

Muscles of the posterior triangle of the neck

Levator scapulae. The levator scapulae can be approached either from an anterior direction in the posterior triangle of the neck (Fig. 7.9a,b) or from a posterior direction at its insertion on the scapula, where it lies deep to the trapezius muscle (Fig. 7.9c). It is often best to perform a preliminary scan using both an anterior and posterior approach to determine which technique provides the best view of and approach to the muscle.

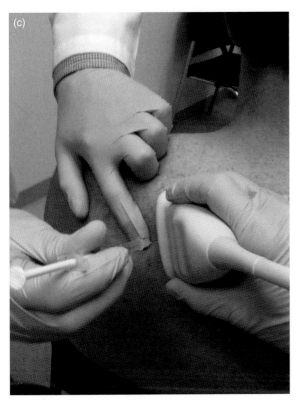

Fig. 7.9 (cont.)

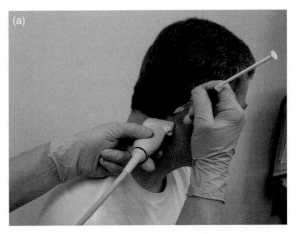

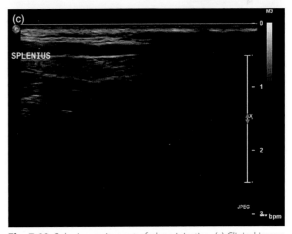

Muscle atrophy, which may occur after repeated injections, may make visualization of the muscle from the anterior approach more challenging.

Splenius capitis. With US guidance, the splenius capitis is generally approached at the level of the mastoid, just distal to its origin from the ligamentum flavu. At this level (i.e. the mastoid), the splenius capitis lies deep to and posterior to the sternocleidomastoid and deep to and anterior to the trapezius (Fig. 7.10).

Posterior cervical muscles

Trapezius. The trapezius is divided into upper, middle and lower sections. For patients with CD, injections are generally directed to the upper and middle sections. The trapezius is the most superficial muscle in the posterior neck. The upper or cervical section of the trapezius is approached from either a longitudinal or a transverse approach (Fig. 7.11). Deep to the trapezius are the underlying cervical paraspinal muscles (Fig. 7.12).

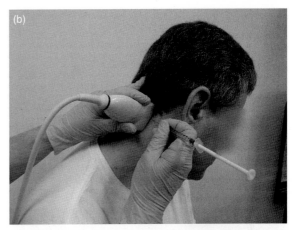

Fig. 7.10 Splenius capitus out-of-plane injection. (a) Clinical image showing transverse scan; (b) clinical image for longitudinal scan; (c) B-mode ultrasound image for this longitudinal scan.

Semispinalis capitis/longissimus capitis. These muscles lie deep to and lateral to the trapezius. As with the trapezius, the muscles are easily

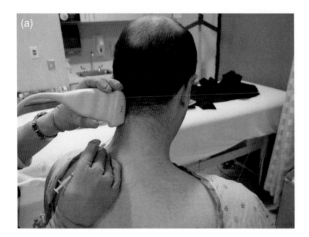

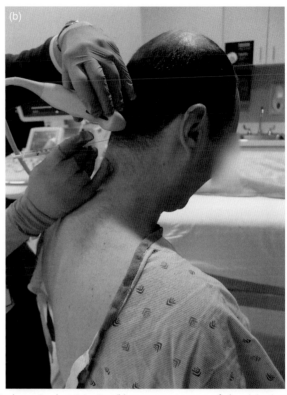

Fig. 7.11 Transducer positions for upper trapezius muscle. (a) Longitudinal scan, in-plane injection; (b) transverse scan, out-of-plane injection.

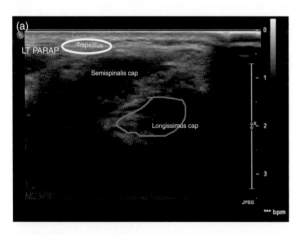

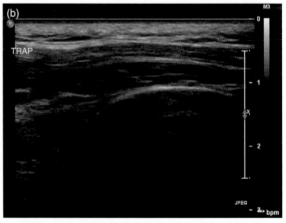

Fig. 7.12 Trapezius and longissimus capitis by B-mode ultrasound. (a) Transverse scan; (b) longitudinal scan.

visualized from longitudinal or transverse scans. The transverse view often provides a better view of the fascial planes between the muscle groups) (Figs. 7.11–7.13).

Oblique capitus inferioris. This muscle lies deep in the upper cervical region and is difficult to isolate with EMG or palpation. On US, this muscle is easily discriminated from the surrounding cervical paraspinal muscles as it runs in a plane nearly in longitudinal axis, the paraspinals will be seen in a transverse view (Fig. 7.14).

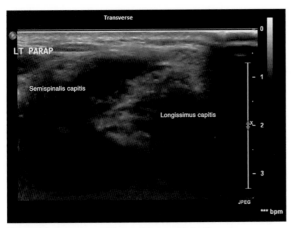

Fig. 7.13 Trapezius and longissimus capitis by B-mode ultrasound in transverse scan.

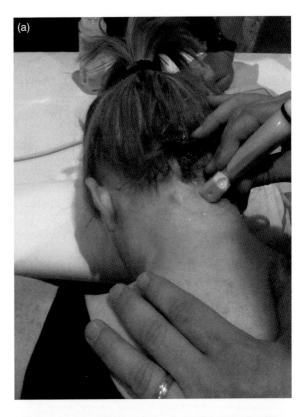

Summary

Using US guidance has a number of advantages over other techniques and increasing evidence supports a higher accuracy for most US-guided procedures. Additional studies are needed to evaluate whether this increased accuracy leads to improved treatment efficacy and reduced risk. In 2013, US guidance seems to be the way forward for guided BoNT injections. The time spent and the effort required to acquire this skill is offset by potential benefits to patients.

Hands-on training at a live course, time spent with an experienced colleague and the use of reference materials can all help physicians to acquire the skills required for US-guided BoNT procedures. The author recommends that physicians begin to use US as an "add on" technique to whatever guidance technique is currently used. This strategy allows the physician to achieve the repeated hands-on practice to acquire the skills needed for US imaging and procedural guidance.

References

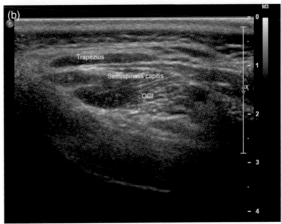

Fig. 7.14 Oblique capitis inferioris (oci). (a) Clinical image showing transducer position; (b) corresponding B-mode ultrasound image.

Alter KE (2010). High-frequency ultrasound guidance for neurotoxin injections. *Phys Med Rehabil Clin N Am*, **21**, 607–30.

Alter KE, Hallett M, Karp B (eds.) (2012). *Ultrasound Guided Chemodenervation Procedures. Text and Atlas*. New York: Demos Medical, pp. 84–107.

Boon AJ, Oney-Marlow TM, Murthy NS *et al.* (2011). Accuracy of electromyography needle placement in cadavers: non-guided vs. ultrasound guided. *Muscle Nerve*, **44**, 45–9.

Botwin KP, Sharma K, Saliba R, Patel BC (2008). Ultrasound-guided trigger point injections in the cervicothoracic musculature: a new and unreported technique. *Pain Physician*, **11**, 885–9.

Brans JW, Lindeboom R, Snoek JW *et al.* (1996). Botulinum toxin versus trihexyphenidyl in cervical dystonia: a prospective, randomized, double-blind controlled trial. *Neurology*, **46**, 1066–72.

Brashear A, Lew MF, Dykstra DD *et al.* (1999). Safety and efficacy of NeuroBloc (botulinum toxin type B) in type A-responsive cervical dystonia. *Neurology*, **53**, 1439–6.

Comella CL, Tanner CM, DeFoor-Hill L, Smith C (1992). Dysphagia after botulinum toxin injections for spasmodic torticollis: clinical and radiologic findings. *Neurology*, **42**, 1307–10.

Comella CL, Jankovic J, Truong DD, Hanschmann A, Grafe S (2011). US. XEOMIN Cervical Dystonia Study Group. Efficacy and safety of incobotulinumtoxinA (NT 201, XEOMINVR, botulinum neurotoxin type A, without accessory proteins) in patients with cervical dystonia. *J Neurol Sci*, **308**, 103–9.

Costa J, Espírito-Santo C, Borges A *et al.* (2005). Botulinum toxin type B for cervical dystonia. *Cochrane Database Syst Rev*, (1), CD004315.

Danielson K, Odderson IR (2008). Botulinum toxin type A improves blood flow in vascular thoracic outlet syndrome. *Am J Phys Med Rehabil*, **87**, 956–9.

Davidson J, Jayaraman S (2011). Guided interventions in musculoskeletal ultrasound: what's the evidence? *Clin Radiol*, **66**, 140–52.

Defazio G, Abbruzzese G, Livrea P, Berardelli A (2004). Epidemiology of primary dystonia. *Lancet Neurol*, **3**, 673–8.

Elovic EP, Esquenazi A, Alter KE *et al.* (2009). Chemodenervation and nerve blocks in the diagnosis and management of spasticity and muscle overactivity. *PM R*, **1**, 842–51.

Glass GA, Ku S, Ostrema JL *et al.* (2009). Fluoroscopic, EMG-guided injection of botulinum toxin into the longus collifor the treatment of anterocollis. *Parkinsonism Relat Disord*, **15**, 610–13.

Henzel KM, Munin MC, Kiyonkuru C *et al.* (2010). Comparison of surface and ultrasound localization to identify forearm flexor muscles for botulinum toxin therapy. *PM R*, **2**, 642–6.

Hong JS, Sathe GG, Niyonkuru C *et al.* (2012). Elimination of dysphagia using ultrasound guidance for botulinum toxin injections in cervical dystonia. *Muscle Nerve*, **46**, 535–9.

Jankovic J (2004). Treatment of cervical dystonia. In Brin MF, Comella CL, Jankovic J (eds.) *Dystonia: Etiology, Clinical Features, and Treatment.* Philadelphia, PA: Lippincott, Williams & Wilkins, pp. 159–66.

Jordan SE, Ahn SS, Gelabert HA (2007). Combining ultrasonography and electromyography for botulinum chemodenervation treatment of thoracic outlet syndrome: comparison with fluoroscopy and electromyography guidance. *Pain Physician* **10**, 541–6.

Kwon JY, Hwang JH, Kim JS (2010). Botulinum toxin A injection into calf muscles for treatment of spastic equinus in cerebral palsy: a controlled trial comparing sonography and electric stimulation-guided injection techniques: a preliminary report. *Am J Phys Med Rehabil*, **89**, 279–86.

Lee IH, Yoon YC, Sung DH, Kwon JW, Jung JY (2009). Initial experience with imaging-guided intramuscular botulinum toxin injection in patients with idiopathic cervical dystonia. *AJR Am J Roentgenol*, **192**, 996–1001.

Lim EC, Quek AM, Seet RC (2011). Accurate targeting of botulinum toxin injections: how to and why. *Parkinsonism Relat Disord*, **17**(Suppl 1), S34–9.

Molloy FM, Shill HA, Kaelin-Lang A, Karp BI (2002). Accuracy of muscle localization without EMG: implications for treatment of limb dystonia. *Neurology*, **58**, 805–7.

Peck E, Finnoff JT, Smith J *et al.* (2011). Accuracy of palpation-guided and ultrasound-guided needle tip placement into the deep and superficial posterior leg compartments. *Am J Sports Med*, **39**, 1968–74.

Picelli A, Tamburin S, Bonetti P *et al.* (2012). Botulinum toxin type A injection into the gastrocnemius muscle for spastic equinus in adults with stroke: a randomized controlled trial comparing manual needle placement, electrical stimulation and ultrasonography-guided injection techniques. *Am J Phys Med Rehabil*, **91**, 957–64.

Schnitzler A, Roche N, Denormandie P *et al.* (2012) Manual needle placement: accuracy of botulinum toxin A injections. *Muscle Nerve*, **46**, 531–4.

Simpson DM, Blitzer A, Brashear A *et al.* (2008). Assessment: botulinum neurotoxin for the treatment of movement disorders (an evidence-based review). Report of the Therapeutics and Technology Assessment Subcommittee of the American Academy of Neurology. *Neurology*, **70**, 1699–706.

Simpson DM, Gracies JM, Graham K *et al.* (2009). Assessment: botulinum neurotoxin for the treatment of spasticity (an evidence-based review). *Neurology*, **73**, 736–7; author reply, 737–8.

Smith J, Finnoff JT (2009a). Diagnostic and interventional musculoskeletal ultrasound: part 1. Fundamentals. *PM R*, **1**, 64–75.

Smith J, Finnoff JT (2009b). Diagnostic and interventional musculoskeletal ultrasound: part 2. Clinical applications. *PM R*, **1**, 162–77.

Speelman JD, Brans JW (1995). Cervical dystonia and botulinum treatment: is electromyographic guidance necessary? *Mov Disord*, **10**, 802.

Torriani M, Gupita R, Donahue DM (2010). Botulinum toxin injection in neurogenic thoracic outlet syndrome: results and experience using a ultrasound-guided approach. *Skeletal Radiol*, **39**, 973–80.

Truong D, Lewitt P, Cullis P (1989). Effects of different injection techniques in the treatment of torticollis with botulinum toxin. *Neurology*, **39**(Suppl), 294.

Truong D, Brodsky M, Lew M *et al.* (2010). Long-term efficacy and safety of botulinum toxin type A (Dysport) in cervical dystonia. *Parkinsonism Relat Disord*, **16**, 316–23.

Useros-Olmo AI, Collado-Vázquez S. (2010). Effects of an hydrotherapy program in the treatment of cervical dystonia. A pilot study. *Rev Neurol*, **51**, 669–76.

Yang EJ, Rha DW, Yoo JK, Park ES (2009). Accuracy of manual needle placement for gastrocnemius muscle in children with cerebral palsy checked against ultrasonography. *Arch Phys Med Rehabil*, **90**, 741–4.

Treatment of blepharospasm

Carlo Colosimo, Dorina Tiple and Alfredo Berardelli

Introduction

Primary blepharospasm is a common adult-onset focal dystonia, characterized by involuntary contractions of the periocular muscles that result in forceful eye closure and impaired opening and closing of the eyes (Marsden, 1976; Berardelli *et al.*, 1985; Defazio *et al.*, 2007). The severity of blepharospasm can vary from repeated frequent blinking, causing only minor discomfort, to persistent forceful closure of the eyelids leading to functional blindness (Fig. 8.1). Blepharospasm can be caused by tonic or phasic contractions of the orbicularis oculi muscles and may also be associated with levator palpebrae muscle inhibition (apraxia of eyelid opening) or involuntary movements in the lower face and masticatory muscles (Meige's syndrome). In most cases, blepharospasm is considered primary and is only occasionally secondary to structural brain lesions or drug therapy (Jankovic, 2006).

Pathophysiology

Neurophysiological recordings of the blink reflex have given important insights into the pathophysiology of blepharospasm. In patients with blepharospasm, the recovery cycle of the R2 component of the blink reflex is enhanced, presumably owing to a lack of brainstem interneuronal inhibition (Berardelli *et al.*, 1985, 1998). Blepharospasm is also associated with an abnormal responsiveness of the blink reflex to sensory stimuli. Studies using magnetic brain stimulation also suggest a loss of inhibition and increased plasticity in the central nervous system of patients with blepharospasm (Defazio *et al.*, 2007; Quartarone *et al.*, 2008).

Anatomy of the periocular muscles

Knowledge of the anatomy of the upper facial muscles is essential for treating patients with blepharospasm. The muscle most commonly involved in blepharospasm is the orbicularis oculi. The orbicularis oculi, a sphincter muscle around the eye, comprises orbital, preseptal and pretarsal parts (Fig. 8.2). The orbital part originates in the medial part of the orbit and runs around the eye via the upper eye cover fold and lid and returns in the lower eyelid to the palpebral ligament. The preseptal or palpebral part originates in the palpebral ligament and runs above and below the eye to the lateral angle of the eye. The orbital and the preseptal muscles form concentric circles around the eye. The pretarsal part lies just around the palpebral margin.

Blepharospasm can also involve the levator palpebrae superioris. This muscle arises from the inferior surface of the sphenoid bone. From this point, it diverges anteriorly to insert into the skin of the upper eyelid and the superior tarsal plate. The levator palpebrae elevates and retracts the upper eyelid. Other

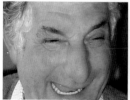 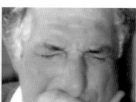 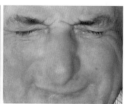

Fig. 8.1 Example of a patient with severe chronic blepharospasm; a disabling spasm of the periocular muscles is observed.

Manual of Botulinum Toxin Therapy, 2nd edition, ed. Daniel Truong, Mark Hallett, Christopher Zachary and Dirk Dressler. Published by Cambridge University Press. © Cambridge University Press 2013.

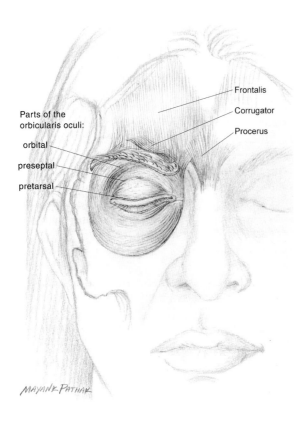

Fig. 8.2 Normal anatomy of the orbicularis oculi muscle. The orbital, preseptal and pretarsal parts are shown.

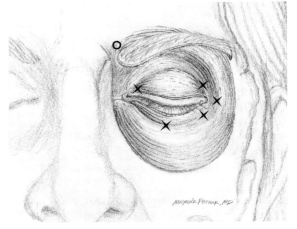

Fig. 8.3 Injection points in patient with blepharospasm. X, onabotulinumtoxinA 5 U/abobotulinumtoxinA 20 U; 0, onabotulinumtoxinA 2.5 U/abobotulinumtoxinA 10 U.

muscles that may also be affected in patients with blepharospasm are the corrugator, the procerus and the frontalis. The corrugator muscle originates at the inner orbit near the root of the nose and inserts into the skin of the forehead above the center of each eyebrow and pulls the eyebrows and skin from the center of each eyebrow to its inner corner medially and down. The procerus muscle originates in the fascia of the nasal bone and upper nasal cartilage, runs through the area of the root of the nose and fans upward to insert in the skin in the center of the forehead between the eyebrows. It acts to pull the skin of the center of the forehead down, forming transverse wrinkles in the glabella region and bridge of the nose. It usually acts together with corrugator or orbicularis oculi, or both. The frontalis muscle is a thin and quadrilateral muscle adherent to the superficial fascia. The frontalis muscle passes through and inserts into the bundles of the orbicularis oculi muscle on the superior border of the eyebrow at the middle and medial side of the upper eyelid. The frontalis muscle intermixes with the bundle of the orbicularis oculi muscle.

Botulinum neurotoxin treatment: techniques and results

In 1989 the US Food and Drug Administration approved botulinum neurotoxin serotype A (BoNT-A; formulation onabotulinumtoxinA [Botox, Allergan, Irvine, CA, USA]) as a therapeutic agent in patients with blepharospasm, and the European approval followed in 1994. Other formats of BoNT-A (abobotulinumtoxinA [Dysport, Ipsen, Paris, France] or incobotulinumtoxinA [Xeomin, Merz, Frankfurt, Germany]) were also shown to be effective and were subsequently approved worldwide (Truong *et al.*, 2008). Treatment of blepharospasm with BoNT-A is usually straightforward and easy. Four injections are usually given in the orbital or preseptal portion of the orbicularis oculi muscle, but the number of injections in the orbicularis oculi can be increased to include the lateral canthus. The BoNT-A can also be injected into the pretarsal portion of the orbicularis oculi (Fig. 8.3) (Albanese *et al.*, 1996; Cakmur *et al.*, 2002). In most patients, pretarsal BoNT-A treatment achieves a significantly higher response rate and longer-lasting maximum response. Injection into the pretarsal part is more painful but produces fewer side effects. Injected into the pretarsal portion of the orbicularis oculi muscle is now considered by several authors the best method for treating involuntary eyelid closure caused by contractions of this muscle and for treating apraxia of eyelid opening (Ward *et al.*, 2006). Different formulations of BoNT-A, such as abobotulinumtoxinA, incobotulinumtoxinA, have similar results, provided that approximate dose ratios

61

of 1:4 (onabotulinumtoxinA: abobotulinumtoxinA) and 1:1 (onabotulinumtoxinA:incobotulinumtoxinA) are utilized. (The use of formal ratios is discouraged.) The total dose of BoNT-A injected per session ranges from 25 to 50 U onabotulinumtoxinA/incobotulinumtoxinA or 100 to 240 U abobotulinumtoxinA. In rare and selected patients with severe blepharospasm refractory to standard treatment regimens, increasing the dose of BoNT-A up to 100 U onabotulinumtoxinA (or equivalent doses) per session may be helpful. The mean treatment interval is around 3–4 months and appears strikingly stable in most patients. In individuals with severe blepharospasm involving other nearby facial muscles, the corrugator, procerus and frontalis can also be injected in addition to orbicularis oculi. The recommended doses are 2.5–5.0 U onabotulinumtoxinA/incobotulinumtoxinA or 10–15 U abobotulinumtoxinA for corrugators; 2.5–5 U onabotulinumtoxinA/incobotulinumtoxinA or 5–7.5 U abobotulinumtoxinA for the procerus muscle; and 15 U onabotulinumtoxinA/incobotulinumtoxinA or 40 U abobotulinumtoxinA for the frontalis muscle.

In practice, the vial of onabotulinumtoxinA or incobotulinumtoxinA with 100 U can be diluted with 2 or 4 ml of normal saline. This results in a dilution to 5 U/0.1 ml or 2.5 U/0.1 ml, respectively. AbobotulinumtoxinA comes in vials of 300 U and 500 U, which are diluted in 1.5 or 2.5 ml, respectively, to come to final concentration of 200 U/ml. In selected patients, a lower concentation may be warranted. For these injections, 0.5 ml of the solution may be drawn and diluted inside the syringe with another 0.5 ml of normal saline. The final concentration used for injection would be 10 U in 0.1 ml. The BoNT is given at different sites as shown in Fig. 8.3.

Botulinum neurotoxin type A is now recognized as the first-choice treatment for the symptomatic control of blepharospasm. Although only few small randomized, controlled studies support the use of BoNT-A in this indication (Jankovic and Orman, 1987), results from several open-label studies suggest that it is highly effective, providing an improvement in 90–95% of the patients with very few side effects. There is little information published on the other BoNT serotypes (B, C and F) and their use offers no advantage over >the common treatment with BoNT-A (Colosimo et al., 2003). Side effects after BoNT injection, including ptosis, diplopia, dry eyes, epiphora, keratitis, lid edema, entropion/ectropion and facial weakness, are transient and usually mild in experienced hands. A meta-analysis concluded that the efficacy of BoNT-A in blepharospasm was already reasonably established and further new placebo-controlled trials might not be useful (Costa et al., 2005). Future trials should explore technical factors such as optimum treatment intervals and doses, different injection techniques (including choice of sites, concentration and speed of injection of the solution) and the applicability of the various BoNT-A formulations (Ward et al., 2006). A recent systematic review critically assessed studies with at least 1 year of follow-up to confirm the long-term efficacy of BoNT-A therapy in blepharospasm (Colosimo et al., 2012). Although BoNT-A has been effectively used for more than three decades for treating blepharospasm, only six studies could be found reporting on its long-term efficacy in blepharospasm, and all were of low quality (Class IV). The review concluded that the efficacy and safety profile of BoNT-A remain substantially unchanged over many years of use.

Surgical treatments, such as facial nerve lysis and orbicularis oculi myectomy, once used extensively in the treatment of blepharospasm, have been essentially abandoned because BoNT-A is highly effective in most cases and does not have the postoperative complications commonly observed after surgery.

References

Albanese A, Bentivoglio AR, Colosimo C et al. (1996). Pretarsal injections of botulinum toxin improve blepharospasm in previously unresponsive patients. *J Neurol Neurosurg Psychiatry*, **61**, 693–4.

Berardelli A, Rothwell JC, Day BL, Marsden CD (1985). Pathophysiology of blepharospasm and oromandibular dystonia. *Brain*, **108**, 593–608.

Berardelli A, Rothwell JC, Hallett M et al. (1998). The pathophysiology of primary dystonia. *Brain*, **121**, 1195–1212.

Cakmur R, Ozturk R, Uzunel F, Donmez B, Idiman F (2002). Comparison of preseptal and pretarsal injections of botulinum toxin in the treatment of blepharospasm and hemifacial spasm. *J Neurol*, **249**, 64–8.

Colosimo C, Chianese M, Contarino F, Giovannelli M, Bentivoglio AR (2003). Botulinum toxin type B in blepharospasm. *J Neurol Neurosurg Psychiatry*, **74**, 687.

Colosimo C, Tiple D, Berardelli A (2012). Efficacy and safety of long-term botulinum toxin treatment in craniocervical dystonia: a systematic review. *Neurotox Res*, **22**, 265–73.

Costa J, Espírito-Santo C, Borges A et al. (2005). Botulinum toxin type A therapy for blepharospasm. *Cochrane Database Syst Rev*, **(1)**, CD004900.

Defazio G, Berardelli A, Hallett M (2007). Do primary adult-onset focal dystonias share aetiological factors? *Brain*, **130**, 1183–93.

Jankovic J (2006). Treatment of dystonia. *Lancet Neurol*, **5**, 864–72.

Jankovic J, Orman J (1987). Botulinum A toxin for cranial-cervical dystonia: A double-blind, placebo-controlled study. *Neurology*, **37**, 616–23.

Marsden CD (1976). Blepharospasm–oromandibular dystonia syndrome (Brueghel's syndrome). A variant of adult-onset torsion dystonia? *J Neurol Neurosurg Psychiatry*, **39**, 1204–9.

Quartarone A, Morgante F, Sant'angelo A *et al.* (2008). Abnormal plasticity of sensorimotor circuits extends beyond the affected body part in focal dystonia. *J Neurol Neurosurg Psychiatry*, **79**, 985–90.

Truong D, C. Comella *et al.* (2008). Efficacy and safety of purified botulinum toxin type A (Dysport) for the treatment of benign essential blepharospasm: a randomized, placebo-controlled, phase II trial. *Parkinsonism Relat Disord*, **14**, 407–14.

Ward AB, Molenaers G, Colosimo C, Berardelli A (2006). Clinical value of botulinum toxin in neurological indications. *European J Neurol*, **13**(Suppl 4), 20–6.

Botulinum neurotoxin in oromandibular dystonia

Roongroj Bhidayasiri, Francisco Cardoso and Daniel Truong

Introduction

Oromandibular dystonia (OMD) is a form of focal dystonia that involves the masticatory, lower facial, labial and lingual musculature. The term "cranial dystonia" is used when oromandibular dystonia occurs in association with blepharospasm. This particular combination is often referred to as Meige's syndrome (reviewed by Bhidayasiri *et al.*, 2006).

Epidemiology, clinical features and etiology

Oromandibular dystonia frequently affects women more than men and the prevalence was estimated to be around 68.9 cases per 1 million in the USA (Bhidayasiri *et al.*, 2006). The mean age at onset is between 50 and 60 years. The involvement of masticatory muscles in OMD may cause jaw closing or jaw opening, lateral deviation, protrusion, retraction, or a combination of these. These movements often result in involuntary biting of the tongue, cheek or lips and difficulty with speaking and chewing. Its appearance is often socially embarrassing and disfiguring. In patients with jaw-closing OMD, dystonic spasms of the temporalis and masseter muscles may result in clenching or trismus and grinding of the teeth or bruxism. Jaw-opening OMD commonly involves the lateral pterygoids, anterior belly of the digastric muscle and other submental muscles; contractions of these muscles may lead to some degree of anterocollis. The effects of OMD may be alleviated by different proprioceptive sensory inputs ("sensory tricks"). These include touching the lips or chin, chewing gum or biting on a toothpick. Coexistence with dystonia in other regions and presences of sensory tricks is more common in jaw-opening than jaw-closing OMD. The contraction of mouth and pharynx muscles may cause

involuntary vocalizations, occasionally confounded with vocal tics. In addition to the dystonic symptoms, many patients with OMD complain of tension-type headache, dental wear, temporomandibular joint syndrome and, more rarely, temperomandibular joint dislocation, resulting in upper airway collapse.

As with most forms of dystonia, most patients with OMD have idiopathic disorder. However, tardive dystonia represents the most common cause of secondary OMD. While most patients with tardive OMD are more likely to have their dystonia confined to the oromandibular region, blepharospasm, cervical dystonia and spasmodic dysphonia are more commonly associated with idiopathic OMD. By comparison, the presence of akathisia, stereotypic movements in the limbs or respiratory dyskinesia strongly suggests prior neuroleptic exposure (Tan and Jankovic, 2000). Less commonly, OMD can occur as an accompanying manifestation of neurodegenerative disorders or focal brain or brainstem lesions. Among degenerative illnesses, neuroacanthocytosis is an important cause of OMD that needs to be excluded whenever patients present with OMD combined with chorea, seizures, amyotrophy and subcortical dementia. More recently, attention has been devoted to OMD characterized by prominent lingual protrusion, a syndrome which can be caused by pantothenate kinase-associated neurodegeneration, Lesch–Nyhan syndrome or anoxia (Schneider *et al.*, 2006).

Treatment options

Several studies suggest that OMD responds poorly to oral medications, which are commonly used to treat other forms of dystonia, including anticholinergics, tetrabenazine, baclofen or clonazepam (reviewed by Bhidayasiri *et al.*, 2006). Muscle afferent block by intramuscular injection of lidocaine and alcohol has

Manual of Botulinum Toxin Therapy, 2nd edition, ed. Daniel Truong, Mark Hallett, Christopher Zachary and Dirk Dressler.
Published by Cambridge University Press. © Cambridge University Press 2013.

Table 9.1 Reports on treatment of oromandibular dystonia

Reference	Type of Study	No. patients	Duration of effect (weeks)	Neurotoxin product	Electromyography guidance
Brin et al. (1987)	Open	4	Not given	Botox	Yes
Jankovic and Orman (1987)	Double	3	5.6	Botox	No
Blitzer et al. (1989)	Open	20	Not given	Botox	Yes
Hermanowicz and Truong (1991)	Open	5	Not given	Botox	Yes
Van den Bergh et al. (1995)	Open	5	27.0 ± 4.5	Dysport	Yes
Tan and Jankovik (1999)	Open	162	16.4 ± 7.1	Botox	No
Laskawi and Rohrbach (2001)	Open	6	14 ± 9.2	Botox	Yes
Wan et al. (2005)	Open	12	13.8 ± 2.9	MyoBloc	No

Botox, onabotulinumtoxinA; Dysport, abobotulinumtoxinA; MyoBloc, rimabotulinumtoxinB.
Source: Bhidayasiri et al., 2006.

been shown to be helpful, but further experience and evaluation is needed to determine the long-term efficacy and benefit of afferent blockade (Yoshida *et al.*, 1998). Lastly, pallidal deep brain stimulation has been performed in a few patients with OMD–blepharospasm with positive results and may be considered as an option in some patients with intractable OMD (Bhidayasiri *et al.*, 2006).

The lack of a significant number of controlled trials has led authors of evidence-based reviews to state that, with the exception of jaw-closing dystonia, it is unclear as to what the role of botulinum neurotoxin (BoNT) injections is in the treatment of OMD (National Institutes of Health, 1991; Bhidayasiri *et al.*, 2006). Nevertheless, many studies as well as clinical experience strongly indicate that BoNT is the first-line treatment for OMD regardless of its clinical presentation (Brin, 1994; Bhidayasiri *et al.*, 2006). Most of the reported literature on OMD has been open studies (Table 9.1) but all have reported improvement with BoNT. In a large prospective open study, Tan and Jankovic (1999) reported a mean total duration of response up to 16.4 (±7.1) weeks. The best response is obtained with jaw-closing OMD.

Dystonia is not a stereotyped disorder and its presentation in OMD is even more colorful. The treatment has to be individualized to accommodate the patient's needs and symptoms. The various subtypes of OMD (jaw closing, jaw opening, jaw deviation,

lingual, pharyngeal and mixed) need to be considered and the function of each muscle needs to be understood when assessing which muscles should be injected. Tables 9.2 and 9.3 (adapted from Bhidayasiri *et al.*, 2006) list the muscle and their respective function.

Injection techniques

Because of the lack of controlled trials and the significant heterogeneity of clinical presentation of OMD, the discussion that follows, which is subdivided according to main clinical types, is primarily based on the clinical experience of the authors.

Jaw-closing oromandibular dystonia

For jaw-closing OMD, often the masseter is the initial muscle selected for denervation (Bhidayasiri *et al.*, 2006). If the response is not adequate, other muscles can be considered, including temporalis and pterygoid medialis. Injection is individualized for each patient and electromyography (EMG) guidance is only used to identify deep muscles that are not available to manual palpation since there is a suggestion that comparable results can be obtained without EMG (Bhidayasiri *et al.*, 2006).

The masseter is a thick quadrilateral muscle with three parts – superficial, intermediate and deep – that arises from the zygomatic arch and inserts into the angle

Table 9.2 Oral muscles and function

Muscle name	Functions
Temporalis	Close the jaw Posterior fibers retract the mandible Move jaw to the same side
Masseter	Close the jaw by elevating the mandible
Medial pterygoid	Close the jaw Protrude the jaw Moving the jaw to the opposite side
Lateral pterygoid	Open the mouth Protrude the jaw Move the jaw to the opposite side
Digastric	Open the jaw Elevate the hyoid bone
Mylohyoid	Open the jaw Raise the floor of the mouth
Geniohyoid	Open the jaw Elevate and draw hyoid bone forward

Source: Bhidayasiri et al., 2006.

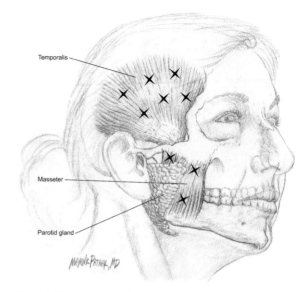

Fig. 9.1 The masseter and temporalis muscles.

Table 9.3 Subtypes of oromandibular dystonia

Subtype	Muscles involved
Jaw closing	Temporalis Masseter Medial pterygoid
Jaw opening	Lateral pterygoid Mylohyoid Digastric Geniohyoid
Jaw deviation	Contralateral lateral pterygoid Ipsilateral medial pterygoid Temporalis

Source: Bhidayasiri et al., 2006.

and the lateral surface of the ramus of the mandible (Clemente, 1984) (Fig. 9.1). It can be easily palpable by instructing the patient to clench the teeth. Very uncommonly, EMG guidance is required to reach it. In this case, it is approached using a teflon-coated needle connected to an EMG machine at 1 cm anterior to the posterior border of the ramus. The muscle discharge when the patient clenches the teeth also helps to confirm that the insertion is not in the parotid gland, which extends from the ear to the masseter and partially covers the posterior part of the muscle. A good starting dose is 50 U onabotulinumtoxinA/incobotulinumtoxinA or 100 U abobotulinumtoxinA. Experience with rimabotulinumtoxinB is not available

from the literature except in two non-English journals (Cardoso, 2003; Wan et al., 2005). In our limited experience, we have used 2500 U rimabotulinumtoxinB for each masseter muscle.

The medial pterygoid occupies the inner aspect of the ramus of the mandible opposite that of the masseter. It arises from the lateral pterygoid plate and the pyramical process of the palatine bone and inserts into the lower and back part of the medial surface of the ramus and angle of the mandible (Clemente, 1984) (Fig. 9.2). Because of its deep location, injection often requires EMG guidance. The medial pterygoid can be approached either intraorally or from below. When approached from below, the needle is inserted about 0.5–1 cm anterior to the angle of the mandible along the interior aspect of the mandible and angled perpendicularly to the mandible until it can be verified by the EMG with the patient clenching the teeth. Care should be taken to avoid the facial artery, which lies anteriorly. A good starting dose here is 20 U onabotulinumtoxinA/incobotulinumtoxinA, 30 U abobotulinumtoxinA Dyport (Bhidayasiri et al., 2006) or 1000 U rimabotulinumtoxinB.

The third muscle involved in jaw-closing OMD is the temporalis muscle (Fig. 9.1). This broad, radiating muscle arises from the temporal fossa. Its tendon inserts into the medial surface, apex and anterior border of the coronoid process and the anterior border of the ramus of the mandible (Clemente, 1984). The temporalis closes the jaws

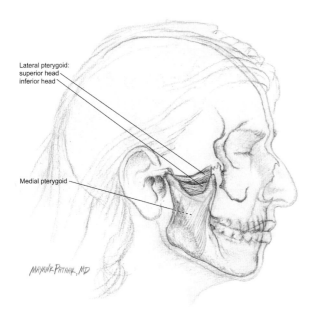

Lateral pterygoid:
superior head
inferior head

Medial pterygoid

MAYANK PATHAK, MD

Fig. 9.2 The pterygoid muscle.

and its posterior fibers retract the mandible. The temporalis is approached perpendicular to its plane and possibly high in the temporal fossa as the lower part of the temporalis is mostly tendon, where the injection is painful. Because of its wide radiation pattern, three to four injections should be given. Recommended dose by the educational committee of WE MOVE is 40 U onabotulinumtoxinA (WE MOVE Spasticity Study Group, 2005). We, however, have opted for a higher dose, 50–100 U onabotulinumtoxinA/incobotulinumtoxinA. Early reports have used smaller doses (Bhidayasiri *et al.*, 2006). Starting dose for abobotulinumtoxinA is about 100 U and adjusted according to patient's response (Van den Bergh *et al.*, 1995).

Jaw-opening oromandibular dystonia

The muscles involved in jaw opening include the lateral pterygoid, mylohyoid, digastric, geniohyoid and platysma (Clemente, 1984). Opening of the jaws is performed primarily by the pterygoid lateralis. In the beginning of the opening, it is assisted by the submentalis complex, which include the mylohyoid, digastric and geniohyoid (Clemente, 1984). The platysma may also play a minor role in the opening of the jaw. Most investigators reported injections of the lateral pterygoid in jaw-opening OMD, although others have

claimed success with injection of the submentalis complex only (Bhidayasiri *et al.*, 2006).

The lateral pterygoid is a short conical muscle arising from two heads: a superior from the great wing of the sphenoid bone and an inferior from the lateral surface of the lateral pterygoid plate of the sphenoid (Clemente, 1984) (Fig. 9.2). The lateral pterygoid can be approached intraorally or laterally through the mandibular notch. The entry point is about 35 mm from the external auditory canal and 10 mm from the inferior margin of the zygomatic arch. Using an EMG-guided technique, the needle is angled upward about 15 degrees to reach the inferior head of the lateral pterygoid. In close vicinity but more rostral is the pterygoid branch of the maxillary artery. The amount of BoNT reported in literature ranges from 20 to 40 U onabotulinumtoxinA (Blitzer *et al.*, 1989; Laskawi and Rohrbach, 2001). The same amount of BoNT may be used for incobotulinumtoxinA. There is limited experience with abobotulinumtoxinA and we recommend a starting dose of about 60 U, titrating up if needed.

The digastric muscle is part of the submental complex. It arises from the mastoid notch of the temporal bone and attaches to the digastric fossa of the mandible (Fig. 9.3). It is divided into anterior and posterior bellies by the middle tendon, which is attached to the hyoid bone (Clemente, 1984). Besides elevating the hyoid bone, the digastric muscle pulls the chin backward and downward in opening the mouth, in conjunction with the lateral pterygoid. In contrast to the posterior belly, which is crowded with many nerves, the sympathetic trunk, arteries and veins, the anterior belly is open to intervention. The geniohyoid arises from the hyoid bone and inserts into the inferior genial tubercle of the mandible. It elevates the hyoid bone and base of the tongue. With the hyoid bone fixed, it depresses the mandible and opens the mouth. The mylohyoid also arises from the hyoid bone and attaches to the mylohyoid line of the mandible (Fig. 9.3). It raises the floor of the mouth during swallowing. The mylohyoid elevates the hyoid bone, thereby pushing the tongue upward (protrusion of the tongue; Clemente, 1984). It assists in opening the mouth. Muscles of the submental complex may be fused together, making it difficult to separate one from another (Clemente, 1984). This muscle group can be palpated with the patient opening his or her mouth. It is approached about 1 cm from mandible tip and injected slightly lateral from the midline (Fig. 9.3). A good starting dose of onabotulinumtoxinA/

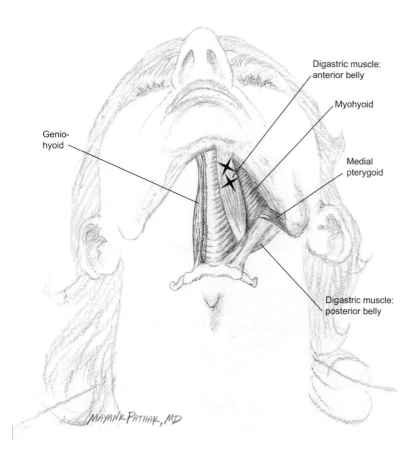

Fig. 9.3 The digastric, geniohyoid and mylohyoid muscles. X, injection site.

Digastric muscle: anterior belly

Myohyoid

Genio-hyoid

Medial pterygoid

Digastric muscle: posterior belly

MAYANK PATHAK, MD

incobotulinumtoxinA is 30 U. These units are divided and injected into the two locations on each side. Higher doses up to 200 U for the submentalis complex have been reported (Tan and Jankovic, 1999) but the risk of severe dysphagia is considerable. For abobotulinumtoxinA, 90 U could be a good starting dose and for rimabotulinumtoxinB about 500 U.

In some patients, injection of the platysma can give additional improvement. This muscle depresses the mandible and soft tissue of the lower face as well as tenses the skin of the neck. The platysma fascicles can be easily identified visually. Often the platysma is injected with 20 U onabotulinumtoxinA/incobotulinumtoxinA, 60 U abobotulinumtoxinA and about 1000 U rimabotulinumtoxinB.

Jaw-deviating oromandibular dystonia

The contralateral lateral pterygoid works in conjunction with the ipsylateral medial pterygoid to deviate the mouth to the opposite side. The temporalis pulls the jaw to the same side. The injections follow the above-mentioned techniques (Figs. 9.1 and 9.2).

Lingual oromandibular dystonia

The extrinsic muscles of the tongue include the genioglossus, hyoglossus, chondroglossus, styloglossus and palatoglossus. Careful examination of the movements of the tongue is paramount for successful treatment. The need to preserve functional activity limits the amount of BoNT that can be used. Tongue thrusting, one of the movements often encountered in OMD, results from the action of posterior fibers of the genioglossus, whereas the anterior fibers draw the tongue back into the mouth (Clemente, 1984). Suggested initial dose is 10 U onabotulinumtoxinA/incobotulinumtoxinA or 30 U abobotulinumtoxinA (Bhidayasiri *et al.*, 2006). There is no known experience of rimabotulinumtoxinB with this muscle but initial therapy with 500 U may be reasonable. The hyoglossus depresses the tongue and draws down its side. Similar doses are used here to those for the genioglossus.

One note of caution in injecting lingual muscles: the therapeutic window is quite narrow, which means that doses slightly above the therapeutic level can induce disabling weakness associated with severe dysphagia.

Pharyngeal oromandibular dystonia

The pharyngeal muscles consist of the three constrictor muscles and the stylo-, salpingo- and palatopharyngei. The three constrictors are superior, middle and inferior constrictors. They exercise general sphincteric and peristaltic action in swallowing. Pharyngeal OMD often involves the constrictor pharynges. The patients often complain of choking and swallowing difficulty. Pharyngeal OMD often occurs with spasmodic dystonia. We have noted that sometimes after treatment of spasmodic dysphonia there is also unexpected improvement of pharyngeal dystonia. As treatment of the pharyngeal constrictors is almost invariably associated with dysphagia, injections of these muscles are seldom performed. Dosage often used is 10 U onabotulinumtoxinA/incobotulinumtoxinA or 30 U abobotulinumtoxinA.

Summary

The development of BoNT has markedly altered the treatment of focal dystonia, including OMD. The difference in potency between different commercially available BoNT products, even when they are from the same class, creates some confusion for practice. The lack of published material in OMD further complicates the ability of physicians for switching from one preparation to another. The data in the chapter have not taken into account the published literature suggesting equivalence of onabotulinumtoxinA and abobotulinumtoxinA, which has been variously reported as between 1:2.5 and 1:6 (reviewed by Bhidayasiri *et al.*, 2006), and for onabotulinumtoxinA and incobotulinumtoxinA of 1:1 (Benecke, 2009) as injections into the oral cavity are limited by the potential side effects of the compound used.

Acknowledgments

The authors thank Dr. Mauro César Quintão Cunningham, Débora Palma Maia and Antônio Lúcio Teixeira for their assistance during the preparation of the manuscript.

References

Benecke R (2009). Xeomin in the treatment of cervical dystonia. *Eur J Neurol*, **16**(Suppl. 2) 6–10.

Bhidayasiri R, Cardoso F, Truong D (2006). Botulinum toxin in blepharospasm and oromandibular dystonia. *Eur J Neurol*, **13**(Suppl 1), 21–9.

Blitzer A, Brin MF, Greene PE, Fahn S (1989). Botulinum toxin injection for the treatment of oromandibular dystonia. *Ann Otol Rhinol Laryngol*, **98**, 93–7.

Brin MF (1994). Oromandibular dystonia: treatment of 96 patients with botulinum toxin type A. In Jankovic J, Hallett M (eds.) *Therapy with Botulinum Toxin*. New York: Marcel Dekker, pp. 429–35.

Brin MF, Fahn S, Moskowitz C *et al.* (1987). Localized injections of botulinum toxin for the treatment of focal dystonia and hemifacial spasm. *Mov Disord*, **2**, 237–54.

Cardoso F (2003). [Botulinum toxin type B in the management of dystonia non-responsive to botulinum toxin type A.] *Arq Neuropsiquiatr*, **61**, 607–10.

Clemente C (1984). Muscles and fasciae. In Clemente C (ed.) *Gray's Anatomy*. Philadelphia, PA: Lea and Feabiger, pp. 429–605.

Hermanowicz N, Truong DD (1991). Treatment of oromandibular dystonia with botulinum toxin. *Laryngoscope*, **101**, 1216–18.

Jankovic J, Orman J (1987). Botulinum A toxin for cranial-cervical dystonia: a double-blind, placebo-controlled study. *Neurology*, **37**, 616–23.

Laskawi R, Rohrbach S (2001). [Oromandibular dystonia. Clinical forms, diagnosis and examples of therapy with botulinum toxin.] *Laryngorhinootologie*, **80**, 708–13.

National Institutes of Health (1991). National Institutes of Health Consensus Development Conference. Clinical use of botulinum toxin. National Institutes of Health Consensus Development Statement, November 12–14, 1990. *Arch Neurol*, **48**, 1294–8.

Schneider SA, Aggarwal A, Bhatt M *et al.* (2006). Severe tongue protrusion dystonia: clinical syndromes and possible treatment. *Neurology*, **67**, 940–3.

Tan EK, Jankovic J (1999). Botulinum toxin A in patients with oromandibular dystonia: long-term follow-up. *Neurology*, **53**, 2102–7.

Tan EK, Jankovic J (2000). Tardive and idiopathic oromandibular dystonia: a clinical comparison. *J Neurol Neurosurg Psychiatry*, **68**, 186–90.

Van den Bergh P, Francart J, Mourin S, Kollmann P, Laterre EC (1995). Five-year experience in the treatment of focal movement disorders with low-dose Dysport botulinum toxin. *Muscle Nerve*, **18**, 720–9.

Wan XH, Vuong KD, Jankovic J (2005). Clinical application of botulinum toxin type B in movement disorders and autonomic symptoms. *Chin Med Sci, J* **20**, 44–7.

WE MOVE Spasticity Study Group (2005). *BTX-A Adult Dosing Guidelines*. New York: WE MOVE (http://www.mdvu.org/classrooms/cme/CHEMD3/ AdultSpastDosing.pdf, accessed 21 May 2013).

Yoshida K, Kaji R, Kubori T *et al.* (1998). Muscle afferent block for the treatment of oromandibular dystonia. *Mov Disord*, **13**, 699–705.

Chapter 10

Treatment of focal hand dystonia

Barbara Illowsky Karp, Chandi Das, Daniel Truong
and Mark Hallett

Introduction

Focal hand dystonia (FHD) is characterized by dystonic hand contractions that are often aggravated by purposeful actions and may be specific to a particular task. For example, a patient may have dystonia when using the hand for writing but not for other tasks such as eating or typing. The term "occupational dystonia" is used when dystonia affecting performance of the job arises in individuals with a particular occupation, usually an occupation requiring repetitive and excessive fine motor activity. The occupations particularly prone to have focal task-specific dystonia are listed in Table 10.1. Most of these hand dystonias fall under the rubric of primary focal dystonias.

This chapter discusses writer's cramp and musician's dystonia (cramp) in detail, the two most common occupational dystonias, followed by a discussion of other focal occupational dystonias.

Pathogenesis

The exact cause of FHD is not yet elucidated. A consistent physiological finding is excessive activation of antagonists and overflow and prolongation of muscle activation. Both of these are thought to reflect deficiency of inhibition at multiple levels of the motor system circuitry (Hallett, 2000, 2006a,b). Dopamine dysfunction has also been implicated. Although FHD is a movement disorder, somatosensory dysfunction is also present, including distorted sensory maps of the affected hand (Bara-Jimenez et al., 1998) and impaired sensory discrimination (Sanger et al., 2001). Structural MRI analyses have shown increased gray matter volume in the basal ganglia of musicians (Granert et al., 2011) and writers (Garraux et al., 2004) with FHD. Functional MRI has shown impaired activation of the primary sensorimotor and supplementary motor cortex during voluntary muscle relaxation and contraction (Oga et al., 2002). A genetic factor in the development of hand dystonia is possible, as up to 20% of patients with writer's cramp have family members with dystonia.

As with other focal dystonias, it is likely that FHD arises from an interaction of proprioceptive, behavioral, genetic, environmental and psychological factors. Hand overuse or repetitive motions using small hand muscles may be a precipitating factor, particularly in the presence of a putative underlying genetic predisposition (Hallett, 1998).

Writer's cramp

Writer's cramp was first reported amongst scribes in the eighteenth century under the term "occupational palsy," where some workers had disabling spasms of their hands only when performing their jobs (Ramazzini, 1713; Solly, 1864). This task-specific FHD may be particularly likely in people whose profession involves excessive writing. The incidence of writer's cramp has been reported at 14 per million in Europe (Epidemiological Study of Dystonia in Europe, 2000) and 2.7 per million in Rochester Minnesota (Nutt et al., 1988). These figures may be underestimates, as suggested by a recent population-based study that found writer's cramp to be the most common focal dystonia (Das et al., 2007). Among the various forms of focal dystonias, writer's cramp is variably reported to be seen in 5% to 19% of cases (Duffey et al., 1998; Epidemiological Study of Dystonia in Europe, 2000). In contrast to other focal dystonias, writer's cramp is seen more frequently in men than in women (Soland et al., 1996; Duffey et al., 1998; Epidemiological Study of Dystonia in Europe, 1999).

Manual of Botulinum Toxin Therapy, 2nd edition, ed. Daniel Truong, Mark Hallett, Christopher Zachary and Dirk Dressler.
Published by Cambridge University Press. © Cambridge University Press 2013.

Table 10.1 Occupations prone to focal hand dystonia

Excessive writers	Musicians	Others
Students	Pianists	Typists
Teachers	Horn player	Telegraphers
Clerks	Clarinetists	Computer operators
	Guitarists	Watch makers
	Violinists	Seamstresses
	Flutists	Surgeons/dentists
	Saxophonists	Golfers
		Fencing masters
		Cobblers
		Tailors
		Bookmakers

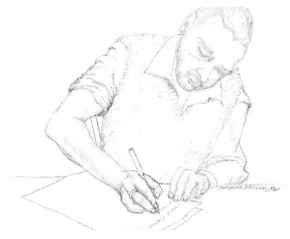

Fig. 10.1 Arm abduction pattern. Arm abduction while writing may be dystonic or compensatory.

Clinical subtypes

In "simple writer's cramp," acts requiring dexterity other than writing, such as buttoning clothes or handling of forks and knives, are unimpaired. Some patients have dystonia elicited by tasks other than writing as well and are said to have "dystonic writer's cramp," but the term "complex writer's cramp" may be more appropriate (Jedynak *et al.*, 2001). Simple writer's cramp can be a prelude to complex writer's cramp, but for many patients the condition remains simple. When severe, dystonic posturing may be present at rest as well as during eliciting tasks.

Dystonic posturing is more often flexor than extensor and can involve the wrist and arm as well as the fingers. Less commonly, there is a combination of flexion and extension in the same hand. Uncontrolled pronation or supination may also be present. Arm abduction may occur while writing, which could be a primary component of the dystonia or a compensatory mechanism (Fig. 10.1).

Disability in writer's cramp

When writing, dystonic muscle activity interferes with normal muscle activation patterns. Not infrequently, muscle aching develops, largely as a consequence of the excessive muscle contractions. The severity of pain usually does not correlate with the severity of writing impairment but may correlate with the handicap score (Jedynak *et al.*, 2001).

In contrast to disability during writing, patients with writer's cramp are often able to conduct most of their other activities without difficulty. In other tasks requiring activation of the same muscle groups, the hand appears normal and performs unremarkably.

Such task specificity is a characteristic feature of writer's cramp and other FHDs.

Frequently patients switch to writing with the non-dominant hand. Unfortunately, writer's cramp tends to develop in the non-dominant hand in 10–15% of the patients. About half of the patients with writer's cramp have "mirror dystonia," with dystonic muscle activity elicited in their dystonic hand when they write with the non-dystonic hand (Jedynak *et al.*, 2001). Occasionally, writer's cramp is associated with other focal dystonias, such as cervical dystonia or oromandibular dystonia. Almost half of those with writer's cramp have postural tremor in the affected hand (Rosenbaum and Jankovic, 1988).

Musician's dystonia

Musician's dystonia (cramp) is the term applied to a focal dystonia localized to hand muscles controlling fine movements of the digits or the embouchure muscles involved in playing instruments (Tubiana, 2003). Similar to writer's cramp, musician's FHD can be task specific, with abnormal spasms or posturing of isolated muscle groups apparent only during playing. Musicians affected with FHD report lack of coordination while playing that is frequently accompanied by involuntary flexion or extension of fingers, particularly during music passages that emphasize rapid and forceful finger movements (Wilson *et al.*, 1993).

In pianists, the fingers most often implicated are the two ulnar digits. These two fingers constitute the power grip part of the hand; they are not designed for the prolonged, rapid, highly complex movements

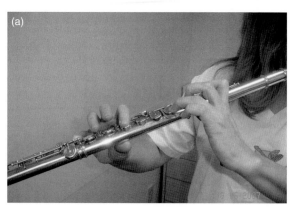 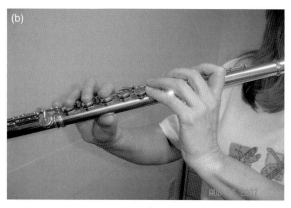

Fig. 10.2 Musician's dystonia. (a) dystonic flexion in the left second, third and fourth fingers and wrist. (b) Non-dystonic hand posture: the hand is relaxed with slight curving of the fingers and the wrist.

demanded in musical performance (Newmark and Hochberg, 1987). However, the radial digits and thumb may also be involved, particularly the thumb of the right hand in pianists. In violinists and viola players, the left, non-bowing, hand is more frequently involved. In wind players, the hand supporting the instrument and doing the fingering at the same time is most often affected (e.g. left hand in flutists and right hand in clarinetists) (Fig. 10.2).

Sometimes the onset of symptoms is found to coincide with a period of intense musical activity and overuse, such as preparation for a competition or obsessive practice in an attempt to increase the speed of a difficult passage. Usually the disorder does not progress beyond the focal task-specific problem, although it sometimes generalizes to other tasks or other parts of the body. The examination of the patient while playing the instrument that elicits the dystonia is important for the diagnosis and to target therapy.

Treatment of writer's cramp

Non-pharmacologic approaches may have some utility in the treatment of FHD. Physical therapy or splints are sometimes helpful. Various pens, such as those with thicker barrels or that place the hand in a different position, may decrease fatigue and enable clearer writing in some patients. Sensory training to try to restore a more normal pattern of sensory representation has been tried. For example, learning Braille reading and practicing for 30–60 minutes per day for up to 1 year has provided some benefit (Zeuner et al., 2002; Zeuner and Hallett, 2003) as well as specific types of motor training (Zeuner et al., 2005). Limb immobilization via a plastic splint for 4–5 weeks has been

proposed, but the value of this has been questioned and would not be recommended. Stereotactic nucleus ventrooralis thalamotomy has shown benefit for up to 29 months in writer's cramp (Taira et al., 2003) and deep brain stimulation is being explored (Cho et al., 2009), but these should be considered experimental at this time. Oral medications, such as trihexyphenidyl or clonazepam play a limited role in the treatment of FHD.

Botulinum neurotoxin therapy

Injection of botulinum neurotoxin (BoNT) has been shown to be safe and effective in the treatment of FHD (Simpson et al., 2008). The first step in using BoNT to treat hand dystonia is careful evaluation and selection of muscles for injection. The patient should be examined at rest and during movements that specifically activate the dystonia: writers should be observed while writing and musicians while playing their instruments. However, the complexity of such movements often makes it difficult to determine which movements are dystonic, which are parts of the normal pattern for that activity and which are compensatory. Patients with writer's cramp should be asked to write without trying to compensate and to describe any abnormal pulling that they experience. It is often helpful also to have the patient perform other activities that may elicit the dystonia without associated movements or compensation. Writing with the non-dominant hand, which can evoke dystonia in the dominant, resting hand (mirror dystonia), is one such strategy. Mirror dystonia can be helpful to identify dystonic muscle activity and to distinguish dystonia from compensatory muscle activity (Singer et al., 2005). The efficacy of treatment depends critically on the correct choice of muscles for injection.

Botulinum neurotoxin is effective in writer's cramp and other occupational dystonias (Karp et al., 1994; Karp, 2004). The onset of benefit starts approximately 1 week after injection, peaks at 2 weeks and lasts approximately 3 months. Benefit can be demonstrated objectively as well as subjectively. A quantitative analysis by Wissell et al. (1996) using the Writer's Cramp Rating Scale performed on 31 patients showed a good response to BoNT. The mean dose injected per session was 133.2 U abobotulinumtoxinA. Of all 124 injection sessions during a mean follow-up of 1 year, 76% produced a good improvement. The most common side effect was weakness with 72% of the injection sessions. The scores on the Writer's Cramp Rating Scale and the speed of the pen movements showed significant improvement after treatment. Other studies have shown more than half of the patients with writer's cramp returned repeatedly and could have sustained benefit for long follow-up periods (Turjanski et al., 1996; Hsuing et al., 2002; Lungu et al., 2011).

In a study of 53 patients by Karp et al. (1994), patients with localized writer's cramp fared better and those with associated tremors fared the worst. In a prospective study on 47 patients, Djebbari et al. (2004) showed that those with a flexion and pronation of the forearm and those with thumb extension have a significantly better response on the Burke–Fahn–Marsden Scale. An earlier placebo-controlled double-blind study by Tsui et al. (1993) also showed better outcome in those with wrist deviation. The restoration of normal motor function in focal task-specific dystonias may be better when treatment is initiated as early as possible and when motor performance deterioration is still mild.

Injection sites are generally chosen based on clinical observation of muscle spasm during the precipitating task, perhaps supplemented with observations of mirror dystonia. The injections are most often given into muscle localization points described in manuals of electromyography (EMG) using specialized EMG/injection needles, so that EMG can be used to ensure that the needle is in the proper muscle. The intended muscle or fascicle may be missed in up to 50% of attempts to place the needle in a forearm muscle without use of EMG (Molloy et al., 2002). Use of EMG for guidance is particularly recommended where deeper muscles are targeted. Ultrasound can also be a valuable tool for accurate

targeting. Injection of BoNT is into one, two or more sites depending on the dose to be injected and the muscle bulk. Data are available on the safety and efficacy of onabotulinumtoxinA and abobotulinumtoxinA for FHD. There have been no FHD studies reported with rimabotulinumtoxinB or incobotulinumtoxinA and there have been no trials directly comparing the efficacy of the different commercially available formulations of BoNT in writer's cramp.

Commonly injected muscles and patterns

Treatment with BoNT relies on recognizing which muscles contribute to different patterns of dystonic movement and a thorough knowledge of arm and hand anatomy.

Focal flexor pattern

In the focal flexor pattern (Fig. 10.3), the thumb and/or the index finger flexes with writing. The flexor pollicis longus and/or brevis are involved in the thumb flexion. Individual fascicles of the flexor digitorum superficialis or profundus can also be involved and are associated with proximal or distal finger flexion, respectively.

Flexor pollicis longus

The flexor pollicis longus originates in the anterior surface of the middle half of the radius and inserts in the palmar surface of the distal phalanx of the thumb (Lee and DeLisa, 2000). The needle is inserted between the middle and the distal third of the flexor side of forearm. The needle is verified by the patient flexing

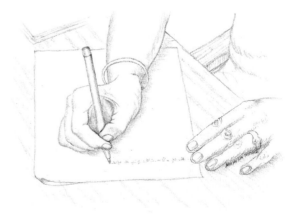

Fig. 10.3 Focal flexor pattern.

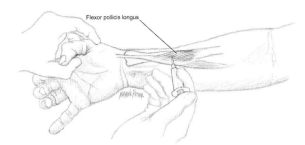

Fig. 10.4 Flexor pollicis longus.

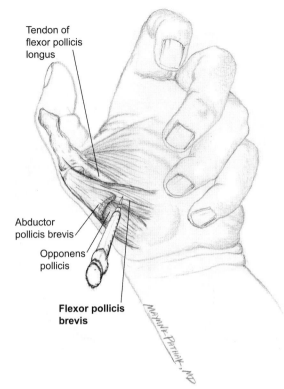

Fig. 10.5 Flexor pollicis brevis.

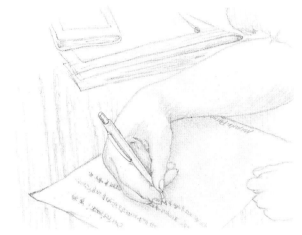

Fig. 10.6 Wrist flexor pattern.

the distal phalanx of the thumb. Prior to needle insertion, the radial artery should be noted (Fig. 10.4).

Flexor pollicis brevis

The flexor pollicis brevis has two heads. One head originates in the flexor retinaculum, trapezium and trapezoid. The other is from the second and third metacarpals. The flexor pollicis brevis inserts into the lateral side of the base of the proximal phalanx of the thumb. The needle is inserted into the medial half of the thenar eminence. The muscle is verified by the patient flexing the thumb (Fig. 10.5) (Lee and DeLisa, 2000).

Generalized flexor pattern

The generalized flexor pattern (Figs. 10.6 and 10.7) is seen when the patient's wrist has the tendency to flex after the start of the writing. The patient complains of aching either in the palm or the flexor forearm muscle group. The flexor carpi radialis and/or flexor carpi ulnaris are often involved. Commonly there is accompanying increased activation of finger flexors (flexor digitorum superficialis or profundus) and possibly

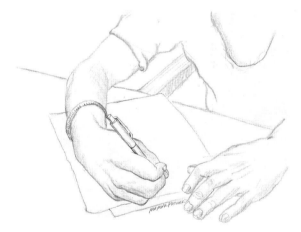

Fig. 10.7 Wrist and finger flexor pattern.

palmaris longus (Fig. 10.8) or the forearm pronator muscles.

Flexor digitorum superficialis

The flexor digitorum superficialis originates from the medial epicondyle and coronoid process of the ulna. It divides into four tendons and inserts into the

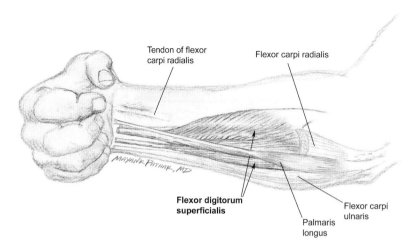

Fig. 10.8 Flexor digitorum superficialis.

middle phalanges of digits 2–5. With the patient's arm supinated, the needle is inserted at the mid forearm in the layer between the palmaris longus and flexor carpi ulnaris (Lee and DeLisa, 2000). These two muscles are identified by following their tendons from the wrist. Each fascicle of the flexor digitorum superficialis can be identified by flexing the respective finger at the middle phalanx (Fig. 10.8).

Flexor digitorum profundus

The flexor digitorum profundus originates in the proximal anterior surface of the ulna and the anterior interosseous membrane. It divides into four tendons and inserts into the palmar surface of the distal phalanges of fingers 2–5. With the patient's hand supinated and the elbow flexed, the needle is inserted at the middle of the forearm, passing through the flexor carpi ulnaris and advanced tangentially toward the radial side. Alternatively, the muscle can be approached from the ulnar aspect of the arm with the arm supinated and the elbow flexed. Each of the muscle fascicles can be identified by having the patient flex the distal phalanx of the second to fifth fingers individually (Fig. 10.9).

Palmaris longus

The palmaris longus muscle, which is medial to the flexor carpi radialis, originates in the medial epicondyle and inserts into the palmar aponeurosis and flexor retinaculum. The needle is inserted into the proximal upper third of the line between the middle of the wrist and the medial epicondyle (Fig. 10.10). As

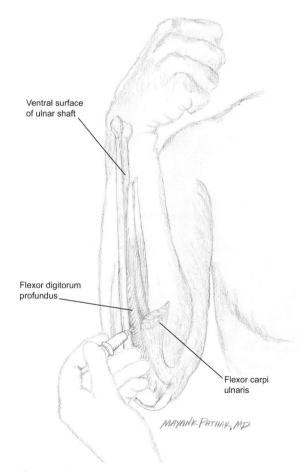

Fig. 10.9 Flexor digitorum profundus.

this is a superficial muscle, caution must be taken not to insert the needle too deeply into the flexor digitorum profundus.

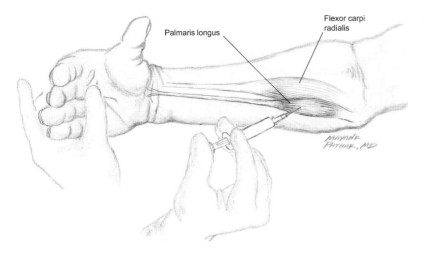

Fig. 10.10 Palmaris longus.

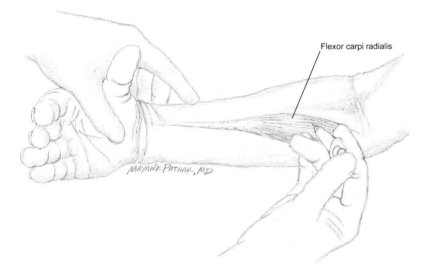

Fig. 10.11 Flexor carpi radialis.

Flexor carpi radialis

The flexor carpi radialis originates in the medial epicondyle of the humerus and inserts at the second metacarpal bone. The needle is inserted at about a third of the distance from the medial epicondyle and the needle tip is verified by asking the patient to flex and adduct the wrist (Fig. 10.11).

Flexor carpi ulnaris

The flexor carpi ulnaris originates in the medial epicondyle of the humerus and inserts in the pisiform and hamate bone and the fifth metacarpal bone. The needle is inserted into the middle of the muscle. The needle tip is verified by the patient flexing with ulnar deviation of the wrist or by simply flexing and abducting the fifth finger (Fig. 10.12).

Pronator teres

The pronator teres originates in the medial epicondyle of the humerus and coronoid process of the ulna. It wraps around the radius and inserts into the lateral surface of the radius. With the patient in supine position and the forearm supinated, the needle is introduced medial to the cubital fossa about two fingers below the elbow. The position of the needle is verified by the patient pronating the forearm with slight elbow flexion (Fig. 10.13).

Pronator quadratus

The pronator quadratus originates in the anteromedial aspect at the distal part of the ulna and inserts into the anteromedial aspect of the distal part of the radius (Fig. 10.13). With the patient in supine position and the forearm pronated, the needle is inserted 3 cm

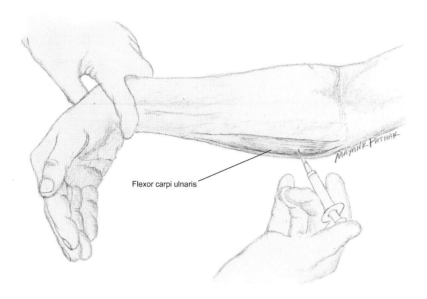

Fig. 10.12 Flexor carpi ulnaris.

Flexor carpi ulnaris

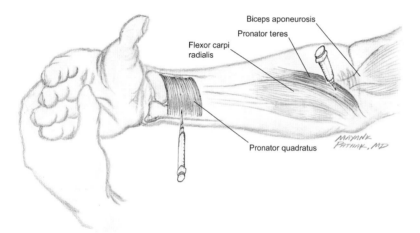

Fig. 10.13 Pronator teres and quadratus.

Biceps aponeurosis
Pronator teres
Flexor carpi radialis
Pronator quadratus

proximal to the ulnar styloid close to the surface of the ulna. Another approach is from the dorsal surface of the distal forearm, the needle is advanced through the interosseous membrane to the pronator quadratus. Pronation of the forearm verifies the needle position.

Focal extensor pattern

In the focal extensor dystonia, the extensor pollicis longus and extensor indicis proprius are often involved (Fig. 10.14).

Extensor indicis proprius

The extensor indicis proprius is often involved in extensor writer's cramp. The patient extends the index finger while holding the pen with the other

fingers. The extensor indicis proprius originates in the dorsal surface of the ulna and inserts in the second finger. The muscle is approached with the hand pronated and the needle is inserted into the distal fourth of the forearm lateral to the radial side of the ulna (Fig. 10.15). The needle is verified by extension of the index finger. Caution must be taken because if the needle is inserted too proximally, it will be in the extensor pollicis longus.

Extensor pollicis longus

The extensor pollicis longus originates from the posterior surface of the middle third of the ulnar shaft and the posterior interosseous membrane (Fig. 10.16). It inserts into the dorsal surface of the base of the distal phalanx of the thumb. The needle is inserted at the middle third of the forearm along the radial side of the ulna. The position of the needle is verified by extension of the distal joint of the thumb.

Generalized extensor pattern

In the generalized extensor pattern, the hand extends with writing (Fig. 10.17). The patient may compensate by flexing the fingers in order to maintain a grip on the pen.

Extensor carpi radialis longus

The extensor carpi radialis longus originates in the distal third of the lateral supracondylar ridge of the humerus and inserts in the dorsal surface and base of the second metacarpal bone. With the forearm pronated, the patient extends and slightly abducts the wrist radially; the needle is inserted 2–3 cm distal to the elbow joint. The position of the needle is verified by the patient extending the wrist toward the radial side (Fig. 10.18).

Extensor carpi radialis brevis

The smaller extensor carpi radialis brevis originates from the lateral epicondyle of the humerus and the radial collateral ligament of the elbow joint. It inserts in the dorsal surface of the base of the third metacarpal bone. For needle insertion, the extensor carpi radialis brevis is slightly distal and lateral to the extensor carpi radialis longus. Both muscles extend the wrist (Fig. 10.18).

Extensor digitorum communis

The extensor digitorum communis originates in the lateral epicondyle by a common extensor tendon and inserts with a central slip into the middle phalanges of fingers 2–5 and two collateral slips to the terminal phalanges of fingers 2–5. Individual finger involvement can be treated by targeting particular fascicles. The needle is inserted in the upper third on the line drawn between the lateral epicondyle and ulnar styloid (Fig. 10.19). The position of the muscle can be verified by activating each finger separately while the other fingers form a fist. The extensor digitorum communis extends and abducts at the wrist as well.

Extensor carpi ulnaris

The extensor carpi ulnaris originates in the lateral epicondyle of the humerus and inserts at the base of the fifth metacarpal. It is activated by the forearm in the prone position slightly extended at the wrist with ulnar deviation. The needle is inserted at the junction of the upper and middle thirds of the forearm. Localization is confirmed by alternate activation by ulnar extension and relaxation of the muscle (Fig. 10.19).

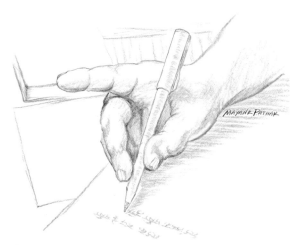

Fig. 10.14 Focal extensor pattern.

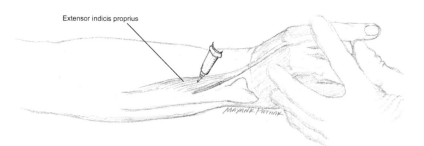

Extensor indicis proprius

Fig. 10.15 Extensor indicis proprius.

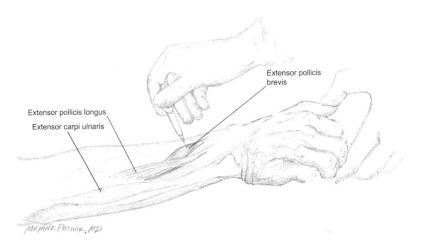

Fig. 10.16 Extensor pollicis longus/brevis.

Extensor pollicis brevis

Extensor pollicis longus

Extensor carpi ulnaris

MAYANK PATHAK, MD

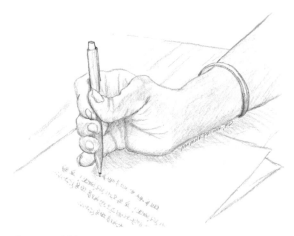

Fig. 10.17 Wrist extensor pattern.

Abductor pollicis longus

The abductor pollicis longus is proximal to the extensor indicis proprius. Patients affected with abductor pollicis longus and extensor indicis proprius spasms are particularly likely to complain of involuntarily losing their pen when writing. The abductor pollicis longus originates in the dorsal surface of the lower half of the ulna, posterior interosseus membrane and the middle third of the radius. It inserts into the radial side of the base of the first metacarpal bone. The needle is inserted at the junction of the middle and lower third of the dorsal surface of the radial bone. Needle position is verified by the patient abducting or extending the thumb at the metacarpal joint (Fig. 10.20).

Extensor pollicis longus

The extensor pollicis longus originates from the posterior surface of the middle third of the ulnar shaft and the posterior interosseous membrane (Fig. 10.20). It inserts into the dorsal surface of the base of the distal phalanx of the thumb. The needle is inserted at the middle of the middle third of the forearm along the radial side of the ulna. The position of the needle is verified by the patient extending the thumb at the distal phalanx.

Extensor pollicis brevis

The extensor pollicis brevis originates at the posterior surface of the radial shaft and the posterior interosseous membrane (Fig. 10.16). It inserts at the dorsal surface of the base of the proximal phalanx of the thumb. The muscle is deep to the extensor pollicis longus. The needle is inserted at the junction of the lower and middle third of the posterior surface of the radial shaft. This thin muscle is verified by extension of the proximal phalanx.

Proximal arm dystonia

In some patients, the upper arm may be abducted (Fig. 10.1) or adducted with attempted writing. Abduction of the arm suggests that the deltoid muscle is involved. Adduction indicates involvement of the pectoralis.

Verification of needle position for botulinum neurotoxin injection

In office practice, needle placement in the selected muscle is guided by surface landmarks and often verified by EMG, hearing an interference pattern with voluntary contraction. Some patients can have difficulty isolating individual movements. Alternative

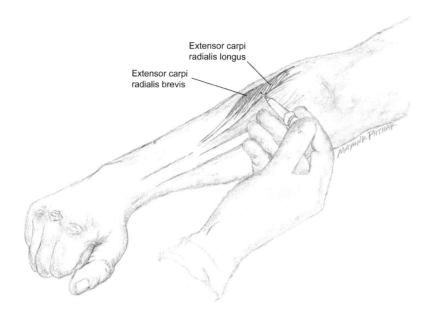

Fig. 10.18 Extensor carpi radialis longus and brevis.

Extensor carpi radialis longus

Extensor carpi radialis brevis

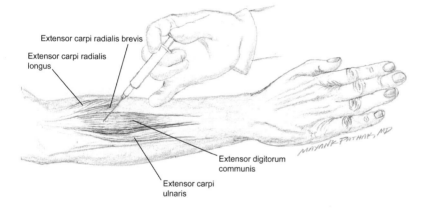

Fig. 10.19 Extensor digitorum communis and extensor carpi ulnaris.

Extensor carpi radialis brevis

Extensor carpi radialis longus

Extensor digitorum communis

Extensor carpi ulnaris

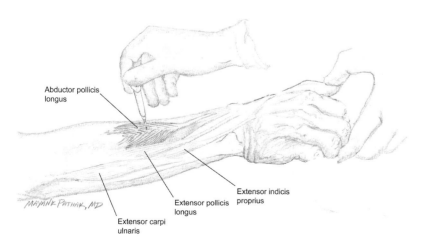

Fig. 10.20 Abductor pollicis longus.

Abductor pollicis longus

Extensor indicis proprius

Extensor pollicis longus

Extensor carpi ulnaris

81

methods for muscle verification include (1) passive movement of the joint with observation of needle movement, (2) stimulation through the needle with observation of movement and (3) ultrasound.

Adverse effects of botulinum neurotoxin injection

Excessive weakness of the target muscle is the most common side effect. Improvement in writer's cramp is almost invariably accompanied by some degree of weakness. The dose of BoNT should be carefully chosen to minimize weakness while maximizing benefit. Weakness may impair non-writing tasks; if severe, it also impairs writing. Atrophy of the injected muscles is commonly seen after repeated injections; however, muscle bulk will recover if injections are stopped. As with any intramuscular injection, the injection may be painful, particularly palmar injections into hand intrinsic muscles and bruising may occur at the injection site.

Neutralizing antibodies may develop against BoNT, particularly when larger doses are required. In this case, further injections with that serotype of BoNT do not cause either benefit or weakness. Benefit may be regained in the presence of antibodies by switching to the other serotype.

Treatment of musician's dystonia

Musician's dystonia is more difficult to treat effectively than writer's cramp. Neurorehabilitation is often the first method tried. One reasonable approach to treatment, given the task specificity of the disorder, is to establish a new sensorimotor program or to reprogram the original motor program. Different methods have been proposed to achieve these goals (Zeuner et al., 2005). A rehabilitation program may include physical and psychological components (Candia et al., 2002; Chamagne, 2003), such as making a musician aware of poor posture and deprogramming non-physiological postures and gestures to ensure that the patient understands the functional anatomy and biomechanics of their dystonia, followed by teaching new movements that respect normal physiology. Such approaches, however, are rarely successful.

Use of BoNT is not as effective for musician's FHD as it is for writer's cramp. Although the degree of improvement in the dystonic symptoms with injection may be similar, the response is still often insufficient to meet the demands for fine motor control of the hand of a professional musician. In addition, weakness from the BoNT may further impair playing. Therefore, musicians have a strong propensity to withdraw from treatment once they find that performance is not sufficiently improved. Despite these considerations and the absence of any more effective alternative, BoNT is the method of choice (Cole et al., 1991). Approach to evaluation and selection of muscles is similar to writer's cramp, but dosing should be conservative.

Other focal hand dystonias

Writer's cramp and musician's dystonia are the most common occupational dystonias; some other less common occupational dystonias deserve mention. Focal hand dystonia affecting golfers is known as "yips." Yips consist of involuntary movements occurring in the course of the execution of focused, finely controlled skilled motor activity (McDaniel et al., 1989). The movements emerge particularly during "putting" and are less evident during "chipping" or "driving." Yips may worsen with anxiety. Compensatory strategies like changing hand preference or handgrip and using a longer putter may ameliorate the symptoms. Recently, EMG studies have documented co-contractions of wrist flexors and extensors in golfers affected with yips, supporting the dystonic nature of this movement disorder. Spontaneous remissions may occur. Benzodiazepines are not helpful in the majority of patients. Botulinum neurotoxin has not been systematically studied in golfer's dystonia.

Typists and telegraphers are also known to develop FHD – known as typist's cramp and telegrapher's cramp, respectively. The affected telegraphers described stiffness, spasm, cramp, tremor and weakness. They also reported that symptoms appeared more in afternoon than morning sessions and on Fridays more often than Sundays, suggesting a relationship to excessive work. Focal hand dystonia has also been described in cobblers, tailors, bookmakers, watch makers, surgeons and dentists, all occupations that involve excessive and repetitive fine motor activity. The pathophysiology of these focal dystonias is likely to be the same as that of writer's cramp, though they have not been studied systematically. The treatment of these conditions is approached similar to that of writer's cramp and musician's dystonia, with a combination of neuromuscular rehabilitation and BoNT.

Table 10.2 Starting range of dosages of botulinum neurotoxin for forearm and hand intrinsic muscles commonly involved in writer's cramp[a]

Muscle	OnabotulinumtoxinA/ incobotulinumtoxinA (U)	AbobotulinumtoxinA (U)	RimabotulinumtoxinB (U)
Finger flexors/extensors[b]	5–20	20–60	250–1000
Wrist flexors/extensors[c]	10–20	50–100	250–1000
Pronator teres	10–30	50–100	500–1500
Hand intrinsic muscles	2.5–10	10–30	250–500

[a] This gives only a rough guide to starting doses. Dosage must be individualized and should be adjusted for subsequent injections based on response. Brands of neurotoxins are not interchangeable and there is no fixed dose ratio between the neurotoxin brands, even within the same serotype.
[b] Flexor digitorum profundus, flexor digitorium superficialis, flexor pollicis longus, extensor digitorum communis, extensor pollicis longus, extensor indicis proprius.
[c] Flexor carpi ulnaris, flexor carpi radialis, extensor carpi ulnaris, extensor carpi radialis.

Table 10.2 gives an approximate guide to BoNT doses. Therapy must be individualized. It should also be noted that the commercially available BoNT products are dosed different and are not interchangeable. Moreover, there is no fixed ratio of potency between the doses of BoNT serotypes, even between onabotulinumtoxinA and incobotulinumtoxinA.

References

Bara-Jimenez W, Catalan MJ, Hallett M, Gerloff C (1998). Abnormal somatosensory homunculus in dystonia of the hand. *Neurology*, **44**, 828–31.

Candia V, Schafer T, Taub E *et al.* (2002). Sensory motor retuning: a behavioral treatment for focal hand dystonia of pianists and guitarists. *Arch Phys Med Rehabil*, **83**, 1342–8.

Chamagne P (2003). Functional dystonia in musicians: rehabilitation. *Hand Clin*, **19**, 309–16.

Cho CB, Park HK, Lee KJ, Rha HK (2009). Thalamic deep brain stimulation for writer's cramp. *J Korean Neurosurg Soc*, **46**, 52–5.

Cole RA, Cohen LG, Hallett M (1991). Treatment of musician's cramp with botulinum toxin. *Med Probl Perform Artists*, **6**, 137–43.

Das SK, Banerjee TK, Biswas A *et al.* (2007). Community survey of primary dystonia in the city of Kolkata India. *Mov Disord*, **22**, 2031–6.

Djebbari R, Dumontcel ST, Sangla S *et al.* (2004). Factors predicting improvement in motor disability in writer's cramp treated with botulinum toxin. *J Neurol Neurosurg Psychiatry*, **75**, 1688–91.

Duffey O, Butler AG, Hawthorne MR, Barnes MP (1998). The epidemiology of the primary dystonias in the north of England. *Adv Neurol*, **78**, 12–15.

Epidemiological Study of Dystonia in Europe (ESDE) Collaborative Group (1999). Sex related influences on the frequency and age of onset of primary dystonia. *Neurology*, **53**, 1871–3.

Epidemiological Study of Dystonia in Europe (ESDE) Collaborative Group (2000). A prevalence study of primary dystonia in eight European countries. *J Neurol*, **247**, 787–92.

Garraux G, Bauer A, Hanakawa T *et al.* (2004). Changes in brain anatomy in focal hand dystonia. *Ann Neurol*, **55**, 736–9.

Granert O, Peller M, Jabusch HC, Altenmuller E, Siebner HR (2011). Sensorimotor skills and focal dystonia are linked to putaminal grey-matter volume in pianists. *J Neurol Neurosurg Psychiatry*, **82**, 1225–31.

Hallett M (1998). Physiology of dystonia. *Adv Neurol*, **78**, 11–18.

Hallett M (2000). Disorder of movement preparation in dystonia. *Brain*. **123**, 1765–6.

Hallett M (2006a). Pathophysiology of dystonia. *J Neural Transm Suppl*. **70**, 485–8.

Hallett M (2006b). Pathophysiology of writer's cramp. *Hum Mov Sci*, **4–5**, 454–63.

Hsuing GY, Das SK, Ranawaya R (2002). Long term efficacy of botulinum toxin A in treatment of various movement disorders over a 10 year period. *Mov Disord*, **17**, 1288–93.

Jedynak PC, Tranchant C, Zegers Debeyl D (2001). Prospective clinical study of writer's cramp. *Mov Disord*, **16**, 494–9.

Karp BI (2004). Botulinum toxin treatment of occupational and focal hand dystonia. *Mov Disord*, **19**(Suppl 8), S116–19.

Karp BI, Cole RA, Cohen LG *et al.* (1994). Long term botulinum toxin treatment of focal hand dystonia. *Neurology*, **44**, 70–6.

Lee H, DeLisa J (2000). *Surface Anatomy for Clinical Needle Electromyography*. New York: Demos Medical Publishing.

Lungu C, Karp BI, Alter K, Zolbrod R, Hallett M (2011). Long-term follow-up of botulinum toxin therapy for focal hand dystonia: outcome at 10 years or more. *Mov Disord*, **26**, 750–3.

McDaniel KD, Cummings JL, Shain H (1989). The "yips": a focal dystonia of golfers. *Neurology*, **39**, 192–5.

Molloy FM, Shill HA, Kaelin-Lang A, Karp BI (2002). Accuracy of muscle localization without EMG: implications for treatment of limb dystonia. *Neurology*, **58**, 805–7.

Newmark J, Hochberg FH (1987). Isolated painless manual incoordination in 57 musicians. *J Neurol Neurosurg Psychiatry*, **50**, 291–5.

Nutt JG, Muenter MD, Aronson A, Kurland LT, Melton LJ (1988). Epidemiology of focal and generalised dystonia in Rochester Minnesota. *Mov Disord*, **50**, 361–5.

Oga T, Honda M, Toma K *et al.* (2002). Abnormal cortical mechanisms of voluntary muscle relaxation in patients with writer's cramp: an MRI study. *Brain*. **125**, 895–903.

Ramazzini B (1713). Diseases of scribes and notaries. In *Diseases of Workers*. New York: Hafner, pp. 421–5.

Rosenbaum F, Jankovic J (1988). Focal task-specific tremor and dystonia: categorization of occupational movement disorders. *Neurology*, **38**, 522–7.

Sanger TD, Tarsy D, Pascual-Leone A (2001). Abnormalities of spatial and temporal sensory discrimination in writer's cramp. *Mov Disord*, **16**, 94–9.

Simpson DM, Blitzer A, Brashear A *et al.* (2008). Assessment: botulinum neurotoxin for the treatment of movement disorders (an evidence-based review): report of the Therapeutics and Technology Assessment Subcommittee of the American Academy of Neurology. *Neurology*, **70**, 1699–706.

Singer C, Papapetropoulos S, Vela L (2005). Use of mirror dystonia as guidance for injection of botulinum toxin in writing dysfunction. *J Neurol Neurosurg Psychiatry*. **76**, 1608–9.

Soland VL, Bhatis KP, Marsden CD (1996). Sex prevalence of focal dystonias. *J Neurol Neurosurg Psychiatry*, **60**, 204–5.

Solly S (1864). Scrivener's palsy, or paralysis of writer's. *Lancet*, **ii**, 709–11.

Taira T, Harashima S, Hori T (2003). Neurosurgical treatment for writer's cramp. *Acta Neurochir*, **87**(Suppl), 129–31.

Tsui JKC, Bhatt M, Calne S, Calne DB (1993). Botulinum toxin in the treatment of writer's cramp. A double blind study. *Neurology*, **43**, 183–5.

Tubiana R (2003). Musician's focal dystonia. *Hand Clin*, **19**, 303–8.

Turjanski N, Pirtosek Z, Quirk J *et al.* (1996). Botulinum toxin in the treatment of writer's cramp. *Clin Neuropharmacol*, **19**, 314–20.

Wilson F, Wagner C, Homberg V (1993). Biomechanical abnormalities in musicians with occupational cramp focal dystonia. *J Hand Ther*, **64**, 234–44.

Wissell J, Kabus C, Wenzel R *et al.* (1996). Botulinum toxin in writer's cramp: objective response evaluation in 31 patients. *J Neurol Neurosurg Psychiatry*, **61**, 172–5.

Zeuner KE, Hallett M (2003). Sensory training as treatment for focal hand dystonia: a 1 year follow up. *Mov Disord*, **18**, 1044–7.

Zeuner KE, Bara-Jimenez W, Noguchi PS *et al.* (2002). Sensory training for patients with focal hand dystonia. *Ann Neurol*, **51**, 593–8.

Zeuner KE, Shill HA, Sohn YH *et al.* (2005). Motor training as a treatment in focal hand dystonia. *Mov Disord*, **20**, 335–41.

Botulinum neurotoxin therapy for laryngeal muscle hyperactivity syndromes

Daniel Truong, Arno Olthoff and Rainer Laskawi

Introduction

Spasmodic dysphonia is a focal dystonia characterized by task-specific, action-induced spasm of the vocal cords. It adversely affects a patient's ability to communicate. It can occur independently, as part of cranial dystonia (Meige's syndrome), or in other disorders such as in tardive dyskinesia.

Clinical features

There are three types of spasmodic dysphonia: the adductor type, the abductor type and the mixed type:

- adductor spasmodic dysphonia (ADSD) is characterized by a strained-strangled voice quality and intermittent voice stoppage or breaks, resulting in a staccato-like voice, caused by overadduction of the vocal folds
- abductor spasmodic dysphonia (ABSD) is characterized by intermittent breathy breaks and associated with prolonged abduction folds during voiceless consonants in speech
- patients with the mixed type have presentations of both.

Symptoms of spasmodic dysphonia begin gradually over several months to years. The condition typically affects patients in their mid-forties and is more common in women (Adler et al., 1997; Schweinfurth et al., 2002).

Spasmodic dysphonia may coexist with vocal tremor. Patients with ADSD show evidence of phonatory breaks during vocalization. The vocal breaks typically occur during phonation associated with voiced speech sounds (Sapienza et al., 2000).

Stress commonly exacerbates speech symptoms; they are absent during laughing, throat clearing, coughing, whispering, humming and falsetto speech productions (Aronson et al., 1968). The voice tends to improve when the patient is emotional.

Botulinum neurotoxin treatment for adductor spasmodic dysphonia

The efficacy of botulinum neurotoxin (BoNT) in the treatment of spasmodic dysphonia has been proven in a double-blind study (Truong et al., 1991). On average, patients treated for ADSD with BoNT experience a 97% improvement in voice. Side effects included breathiness, choking and mild swallowing difficulty (Truong et al., 1991). The duration of benefit averages about 3–4 months depending on the dose used.

Muscles injected with botulinum neurotoxin

Treatment of ADSD involves mostly injection of BoNT into the thyroarytenoid muscles. A study using fine-wire electromyography (EMG) (Klotz et al., 2004) indicated that:

- both the thyroarytenoid and the lateral cricoarytenoid muscle may be affected in ADSD, although the involvement of thyroarytenoid is more predominant
- the thyroarytenoid and lateral cricoarytenoid muscles are equally involved in tremorous spasmodic dysphonia
- interarytenoid muscle may be involved in some patients in both ADSD and in tremorous spasmodic dysphonia.

Successful injections of BoNT into the ventricular folds indicated the involvement of the ventricular muscles in ADSD (Schönweiler et al., 1998).

Manual of Botulinum Toxin Therapy, 2nd edition, ed. Daniel Truong, Mark Hallett, Christopher Zachary and Dirk Dressler. Published by Cambridge University Press. © Cambridge University Press 2013.

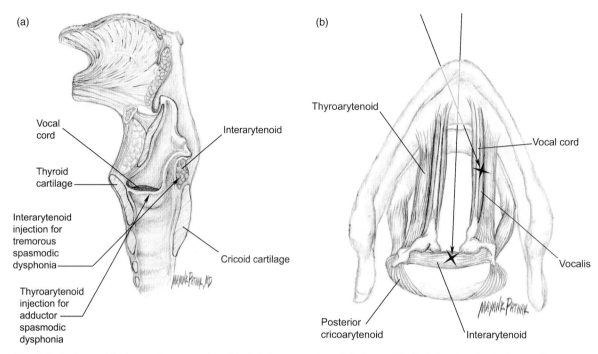

(a)

Vocal cord

Interarytenoid

Thyroid cartilage

Interarytenoid injection for tremorous spasmodic dysphonia

Cricoid cartilage

Thyroarytenoid injection for adductor spasmodic dysphonia

(b)

Thyroarytenoid

Vocal cord

Vocalis

Posterior cricoarytenoid

Interarytenoid

Fig. 11.1 Anatomy of the laryngeal muscles relevant for botulinum neurotoxin injections. (a) Sagittal view showing the laryngeal structure. The arrows denote the direction for injection into the thyroarytenoid muscle for adductor spasmodic dysphonia and into the interarytenoid muscle for the tremorous spasmodic dysphonia. (b) Superior view showing the laryngeal structure and these technical aspects looking from superior angle.

Injection of BoNT can be made into the thyroarytenoid muscle, either unilaterally or bilaterally. Unilateral injection may result in fewer adverse events such as breathiness, hoarseness, swallowing difficulty after the injection (Bielamowicz et al., 2002), but the strong voice intervals are also reduced.

The patient may experience breathiness for up to 2 weeks, followed by the development of a strong voice. After an effective period of a few months, the spasmodic symptoms slowly return as the clinical effect of BoNT wears off. The duration of effect is dose related.

Injection techniques

The BoNT is injected intramuscularly. Different techniques of injection have been proposed, including the percutaneous approach (Miller et al., 1987), the transoral approach (Ford et al., 1990), the transnasal approach (Rhew et al., 1994) and point touch injections (Green et al., 1992).

Percutaneous technique

A teflon-coated needle connected to an EMG machine is inserted through the space between the cricoid and thyroid cartilages and pointing toward the thyroarytenoid muscle (Fig. 11.1). The localization of the needle is verified by high-frequency muscle discharges on the EMG when the patient performs a long "/i/" (Miller et al., 1987). The BoNT is then injected (Fig. 11.2).

For patients with excessive gag reflex, 0.2 ml 1% lidocaine can be injected either through the cricothyroid membrane or underneath into the airway. The resulting cough would anesthetize the undersurface area of the vocal cord as well as the endotracheal structures, enabling the patients to tolerate the gag reflex (Truong et al., 1991).

Transoral technique

In the transoral approach, the vocal folds are indirectly visualized and the injections are performed using a device originally designed for collagen injection. Indirect laryngoscopy is used to direct the needle in an attempt to cover a broad area of motor endplates (Figs. 11.3 and 11.4) (Ford et al., 1990).

A large wastage of the BoNT because of the large dead volume of the long needle is a drawback of this technique.

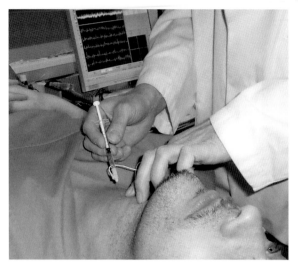

Fig. 11.2 Transcutaneous injection technique. The injection should be done using electromyography control.

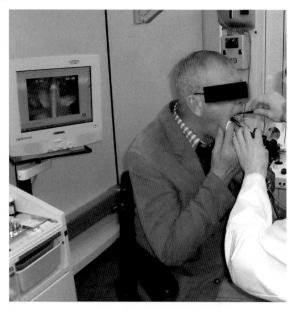

Fig. 11.3 The transoral appproach using a 90° video-endoscope.

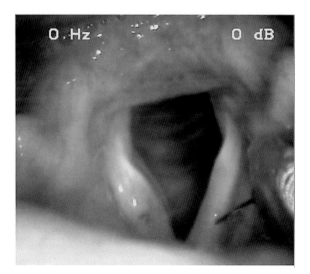

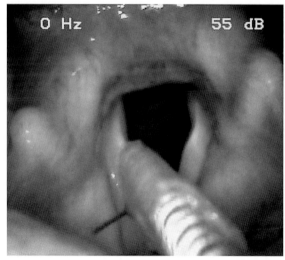

Fig. 11.4 Endoscopic view during transoral botulinum neurotoxin application (see Fig. 11.3). (a) Injection into the left vocal fold. (b) Injection into the right ventricular muscle (ventricular fold).

In patients who cannot tolerate the gag reflex, a direct laryngoscopic injection can be performed under short total anesthesia (Fig. 11.5).

Transnasal technique

In the transnasal approach, BoNT is injected through a channel running parallel to the laryngoscope with a flexible catheter needle. This technique requires prior topical anesthesia with lidocaine spray (Rhew *et al.*, 1994). The location of the injection is lateral to the true vocal fold in order to avoid damaging the vocal fold mucosa.

Point touch injections

In the point touch technique, the needle is inserted through the surface of the thyroid cartilage halfway between the thyroid notch and inferior edge of the thyroid cartilage. The BoNT is given once the needle is passed into the thyroarytenoid muscle (Green *et al.*, 1992).

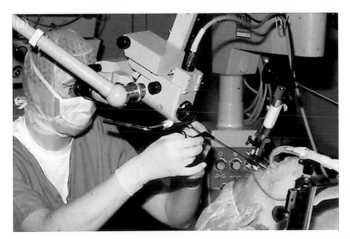 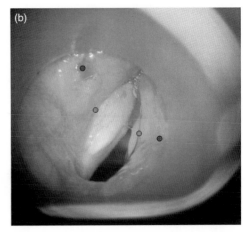

Fig. 11.5 Injection during microlaryngoscopy with a short general anesthetic. (a) The procedure, which normally does not use a tracheal tube and the injection is made during a short period of apnea. (b) Microscopical view of the larynx during microlaryngoscopy, the dots mark the typical injection points.

For injections into the ventricular folds, a transoral or transnasal approach is required (Fig. 11.4). Because EMG signals cannot be received from the ventricular muscle, a percutaneous technique is not recommended.

Botulinum neurotoxin doses

Doses of BoNT used for the treatment of spasmodic dysphonia vary depending on the particular brand of BoNT used. In general, although there are correlations between the doses, the appropriate dose for a given BoNT product is dictated by the possible side effects of the BoNT on the adjacent organs or muscles. The approximate dose relation between onabotulinumtoxinA, incobotulinumtoxinA, abobotulinumtoxinA and rimabotulinumtoxinB is 1: 1: 3: 50. This dose relationship should not be used as a guideline as the diffusion rates of these BoNTs differ and the close proximity of the muscle involved in swallowing should be the defining factor for the dose chosen.

In the early literature, the doses of BoNT (onabotulinumtoxinA) used for ADSD ranged from 3.75 to 7.5 U for bilateral injections (Brin *et al.*, 1988a, b, 1989; Truong *et al.*, 1991) to 15 U for unilateral injections (Miller *et al.*, 1987; Ludlow *et al.*, 1988). Later literature and common practice have recommended the use of lower doses (Blitzer and Sulica, 2001). We recommend starting with 0.5 U onabotulinumtoxinA/incobotulinumtoxinA, 1.5 U abobotulinumtoxinA or 200 U rimabotulinumtoxinB when injected bilaterally and to adjust the dose as needed. Our estimated average dose is 0.5 U

onabotulinumtoxinA/incobotulinumtoxinA, 2–3 U abobotulinumtoxinA or 300 U rimabotulinumtoxinB.

Beneficial effects last about 3–4 months in our patients treated with onabotulinumtoxinA, incobotulinumtoxinA or abobotulinumtoxinA. They last about 8 weeks with rimabotulinumtoxinB (Adler *et al.*, 2004a) but may be longer with higher doses (Guntinas-Lichius, 2003). In patients who received BoNT serotype B after type A failure, the duration was only about 2 months despite higher doses up to 1000 U per cord.

Botulinum neurotoxin treatment for abductor spasmodic dysphonia

Injection technique and muscles injected

With the thyroid lamina rotated forward, the needle is inserted behind the posterior edge and directed toward the posterior cricoarytenoid muscle. Location is verified by maximal muscle discharge when patients perform a sniff (Figs. 11.6 and 11.7) (Blitzer *et al.*, 1992).

The average onset of effect is 4 days and duration of benefit is 10.5 weeks.

Adverse effects include exertional wheezing and dysphagia.

In another approach, the needle is directed along the superior border of the posterior cricoid lamina and between the arytenoid cartilages. For anatomical reasons, the BoNT is injected at a high location and allowed to diffuse down into the muscle for therapeutic effects (Fig. 11.8).

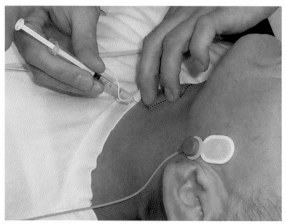

Fig. 11.7 Injection into the posterior cricoarytenoid muscle in a patient using a lateral approach.

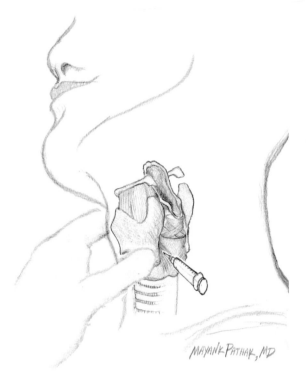

Fig. 11.6 Anterolateral view of the larynx and posterior cricoarytenoid muscle with the thyroid lamina rotated forward and to the other side.

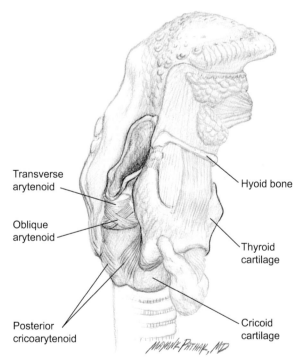

Transverse arytenoid

Oblique arytenoid

Posterior cricoarytenoid

Hyoid bone

Thyroid cartilage

Cricoid cartilage

Fig. 11.8 Dorsolateral view showing the anatomy of posterior cricoarytenoid, oblique arytenoids and transverse arytenoid muscles.

A refined technique with the needle penetrating through the posterior cricoid lamina into the posterior cricoarytenoid muscle seems to be simpler and has the advantage of direct injection into the muscle (Meleca *et al.*, 1997).

Between 2 and 4 U onabotulinumtoxinA/incobotulinumtoxinA or 12 U abobotulinumtoxinA on one side and 1 U onabotulinumtoxinA/3 U abobotulinumtoxinA on the opposite side are used. If a higher dose is required for each side, the injection of the opposite side should be delayed for about 2 weeks to avoid compromising the airway.

Spasmodic laryngeal dyspnea

Spasmodic laryngeal dystonia results in laryngopharyngeal spasm primarily during respiration. Patients' breathing problems are even improved with speaking (Zwirner *et al.*, 1997). Dyspnea is caused by an intermittent glottic and supraglottic airway obstruction from both laryngeal and supralaryngeal/pharyngeal muscle spasms. Treatment includes injections with BoNT into the thyroarytenoid and ventricular folds (Zwirner *et al.*, 1997). These improvements last from 9 weeks to 6 months.

Vocal tremors

Patients with essential tremor also demonstrate tremors of the voice. The intrinsic laryngeal muscles are tremulous during respiration and speech, with the thyroarytenoid muscles most often involved (Koda and Ludlow, 1992).

Table 11.1 Doses of various botulinum neurotoxin products

Diagnosis and treatment technique	OnabotulinumtoxinA (U)	IncobotulinumtoxinA (U)	AbobotulinumtoxinA (U)	RimabotulinumtoxinB (U)
ADSD, unilateral injections	5–15	5–15	15–45	250–500
ADSD, bilateral injections	0.5–3	0.5–3	1.5–9	100–250
ABSD, unilateral injections	15	15	45	Not known
ABSD, bilateral injections	1.25–1.75	1.25–1.75	4.5–6	Not known
Vocal tremor	2	2	7.5	100–250
Spasmodic laryngeal dyspnea	2.5	2.5	7.5	100–250

ADSD, adductor spasmodic dysphonia; ABSD, abductor spasmodic dysphonia.
Source: modified from Truong and Bhidayasiri, 2006.

Patients report subjective reduction in vocal effort and improvement in voice tremors following injection with BoNT into the vocal cord (Adler *et al.*, 2004b).

Improvement may also occur with treatment of the lateral cricoarytenoid and interarytenoid muscles (Klotz *et al.*, 2004).

For the treatment of vocal tremors, the thyroarytenoid muscles are often injected using a technique similar to that used for ADSD.

The average doses used are about 2 U onabotulinumtoxinA/incobotulinumtoxinA or 8 U abobotulinumtoxinA. For rimabotulinumtoxinB, about 200 U would be needed.

References

Adler CH, Edwards BW, Bansberg SF (1997). Female predominance in spasmodic dysphonia. *J Neurol Neurosurg Psychiatry*, **63**, 688.

Adler CH, Bansberg SF, Hentz JG *et al.* (2004a). Botulinum toxin type A for treating voice tremor. *Arch Neurol*, **61**, 1416–20.

Adler CH, Bansberg SF, Krein-Jones K, Hentz JG (2004b). Safety and efficacy of botulinum toxin type B (Myobloc) in adductor spasmodic dysphonia. *Mov Disord*, **19**, 1075–9.

Aronson AE, Brown JR, Litin EM, Pearson JS (1968). Spastic dysphonia. II. Comparison with essential (voice) tremor and other neurologic and psychogenic dysphonias. *J Speech Hear Disord*, **33**, 219–31.

Bielamowicz S, Stager SV, Badillo A, Godlewski A (2002). Unilateral versus bilateral injections of botulinum toxin in patients with adductor spasmodic dysphonia. *J Voice*, **16**, 117–23.

Blitzer A, Sulica L (2001). Botulinum toxin basic science and clinical uses in otolaryngology. *Laryngoscope* **111**, 218–26.

Blitzer A, Brin MF, Stewart C, Aviv JE, Fahn S (1992). Abductor laryngeal dystonia: a series treated with botulinum toxin. *Laryngoscope*, **102**, 163–7.

Brin MF, Fahn S, Moskowitz C *et al.* (1988a). Localized injections of botulinum toxin for the treatment of focal dystonia and hemifacial spasm. *Adv Neurol*, **50**, 599–608.

Brin MF, Blitzer A, Stewart C (1988b). Laryngeal dystonia (spasmodic dysphonia): observations of 901 patients and treatment with botulinum toxin. *Adv Neurol*, **78**, 237–52.

Brin MF, Blitzer A, Fahn S, Gould W, Lovelace RE (1989). Adductor laryngeal dystonia (spastic dysphonia): treatment with local injections of botulinum toxin (Botox). *Mov Disord*, **4**, 287–96.

Ford CN, Bless DM, Lowery JD (1990). Indirect laryngoscopic approach for injection of botulinum toxin in spasmodic dysphonia. *Otolaryngol Head Neck Surg*, **103**, 752–8.

Green DC, Berke GS, Ward PH, Gerratt BR (1992). Point-touch technique of botulinum toxin injection for the treatment of spasmodic dysphonia. *Ann Otol Rhinol Laryngol*, **101**, 883–7.

Guntinas-Lichius O (2003). Injection of botulinum toxin type B for the treatment of otolaryngology patients with secondary treatment failure of botulinum toxin type A. *Laryngoscope*, **113**, 743–5.

Klotz DA, Maronian NC, Waugh PF *et al.* (2004). Findings of multiple muscle involvement in a study of 214 patients with laryngeal dystonia using fine-wire electromyography. *Ann Otol Rhinol Laryngol*, **113**, 602–12.

Koda J, Ludlow CL (1992). An evaluation of laryngeal muscle activation in patients with voice tremor. *Otolaryngol Head Neck Surg*, **107**, 684–96.

Ludlow CL, Naunton RF, Sedory SE, Schulz GM, Hallett M (1988). Effects of botulinum toxin injections on speech in adductor spasmodic dysphonia. *Neurology*, **38**, 1220–5.

Meleca RJ, Hogikyan ND, Bastian RW (1997). A comparison of methods of botulinum toxin injection for abductory spasmodic dysphonia. *Otolaryngol Head Neck Surg*, **117**, 487–92.

Miller RH, Woodson GE, Jankovic J (1987). Botulinum toxin injection of the vocal fold for spasmodic dysphonia.

A preliminary report. *Arch Otolaryngol Head Neck Surg*, **113**, 603–5.

Rhew K, Fiedler DA, Ludlow CL (1994). Technique for injection of botulinum toxin through the flexible nasolaryngoscope. *Otolaryngol Head Neck Surg*, **111**, 787–94.

Sapienza CM, Walton S, Murry T (2000). Adductor spasmodic dysphonia and muscular tension dysphonia: acoustic analysis of sustained phonation and reading. *J Voice*, **14**, 502–20.

Schönweiler R, Wohlfarth K, Dengler R, Ptok M (1998). Supraglottal injection of botulinum toxin type A in adductor type spasmodic dysphonia with both intrinsic and extrinsic hyperfunction. *Laryngoscope*, **108**, 55–63.

Schweinfurth JM, Billante M, Courey MS (2002). Risk factors and demographics in patients with spasmodic dysphonia. *Laryngoscope*, **112**, 220–23.

Truong D, Bhidayasiri R (2006) Botulinum toxin in laryngeal dystonia. *Eur J Neurol*, **13**(Suppl 1), 36–41.

Truong DD, Rontal M, Rolnick M, Aronson AE, Mistura K (1991). Double-blind controlled study of botulinum toxin in adductor spasmodic dysphonia. *Laryngoscope*, **101**, 630–4.

Zwirner P, Dressler D, Kruse E (1997). Spasmodic laryngeal dyspnea: a rare manifestation of laryngeal dystonia. *Eur Arch Otorhinolaryngol*, **254**, 242–5.

The use of botulinum neurotoxin in otorhinolaryngology

Rainer Laskawi, Arno Olthoff and Oleg Olegovich Ivanov

Introduction

Various disorders affecting the ears, nose and throat (ENT) are suited for treatment with botulinum neurotoxin (BoNT). They can be divided into two general groups:

- disorders concerning head and neck muscles (movement disorders)
- disorders caused by a pathological secretion of glands located in the head and neck region.

Table 12.1 summarizes the diseases relevant to otolaryngology. The focus in this chapter lies on indications that are *not* reviewed in other chapters; therefore, laryngeal dystonia, hemifacial spasm, blepharospasm and synkinesis following defective healing of the facial nerve will not be covered here.

Table 12.1 Diseases treated with botulinum neurotoxin type A in otorhinolaryngology[a]

Movement disorders	Disorders of the autonomous nerve system
Facial nerve paralysis	Gustatory sweating (Frey's syndrome)
Hemifacial spasm	Hypersalivation (sialorrhea)
Blepharospasm (Meige's syndrome)	Intrinsic rhinitis
Synkinesis following defective healing of the facial nerve	Hyperlacrimation, tearing
Oromandibular dystonia	
Laryngeal dystonia	
Palatal tremor	
Dysphagia	

[a] Diseases in italics are not reviewed in this chapter.

Dysphagia and speech problems following laryngectomy

Some patients are unable to achieve an adequate speech level for optimal communication after laryngectomy. One of the causes is spasms of the cricopharyngeal muscle. In this condition, BoNT can reduce the muscle activity and improve the quality of speech (Chao *et al.*, 2004). Swallowing disorders in neurological patients can result from a disturbed coordination of the relaxation of the upper esophageal sphincter and can lead to pulmonary aspiration. The cricopharyngeal muscle is a sphincter between the inferior constrictor muscle and the cervical esophagus and is primarily innervated by the vagus nerve.

The following procedure can be used as a test prior to a planned myectomy or as a single therapeutic option that has to be repeated. Botulinum neurotoxin can be injected into the cricopharyngeal muscle at three injection sites under general anesthesia, using 10–20 U onabotulinumtoxinA/incobotulinumtoxinA (or 50–100 U abobotulinumtoxinA or 500–1000 U rimabotulinumtoxinB [BoNT-B]) (Fig. 12.1).

In dysphagia caused by spasms or insufficient relaxation of the upper esophageal sphincter, injection of BoNT as described can improve the patients' complaints (Fig. 12.2). Patients should be evaluated for symptoms of concomitant gastroesophageal reflux to avoid side effects such as "reflux-laryngitis." If there is gastroesophageal reflux, the etiology and treatment should be clarified prior to initiation of BoNT therapy.

Palatal tremor

Repetitive contractions of the muscles of the soft palate (palatoglossus, palatopharyngeus, salpingopharyngeus, tensor and levator veli palatini muscles)

Manual of Botulinum Toxin Therapy, 2nd edition, ed. Daniel Truong, Mark Hallett, Christopher Zachary and Dirk Dressler. Published by Cambridge University Press. © Cambridge University Press 2013.

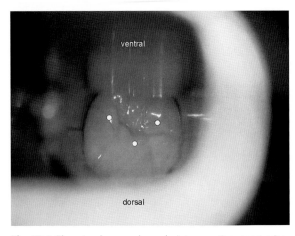

Fig. 12.1 The cricopharyngeal muscle. Intraoperative aspect prior to injection of botulinum neurotoxin into the cricopharyngeal muscle. The dots mark the injection sites (20 U onabotulinumtoxinA at each point).

lead to a rhythmic elevation of the soft palate. This disorder has two forms, symptomatic palatal tremor and essential palatal tremor. Symptomatic palatal tremor can cause speech and also swallowing disorders through velopharyngeal insufficiency. Most patients suffering from essential palatal tremor complain of "ear clicking." This rhythmic tinnitus is caused by a repetitive opening and closure of the orifice of the eustachian tube. A particular sequel of pathological activity of soft palate muscles is the syndrome of a patulous eustachian tube. These patients suffer from "autophonia" caused by an open eustachian tube due to the increased muscle tension of the paratubal muscles (salpingopharyngeus, tensor and levator veli palatini muscles) (Olthoff *et al.*, 2007).

For the first treatment session, the injection of in total 5 U onabotulinumtoxinA/incobotulinumtoxinA

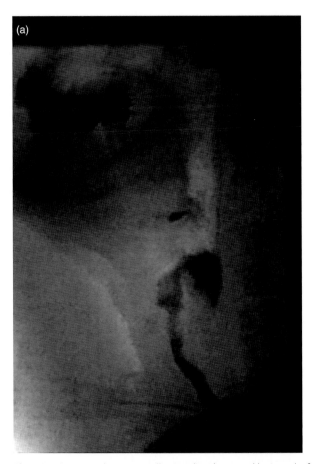

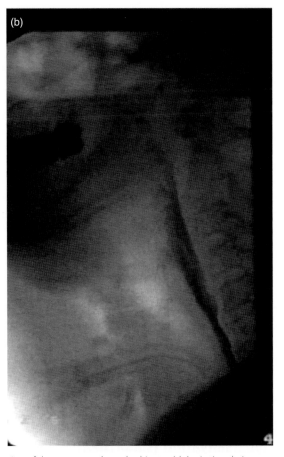

Fig. 12.2 Patient with severe swallowing disorder caused by irregular function of the upper esophageal sphincter. (a) Aspiration during swallowing. (b) Following three injections of botulinum neurotoxin (20 U onabotulinumtoxinA), the pharyngoesophageal passage is normalized.

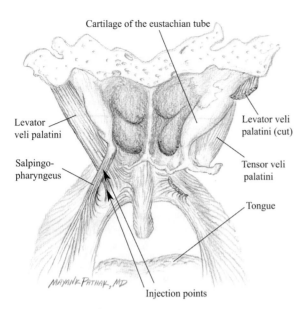

Fig. 12.3 Dorsal view of the nasopharynx and soft palate (modified after Tillmann, 2005). The arrows mark the possible sites of onabotulinumtoxinA injections. The salpingopharyngeal fold is used as a landmark.

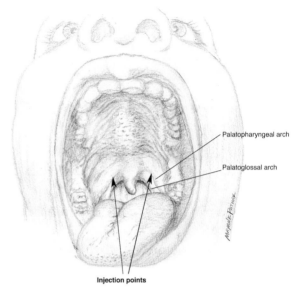

Fig. 12.4 Transoral view of injection sites in patients with palatal tremor. The insertion of the tensor veli palatini muscle is used as landmark.

(uni- or bilaterally) (25 U abobotulinumtoxinA; 250 U rimabotulinumtoxinB) into the soft palate (Figs. 12.3 and 12.4) is adequate in most patients. If necessary, this can be increased to 15 U onabotulinumtoxinA/ incobotulinumtoxinA (75 U abobotulinumtoxinA; 750 U rimabotulinumtoxinB) on each side. The application is normally performed transorally (transpalatinal or via postrhinoscopy) under endoscopic control. The insertion of the tensor veli palatini muscle is used as landmark for the treatment of palatal tremor and the salpingopharyngeal fold as landmark for the treatment of a patulous eustachian tube (Figs. 12.3 and 12.4). To optimize detection of the target muscle, injection under electromyographic control is recommended.

Landmarks are given to avoid vascular injections and to indicate the most "responsible" muscle. The synergistic function of targeted soft palate and paratubal muscles (salpingopharyngeus, tensor and levator veli palatini) often interferes with clinical and therapeutical separation. To avoid side effects such as iatrogenic velopharyngeal insufficiency, treatment should be started with low doses, as described above.

Hypersalivation (sialorrhea)

Hypersalivation can be caused by various conditions such as tumour surgery, neurological and pediatric disorders and disturbances of wound healing following ENT surgery.

Hypersalivation also is of relevance for a number of reasons in patients suffering from head and neck cancers. Some of these patients are unable to swallow their saliva because of a stenosis of the upper esophageal sphincter caused by scar formation after tumor resection. In other patients, there are disturbances of the sensory control of the "entrance" of the supraglottic tissues of the larynx, allowing saliva to pass into the larynx. In patients with Parkinson's disease, decreased swallowing also leads to hypersalivation as it interferes with saliva clearance. This may lead to continuous aspiration and aspiration pneumonia. In a third group of patients, complications of impaired wound healing after extended surgery can occur, such as fistula formation following laryngectomy. Saliva is a very aggressive agent and can inhibit the normal healing process.

Both the parotid and submandibular glands are of interest in this context. The parotid gland is the largest of the salivary glands. It is located in the so-called parotid compartment in the pre- and subauricular region, with a large compartment lying on the masseter muscle. The gland also has contact with the sternocleidomastoid muscle (Fig. 12.5).

The submandibular gland (Figs. 12.6 and 12.7) lies between the two bellies of the digastric muscle and the

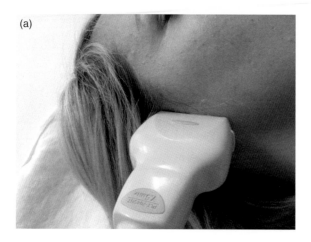

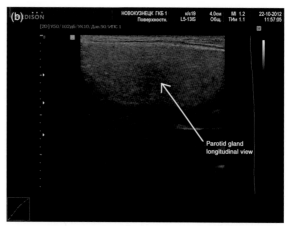

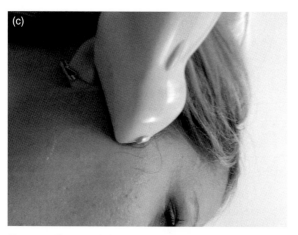

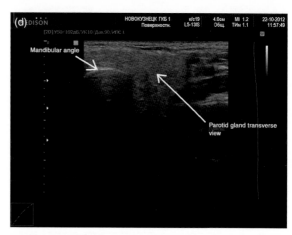

Fig. 12.5 The parotid gland under ultrasound. The presentation depends on the position of the probe. (a,b). Probe in the vertical position (a) to give a longitudinal view of the parotid (b). (c,d) Probe in the horizontal position (c) to give a transverse view of the parotid (d).

inferior margin of the mandible, which form the sub-mandibular triangle. The gland is divided into two parts – the superficial lobe and the deep lobe – by the mylohyoid muscle (Fig. 12.6c).

To reduce saliva flow, we inject 22.5 U onabotulinumtoxinA/incobotulinumtoxinA into each parotid gland under ultrasound guidance at three locations (Ellies *et al.*, 2004) (Figs. 12.8 and 12.9). Each submandibular gland is treated with 15 U onabotulinumtoxinA/incobotulinumtoxinA at one or two sites (Fig. 12.10). Injection of botulinum neurotoxin type A (BoNT-A) has been shown to be effective in reducing saliva flow (Fig. 12.11). Side effects such as local pain, diarrhea, luxation of the mandible and a "dry mouth" are quite rare.

Gustatory sweating (Frey's syndrome)

Gustatory sweating is a common sequel of parotid gland surgery (Laskawi and Rohrbach, 2002). The clinical picture is characterized by extensive production of sweat in the lateral region of the face. The sweating can be intense and become a cause of a serious social stigma. Injection with BoNT has become the first-line treatment (Laskawi and Rohrbach, 2002).

For an optimal outcome, the affected area should be marked with Minor's test (Fig. 12.12). First, the face is divided into regional "boxes" using a waterproof pen (Fig. 12.12b). The affected skin is covered with iodine solution before starch powder is applied. The sweat produced by

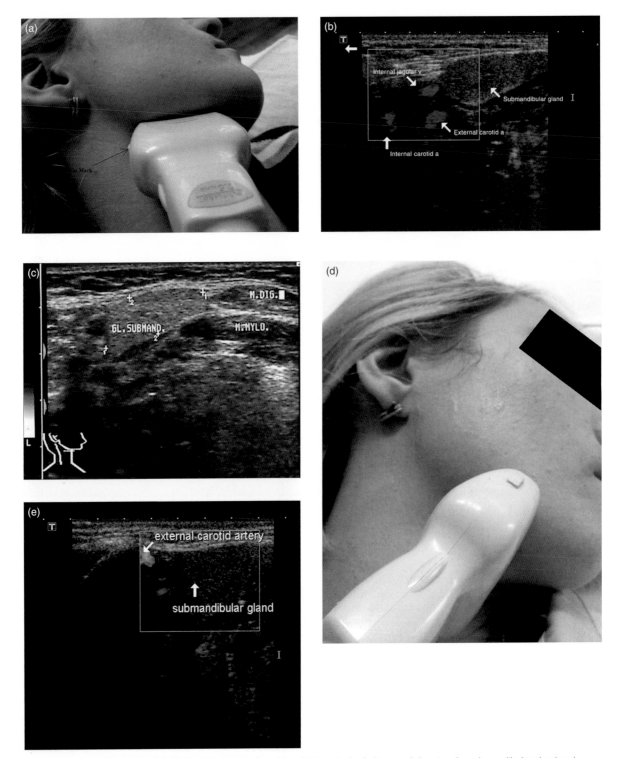

Fig. 12.6 Submandibular gland. (a) Probe in longitudinal position. (b) Longitudinal ultrasound showing the submandibular gland and other structures. Note the location of the internal and external carotid artery and the internal jugular vein. (c) The submandibular gland (GL.SUBMAND.; borders of the gland clearly marked by the four crosses) and the surrounding structures (mylohyoid muscle [M.MYLO.] and digastric muscle [M.DIG]. (d) Probe in transverse position. (e) Transverse ultrasound probe showing the submandibular gland and other structures. Note the location of the external carotid artery.

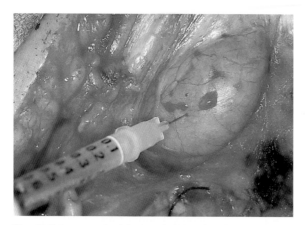

Fig. 12.7 Intraoperative injection of 15 U onabotulinumtoxinA into the submandibular gland during laryngectomy showing the anatomical position of the gland in the submandibular fossa.

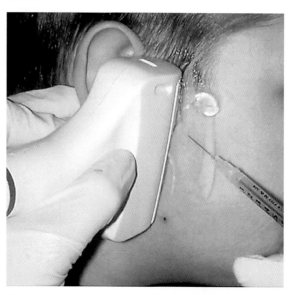

Fig. 12.8 Injection of botulinum neurotoxin type A into the parotid and submandibular glands (same technique used for both). We prefer to inject both glands, with 7.5 U onabotulinumtoxinA into each of the three points of each parotid gland and with 15 U onabotulinumtoxinA into each submandibular gland. Ultrasound-guided injection is recommended.

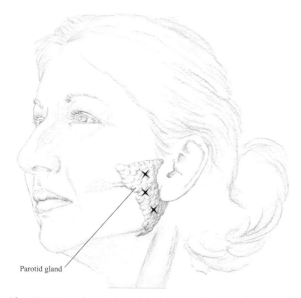

Parotid gland

Fig. 12.9 Frontolateral view of the left parotid gland with typical injections sites for botulinum neurotoxin.

The total dose required depends on the extent of the affected area, and up to 100 U onabotulinumtoxinA/incobotulinumtoxinA (500 U abobotulinumtoxinA, 5000 U rimabotulinumtoxinB) can be necessary. The duration of improvement persists longer than that seen in patients with movement disorders (Laskawi and Rohrbach, 2002), and some patients have a symptom-free interval of several years.

Rhinorrhea, intrinsic rhinitis

In the last few years, BoNT-A has been used in intrinsic or allergic rhinitis (Özcan *et al.*, 2006). The main symptom in these disorders is extensive rhinorrhea with secretions dripping from the nose.

There are two approaches for applying BoNT-A in these patients: it can either be injected into the middle and lower nasal turbinates or applied with soaked on a sponge (Fig. 12.13). For the injection approach, 10 U onabotulinumtoxinA/incobotulinumtoxinA (50 U abobotulinumtoxinA, 500 U rimabotulinumtoxinB) is injected into each middle or lower turbinate. For the

masticating an apple induces a reaction between the iodine solution and the starch powder, resulting in an apparent deep blue color (Laskawi and Rohrbach, 2002).

Intracutaneous injections of BoNT (for 4 cm², approximately 2.5 U onabotulinumtoxinA/incobotulinumtoxinA, 12.5 U abobotulinumtoxinA, 125 U rimabotulinumtoxinB) (Fig. 12.12c). Side effects are rare with some patients experiencing none of the possible sequelae, such as dryness of the skin or eczema.

sponge technique, a sponge is soaked with a solution containing 40 U onabotulinumtoxinA and a sponge is applied into each nostril.

The effect of the injections has been demonstrated in placebo-controlled studies (Özcan *et al.*, 2006). Nasal secretion is reduced for about 12 weeks (Fig. 12.14). Side effects such as epistaxis or nasal crusting are uncommon.

Hyperlacrimation

Hyperlacrimation can be caused by stenoses of the lacrimal duct, misdirected secretory fibers following a degenerative paresis of the facial nerve (crocodile tears) or mechanical irritation of the cornea (in patients with lagophthalmus).

The application of BoNT is useful in reducing pathological tearing in these patients (Whittaker *et al.*, 2003; Meyer, 2004). The lacrimal gland is located in the lacrimal fossa in the lateral part of the upper orbit and is divided into two sections (Fig. 12.15). Usually 5–7.5 U onabotulinumtoxinA/incobotulinumtoxinA (25–37.5 U abobotulinumtoxinA, 250–375 U rimabotulinumtoxinB) is injected into the pars palpebralis of the lacrimal gland, which is accessible under the lateral upper lid (Fig. 12.16). Medial injection may result in ptosis as a possible side effect. The reduction of tear production lasts about 12 weeks (Fig. 12.17) (Meyer, 2004).

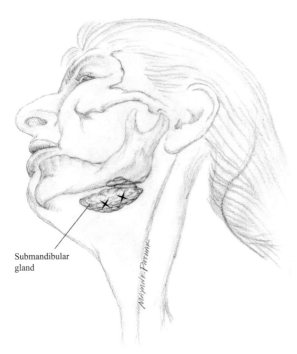

Submandibular gland

Fig. 12.10 Laterocaudal view of the left submandibular gland with typical injections sites for botulinum neurotoxin.

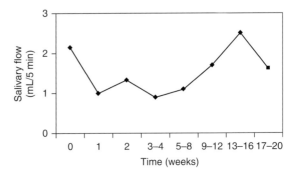

Fig. 12.11 The effect of botulinum neurotoxin injection on saliva flow in patients with hypersalivation. Pretreatment status returns after 12 weeks (Ellies *et al.*, 2004).

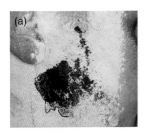 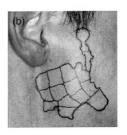 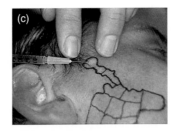 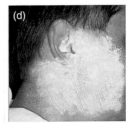

Fig. 12.12 Treatment of gustatory sweating (Frey's syndrome) with botulinum neurotoxin. (a) Patient with extensive gustatory sweating following total parotidectomy. The affected area is marked by Minor's test, showing a deep blue color. (b) The affected area is marked with a waterproof pen and divided into "boxes" to guarantee that the whole plane is treated. (c) Intracutaneous injections of onabotulinumtoxinA are performed. The white color of the skin can be seen during the intracutaneous application of onabotulinumtoxinA. (d) Patient eating an apple 2 weeks after treatment. The marked area that was sweating prior to treatment is now completely dry.

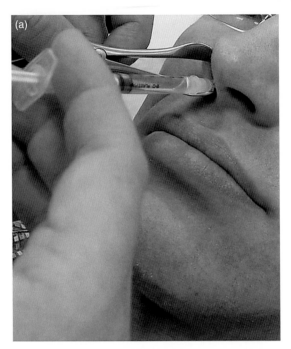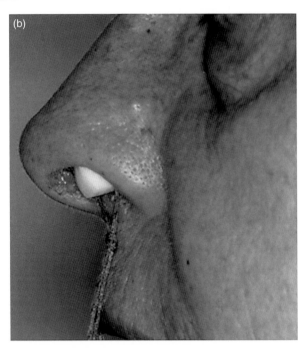

Fig. 12.13 Botulinum neurotoxin is injected into the middle and lower turbinates to treat rhinorrhea (a) or applied with a sponge soaked with a solution of botulinum neurotoxin (b).

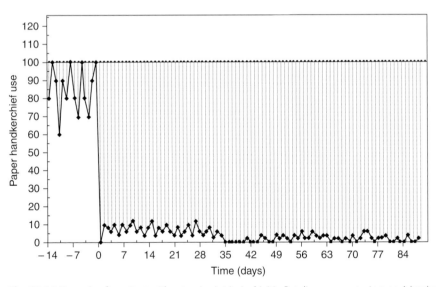

Fig. 12.14 Example of a patient with extensive intrinsic rhinitis. Botulinum neurotoxin type A has been applied with sponges. The consumption of paper handkerchiefs (number shown on vertical axis) is reduced dramatically for a long period after the application (horizontal axis).

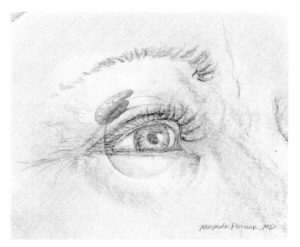

Fig. 12.15 The localization of the lacrimal gland and the upper lid/orbit.

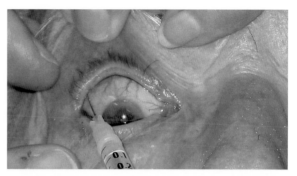

Fig. 12.16 Injection into the pars palpebralis of the lacrimal gland. With the patient looking strongly in the medial direction; the upper lid is lifted and a little "lacrimal prominence" becomes evident. Entering here in a lateral direction, the gland tissue can be approached easily.

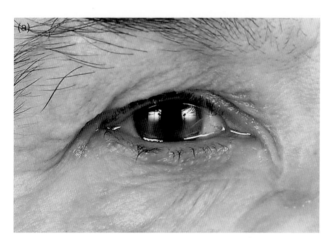

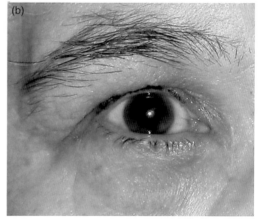

Fig. 12.17 Patient with extensive tearing caused by a stenosis of the lacrimal duct after resection of a malignant tumor of the right maxilla. (a) Pretreatment; (b) post-treatment.

References

Chao SS, Graham SM, Hoffman HT (2004). Management of pharyngoesophageal spasm with Botox. *Otolaryngol Clin North Am*, **37**, 559–66.

Ellies M, Gottstein U, Rohrbach-Volland S, Arglebe C, Laskawi R (2004). Reduction of salivary flow with botulinum toxin: extended report on 33 patients with drooling, salivary fistulas, and sialadenitis. *Laryngoscope*, **114**, 1856–60.

Laskawi R, Rohrbach S (2002). Frey's syndrome: treatment with botulinum toxin. In Kreyden OP, Böni R, Burg G (eds.) *Hyperhidrosis and Botulinum Toxin in Dermatology*. Basel: Karger, pp. 170–7.

Meyer M (2004). Störungen der Tränendrüsen. In Laskawi R, Roggenkämper P (eds.) *Botulinumtoxintherapie im Kopf-Hals-Bereich*. Munich: Urban & Vogel.

Olthoff A, Laskawi R, Kruse E (2007). Successful treatment of autophonia with botulinum toxin: case report. *Ann Otol Rhinol Laryngol*, **116**, 594–8.

Özcan C, Vayisoglu Y, Dogu O, Gorur K (2006). The effect of intranasal injection of botulinum toxin A on the symptoms of vasomotor rhinitis. *Am J Otolaryngol*, **27**, 314–18.

Tillmann B (2005). *Atlas der Anatomie des Menschen*. Berlin: Springer-Verlag, p. 180.

Whittaker KW, Matthews BN, Fitt AW, Sandramouli S (2003). The use of botulinum toxin A in the treatment of functional epiphora. *Orbit*, **22**, 193–8.

Treatment of hemifacial spasm

Karen Frei

Introduction

Hemifacial spasm (HFS) is characterized as involuntary irregular clonic or tonic movements of the facial muscles innervated by cranial nerve VII on one side of the face and is most often a result of vascular compression of the facial nerve at the root exit zone (Wang and Jankovic, 1998). Facial muscle twitches usually begin in the periocular region and can progress to involve the cheek and perioral muscles. Hemifacial spasm is almost always unilateral; however, when bilateral, the two sides are always asynchronous. Atypical cases have been reported to initiate in the orbicularis oris and buccinator muscles and gradually spread upward to involve the orbicularis oculi (Ryu *et al.*, 1998). At times, with involvement of the platysma muscle, a tremor-like appearance of the head can develop (Frei and Truong, 2008). Muscles involved in HFS include the orbicularis oculi, frontalis (rarely), corrugator, nasalis, zygomaticus, risorius, orbicularis oris and sometimes the platysma (Fig. 13.1).

Hemifacial spasm is more prevalent in females, commonly begins in the fifth decade and tends to have a fluctuating course. In contrast to essential blepharospasm, symptoms often continue during sleep and can provoke insomnia. Emotion and stress tend to exacerbate facial twitching. Ear clicks can occur which resolve with treatment of the HFS (Rudzinska *et al.*, 2010). Although benign, HFS can be disabling because of social embarrassment and excessive closure of the affected eye, interfering with vision. Symptoms can progress over time and facial weakness may develop independent from botulinum neurotoxin (BoNT) therapy. Hypertension is thought to be a risk factor for the development of HFS (Oliveira *et al.*, 1999).

Imaging studies have confirmed that the most frequent cause of HFS is vascular compression of the facial nerve at the root exit zone. The severity of compression correlates with the severity of HFS symptoms (Banik and Miller, 2004). Vascular compression generally involves the anterior inferior cerebellar artery, the posterior inferior cerebellar artery, the vertebral basilar artery and the internal auditory artery. The internal auditory artery can be tortuous or ectatic. The offending vessel is ipsilateral to the facial nerve and side of the HFS. Non-vascular origins of HFS occur less commonly and include demyelination, various tumors and space-occupying lesions in the cerebellopontine angle. Evidence suggests that there may be a genetic susceptibility toward vascular anomaly resulting in HFS (Miwa *et al.*, 2002; Lagalla *et al.*, 2010).

Hemifacial spasm must be distinguished from other conditions involving the facial musculature, including blepharospasm, facial myokymia, oromandibular dystonia, facial tic, hemimasticatory spasm, post-Bell's palsy synkinesis and focal seizures. Blepharospasm usually occurs bilaterally at onset and concerns only the eyelids (with the exception that it can be part of involvement of other facial muscles in Meige's syndrome). Blepharospasm is a form of dystonia that causes involuntary closure of the eyes by muscle spasm, or without spasms in a form called apraxia of eyelid opening. Bright light can exacerbate the condition, which subsides during sleep. Blepharospasm may uncommonly coexist with HFS, complicating the diagnosis. One study found blepharospasm to occur following the onset of HFS (Tan *et al.*, 2004). Facial myokymia, a fine rippling movement of the facial muscles, is associated with an abnormality of the brainstem such as that seen in multiple sclerosis. Oromandibular dystonia, another form of dystonia

Manual of Botulinum Toxin Therapy, 2nd edition, ed. Daniel Truong, Mark Hallett, Christopher Zachary and Dirk Dressler. Published by Cambridge University Press. © Cambridge University Press 2013.

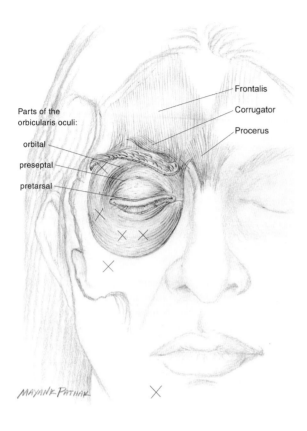

Parts of the orbicularis oculi:

Frontalis

Corrugator

Procerus

orbital

preseptal

pretarsal

MAYANK PATHAK

Fig. 13.1 Proposed sites for injection in treatment of hemifacial spams. The corrugator, orbital orbicularis oculi, frontalis and procerus are marked. Starting doses are from 2.5 to 3.75 U onabotulinumtoxinA depending upon the severity of facial twitching.

involving only the lower facial muscles, subsides during sleep, similar to other dystonias. Facial tics tend to be multifocal and not unilateral, have more complex movements and are usually associated with premonitory sensations and mild voluntary suppression. Hemimasticatory spasm affects jaw closure, with painful muscle contractions. Facial synkinesiae are caused by a misdirected axonal sprouting after facial nerve lesions. Periocular muscle activation would be associated with perioral movements and vice versa. They may be mistaken for HFS; orbicular synkinesis can be treated similar to HFS with BoNT injections (Roggenkamper et al., 1994). Finally, focal seizures, including epilepsia partialis continua, may be erroneously diagnosed as HFS (Wang and Jankovic, 1998).

Diagnostic tests for HFS include a brain MRI with attention to the cerebellopontine angle, with and without contrast, which will detect any space-occupying lesion requiring neurosurgical intervention. Magentic resonance angiography of the intracranial vessels may help to define the site of vascular compression. Electromyography can help with the differential diagnosis in difficult cases, and electroencephalography may be able to detect epileptiform discharges characteristic of a focal seizure.

Treatment

Treatment of HFS has included medications, microvascular decompression and BoNT injections. Medications such as baclofen, clonazepam, carbamazepine and phenytoin may provide mild improvement at the expense of side effects. Microvascular decompression (Janetta's operation) involves placing surgical gauze inbetween the facial nerve and the compressing blood vessel. Success rates from microvascular decompression vary from 88 to 97%, and a small percentage of patients may experience recurrence of HFS following surgery (Miller and Miller, 2012). Surgical complications include hearing loss and facial weakness, in addition to the accepted surgical risk of intracranial hemorrhage, stroke and even death.

Injections of BoNT are the preferred treatment of HFS. They are successful in over 90% of patients. Patients with HFS tend to require a lower dose, with a longer duration of effect compared with that in those with blepharospasm (Cannon et al., 2010). Injections of BoNT provide relief from symptoms for a period of approximately 12 weeks, and repeated injections have been found to be effective for many years. They can provide relief from symptoms without the adverse effects of neurosurgery. Serotype A BoNT, in the forms of onabotulinumtoxinA, abobotulinumtoxinA and incobotulinumtoxinA, and serotype B (rimabotulinumtoxinB) have all been used in the treatment of HFS. Use of EMG guidance during injection is not necessary.

Side effects of BoNT injections tend to be those associated with other facial injections: erythema and ecchymosis of the region injected, dry eyes, mouth droop, ptosis, lid edema and facial muscle weakness (Elston, 1986; Yoshimura et al., 1992; Park et al., 1993). Ptosis and facial muscle weakness are transient and will resolve within 1 to 4 weeks. Ptosis could be caused by local diffusion of the BoNT to affect the levator palpabrea (Brin et al., 1987).

The beneficial effect of BoNT injections occurs within 3 days to 2 weeks, with a peak effect at approximately 2–3 weeks. The effects are transient, with a mean duration of improvement of approximately 2.8 months (Yoshimura et al., 1992). There is a high

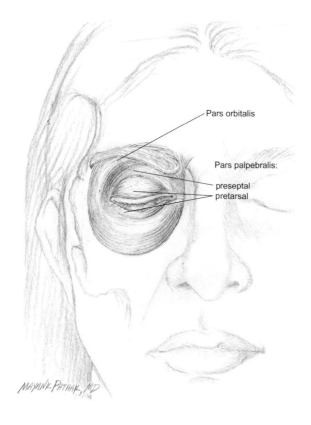

Pars orbitalis

Pars palpebralis:

preseptal
pretarsal

MAYANK PATHAK, MD

Fig 13.2 The orbicularis oculi and its parts..

variability of duration of the beneficial effect among patients.

The muscles injected to treat HFS may be the orbicularis oculi, corrugator, frontalis, risorius, buccinator and depressor anguli oris. The orbicularis oculi is composed of two parts: the pars palpebralis, which ordinarily closes the eyelid, and the pars orbitalis, which squeezes the eye shut with stronger contractions. The pars palpebralis also has two parts: a preseptal and a pretarsal region (Fig. 13.2).

The sites of injection should be decided with the patient's goals in mind. Occasionally, the preferred degree of control of the facial twitches occurs only at the expense of an ipsilateral upper lip droop of varying severity when the levator muscle is also affected (Boghen and Lesser, 2000). The BoNT is injected into four sites in the orbicularis oculi; typically in the lateral and medial part of the upper lid, as well as lateral and at the level of the pupil in the middle of the lower lid (Fig. 13.3). Injection into the brow area has an equally long duration

of effect as injection into the pretarsal region but results in fewer side effects (Price *et al.*, 1997). Lower frequencies of ptosis have been reported with injection either into the lateral (Jitpimolmard *et al.*, 1998) or the pretarsal region than into the preseptal region (Cakmur *et al.*, 2002) of the orbicularis oculi. The middle part of the upper lid is avoided in order to prevent ptosis. The orbicularis oris is avoided to prevent paralysis of the mouth. Injection into the lower facial muscles tends to be beneficial in those with more severe HFS (Colakoglu *et al.*, 2011). In rare cases, the platysma may need to be injected as well.

When injecting facial muscles, there needs to be some concern about cosmetic outcome. For example, weakening zygomaticus leads to a reduction in the elevation of the corner of mouth with smiling. On some occasions, consideration might be given to injections on the good side of the face in the interests of symmetry.

Total doses of BoNT used per hemifacial spasm treatment have been reported from 10 to 34 U onabotulinumtoxinA (Flanders *et al.*, 1993; Mezaki *et al.*, 1999). Total doses of abobotulinumtoxinA used per treatment range from 53 to 160 U (Elston, 1992; Yu *et al.*, 1992; Van den Bergh *et al.*, 1995; Jitpimolmard *et al.*, 1998) and for rimabotulinumtoxinB doses range from 1250 to 4000 U, with a mean effective dose of 2039 U (Tousi *et al.*, 2004). Table 13.1 lists the dosages of each BoNT and the muscles commonly injected (Frei *et al.*, 2006). In practice, the 100 U vial of onabotulinumtoxinA or incobotulinumtoxinA could be diluted with 4 or 5 ml of normal saline. This results in a dilution to 2.5 U/0.1 ml or 2.0 U/0.1 ml, respectively.

Dysport comes in 300 U and 500 U vials, which when diluted in 1.5 or 2.5 ml, respectively, give a dilution of 200 U/ml. For the injection, 0.5 ml of the solution is drawn and diluted inside the syringe with another 0.5 ml of normal saline. The final concentration then would be 10 U in 0.1 ml. This solution is then used for injection into different sites (Fig. 13.3).

To minimize side effects, initial injections usually involve a lower dose of BoNT beginning in the lateral orbital rim, just below the level of the eyebrow and facial muscles as appropriate. The patient should be re-evaluated approximately 1 month later to assess the effects of the initial injections. At that time further modification of the injections, either increasing dose or additional injection sites, can be determined for the next set of injections. Figure 13.3 shows one plan for initial injections.

Table 13.1 Dosages of neurotoxin and muscles commonly injected

Toxin	Dose (U)								
	Frontalis	Corrugator	Procerus	Orbicularis oculi	Zygomaticus minor	Buccinator	Depressor angularis oris	Depressor labii oris	Platysma
OnabotulinumtoxinA/ incobotulinumtoxinA	10	2.5–4	2–3	20	1–1.5	2	1–1.5	1–1.5	15
AbobotulinumtoxinA	30	7.5–10	5–7.5	60–120	2.5	5–7.5	2.5–5	2.5–5	50
RimabotulinumtoxinB	500	50–75	50–75	1000	50	100	50	50	500

Source: modified from Frei et al., 2006.

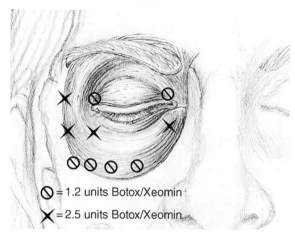

= 1.2 units Botox/Xeomin

= 2.5 units Botox/Xeomin

Fig. 13.3 Orbicularis oculi anatomy and botulinum neurotoxin injection sites used for treatment of hemifacial spasm.

Injection pain can be reduced either with skin cooling using ice or with EMLA cream (lidocaine 2.5% and prilocaine 2.5%) (Linder *et al.*, 2002; Soylev *et al.*, 2002). Treatment with BoNT appears to remain effective over long-term use, ranging from 4 to 20 years, and in most cases will not require dosage increase (Jitpimolmard *et al.*, 1998). If required, the dosage increase usually occurs within the first 2 years of treatment.

References

Banik R, Miller NR (2004). Chronic myokymia limited to the eyelid is a benign condition. *J Neuroophthalmol*, **24**, 290–2.

Boghen DR, Lesser RL (2000). Blepharospasm and hemifacial spasm. *Curr Treat Options Neurol* **2**, 393–400.

Brin MF, Fahn S, Moskowitz C *et al.* (1987). Localized injections of botulinum toxin for the treatment of focal dystonia and hemifacial spasm. *Mov Disord*, **2**, 237–54.

Cakmur R, Ozturk V, Uzunel F, Donmez B, Idiman F (2002). Comparison of preseptal and pretarsal injections of botulinum toxin in the treatment of blepharospasm and hemifacial spasm. *J Neurol*, **249**, 64–8.

Cannon PS, MacKenzie KR, Cook AE, Leatherbarrow B (2010). Difference in response to botulinum toxin type A treatment between patients with benign essential blepharospasm and hemifacial spasm. *Clin Exp Ophthalmol*, **38**, 688–91.

Colakoglu BD, Cakmur R, Uzunel F (2011). Is it always necessary to apply botulinum toxin into the lower facial muscles in hemifacial spasm?: a randomized, single - blind, crossover trial. *Eur Neurol*, **65**, 286–90.

Elston JS (1986). Botulinum toxin treatment of hemifacial spasm. *J Neurol Neurosurg Psychiatry*, **49**, 827–9.

Elston JS (1992). The management of blepharospasm and hemifacial spasm. *J Neurol*, **239**, 5–8.

Flanders M, Chin D, Bogden D (1993). Botulinum toxin: preferred treatment for hemifacial spasm. *Eur Neurol*, **33**, 316–19.

Frei KP, Truong DD (2008). Hemifacial spasm producing tremor-like movements of the head. *J Neurol Sci*, **273**, 133–4.

Frei K, Truong DD, Dressler D (2006). Botulinum toxin therapy of hemifacial spasm: comparing different therapeutic preparations. *Eur J Neurol*, **13**(Suppl 1), 30–5.

Jitpimolmard S, Tiamkao S, Laopaiboon M (1998). Long term results of botulinum toxin type A (Dysport) in the treatment of hemifacial spasm: a report of 175 cases. *J Neurol Neurosurg Psychiatry*, **64**, 751–7.

Lagalla G, Logullo F, DiBella P, Highishipour R, Provinciali L (2010). Familial hemifacial spasm and determinants of late onset. *Neurol Sci*, **31**, 17–22.

Linder JS, Edmonson BC, Laquis SJ, Drewry RD, Jr., Fleming JC (2002). Skin cooling before periocular botulinum toxin A injection. *Ophthal Plast Reconstr Surg*, **18**, 441–2.

Mezaki T, Kaji R, Kimura J, Ogawa N (1999). Treatment of hemifacial spasm with type A botulinum toxin (AGN 191622): a dose finding study and the evaluation of clinical effect with electromyography. *No To Shinkei*, **51**, 427–32.

Miller LE, Miller VM (2012). Safety and effectiveness of microvascular decompression for treatment of hemifacial spasm: a systematic review. *Br J Neurosurg*, **26**, 438–44.

Miwa H, Mizuno Y, Kondo T (2002). Familial hemifacial spasm: report of cases and review of the literature. *J Neurol Sci*, **193**, 97–102.

Oliveira LD, Cardoso F, Vargas AP (1999). Hemifacial spasm and arterial hypertension. *Mov Disord*, **14**, 832–5.

Park YC, Lim JK, Lee DK, Yi SD (1993). Botulinum a toxin treatment of hemifacial spasm and blepharospasm. *J Korean Med Sci*, **8**, 334–40.

Price J, Farish S, Taylor H, O'Day J (1997). Blepharospasm and hemifacial spasm. Randomized trial to determine the most appropriate location for botulinum toxin injections. *Ophthalmology*, **104**, 865–8.

Roggenkamper P, Laskawi R, Damens W, Schroeder M, Nuessgens Z (1994). Orbicular synkinesis after facial paralysis: treatment with botulinum toxin. *Doc Ophthalmol*, **86**, 395–402.

Rudzinska M, Wojcik M, Szczudilik A (2010). Hemifacial spasm non-motor and motor-related symptoms and their response to botulinum toxin therapy. *J Neural Transm*, **117**, 765–72.

Ryu H, Yamamoto S, Miyamoto T (1998). Atypical hemifacial spasm. *Acta Neurochir (Wien)*, **140**, 1173–6.

Soylev MF, Kocak N, Kuvaki B, Ozkan SB, Kir E (2002). Anesthesia with EMLA cream for botulinum A toxin injection into eyelids. *Ophthalmologica*, **216**, 355–8.

Tan EK, Chan LL, Koh KK (2004). Coexistent blepharospasm and hemifacial spasm: overlapping pathophysiologic mechanism? *J Neurol Neurosurg Psychiatry*, **75**, 494–6.

Tousi B, Perumal JS, Ahuja K, Ahmed A, Subramanian T (2004). Effects of botulinum toxin-B (BTX-B) injections for hemifacial spasm. *Parkinsonism Relat Disord*, **10**, 455–6.

Van den Bergh P, Francart J, Mourin S, Kollman P, Laterre EC (1995). Five-year experience in the treatment of focal movement disorders with low-dose Dysport botulinum toxin. *Muscle Nerve*, **18**, 720–9.

Wang A, Jankovic J (1998). Hemifacial spasm: clinical findings and treatment. *Muscle Nerve*, **21**, 1740–7.

Yoshimura DM, Aminoff MJ, Tami TA, Scott AB (1992). Treatment of hemifacial spasm with botulinum toxin. *Muscle Nerve*, **15**, 1045–9.

Yu YL, Fong KY, Chang CM (1992). Treatment of idiopathic hemifacial spasm with botulinum toxin. *Acta Neurol Scand*, **85**, 55–7.

Spasticity

Mayank S. Pathak and Allison Brashear

Introduction

Spasticity is part of the upper motor neuron syndrome produced by conditions such as stroke, multiple sclerosis, traumatic brain injury, spinal cord injury or cerebral palsy that affect upper motor neurons or their efferent pathways in the brain or spinal cord. It is characterized by increased muscle tone, exaggerated tendon reflexes, repetitive stretch reflex discharges (clonus) and released flexor reflexes (great toe extension; flexion at the ankle, knee and hip) (Lance, 1981). Late sequelae may include contracture, pain, fibrosis and muscle atrophy.

Chemodenervation by intramuscular injection of botulinum neurotoxin (BoNT) can reduce spastic muscle tone (usually measured by the Ashworth Scale or Modified Ashworth Scale), normalize limb posture, ameliorate pain, modestly improve motor function (measured by performance of standardized motor tasks or activities of daily living) and prevent contractures. Such efficacy is best documented for the upper limbs (Bhakta *et al.*, 2000; Sheean, 2001; Brashear *et al.*, 2002; Childers *et al.*, 2004; Suputtitada and Suwanwela, 2005; Bergfeldt *et al.*, 2006; Kaňovský *et al.*, 2009; Barnes *et al.*, 2010; Ryuji *et al.*, 2010a; Shaw *et al.*, 2011). In the lower limbs, efficacy is more limited, although rectification of plantar-flexed foot posture is documented (Baricich *et al.*, 2008), and there is a modicum of evidence for amelioration of gait (Bleyenheuft *et al.*, 2009; Ryuji *et al.*, 2010b). In 2008, a large evidence-based review concluded that BoNT should be offered for treatment of spasticity in adults, with level A evidence for improvement of muscle tone and level B for improvement of motor function (Simpson *et al.*, 2008; Elia *et al.*, 2009).

Preparation and dosing

Dilution

OnabotulinumtoxinA and incobotulinumtoxinA 1–4 ml of preservative-free normal saline per 100 U vial, and abobotulinumtoxinA with 2.5 ml per 500 U vial, while rimabotulinumtoxinB is pre-diluted. Higher and lower dilutions are used by practitioners. In general, higher volume dilutions are used for larger muscles or for muscles with diffuse and variable motor points (Wissel *et al.*, 2009). Since the various BoNT products are available in different doses per vial, the dilution ranges in Table 14.1 are expressed in terms of units per milliliter of solution.

Maximum doses

Although there are no absolutes, the usual dose maximums found in literature for a single injection session are also presented in Table 14.1. Higher doses in a single session may increase the risk of both local and diffuse side effects and adverse reactions (Francisco, 2004). However, studies in large series of patients receiving onabotulinumtoxinA and incobotulinumtoxinA did not reveal systemic adverse effects (Dressler and Adib Saberi, 2006). In patients treated with BoNT serotype B, systemic autonomic adverse effects may occur at intermediate doses (Dressler and Benecke, 2003).

Individual muscle doses

The dose of BoNT for individual muscles depends mainly on their size and the degree of spastic contraction. Consideration must also be given to the total number of muscles to be injected and the maximum recommended dose per injection session of the

---

Manual of Botulinum Toxin Therapy, 2nd edition, ed. Daniel Truong, Mark Hallett, Christopher Zachary and Dirk Dressler. Published by Cambridge University Press. © Cambridge University Press 2013.

Table 14.1 Dilutions and maximum dose/session of botulinum neurotoxins

Neurotoxin	Dilution (U/ml saline)	Maximum dose
OnabotulinumtoxinA	25–100	400 U/limb; 600 U/session
AbobotulinumtoxinA	200–500	1500 U/upper limb; 2000 U/lower limb; 2000 U/session
RimabotulinumtoxinB	Pre-diluted	10 000 U/upper limb; 17 500 U/session
IncobotulinumtoxinA[a]	25–100	400 U/limb; 495 U/session

[a] Published spasticity studies for incobotulinumtoxinA are limited, and so far address only the upper limb (Kaňovský *et al.*, 2009; Barnes *et al.*, 2010).
Sources: Hesse *et al.*, 1995; Hyman *et al.*, 2000; Brashear *et al.*, 2003, 2004; Francisco, 2004; Suputtitada and Suwanwela, 2005; WE MOVE Spasticity Study Group, 2005a,b; Wissel *et al.*, 2009; Kaňovský *et al.*, 2009; Barnes *et al.*, 2010.

particular BoNT preparation used. Based on these considerations, Table 14.2 gives the dose ranges usually employed for individual muscles in clinical practice. Spasticity trials using incobotulinumtoxinA have, to date, employed published dosing guidelines for the onabotulinumtoxinA preparation, and a 1:1 dosing ratio for these two preparations is used in general practice (Dressler *et al.*, 2012).

Guidance techniques

Palpation and anatomical landmarks may be used to place injections. However, the use of various guidance techniques increases precision and may improve safety, decrease side effects and possibly increase efficacy (O'Brien, 1997; Traba Lopez and Esteban, 2001; Childers, 2003; Monnier *et al.*, 2003). Guidance is recommended for injecting cervical muscles and deep pelvic or small limb muscles; it is optional for larger easily palpated muscles. The principal guidance techniques are electromyography (EMG), electrical stimulation, ultrasound and fluoroscopy.

In EMG guidance, injections are made through a cannulized, Teflon-coated monopolar hypodermic needle attached to an EMG machine. If able, the patient is asked to voluntarily contract the target muscle. When the bare needle tip is within the target muscle belly, the crisp staccato of motor units firing close to the tip should be heard, and sharp motor units with short rise times are seen on the video monitor. If the needle tip is outside the muscle or in a tendinous portion, only a distant rumbling will be heard, and dull indistinct motor units seen. Tapping the tendon or passively moving the joint may elicit motor units in paralyzed patients.

In patients who are either paralyzed or unable to follow commands, low-amperage electrical stimulation directly through the bare tip of the insulated hypodermic needle may be used to produce visible contraction in the target muscle (O'Brien, 1997; Childers, 2003; Chin *et al.*, 2005). The needle is repositioned until contractions may be reproduced by the lowest stimulation intensities.

Ultrasonography has been used to guide injections in the urinary system and salivary glands and is becoming more popular for skeletal muscles (Berweck *et al.*, 2002; Westhoff *et al.*, 2003). Fluoroscopy is utilized mainly for injection of deep pelvic girdle muscles in nerve entrapment and pain syndromes (Raj, 2004).

Injection placement

Smaller muscles generally require only one injection site anywhere within the muscle belly. Larger, longer or wider muscles are best injected at two to four sites. Although the BoNT works only at endplates, it is not necessary to identify the motor point or endplate region, since this region is generally broad and the BoNT diffuses. Identifying the motor point usually requires repeated repositioning of the needle under electrical stimulation or EMG guidance (Traba Lopez and Esteban, 2001), is painful and any advantage in efficacy appears minimal.

Spasticity patterns

The most common pattern of spasticity in the upper limb involves flexion of the fingers, wrist and elbow, adduction with internal rotation at the shoulder, and sometimes thumb curling across the palm or fist (Mayer *et al.*, 2002) (Fig. 14.1). Wrist or elbow extension is less common. There may sometimes be a combination of metacarpophalangeal flexion and proximal interphalangeal extension.

Table 14.2 Recommended botulinum neurotoxin doses for individual muscles and groups[a]

Muscle	OnabotulinumtoxinA/ incobotulinumtoxinA (U)	AbobotulinumtoxinA (U)	RimabotulinumtoxinB (U)	No. injection sites
Shoulder				
Pectoralis major and minor	50–150	150–300	2500–7500	2–4
Latissimus dorsi	50–150	150–300	2500–7500	2–4
Teres major	25–50	75–150	1500–2500	1–2
Upper limb flexors				
Biceps/brachialis	25–100	100–300	1500–5000	2–4
Brachioradialis	25–50	75–150	1000–2500	1
Flexor carpi radialis	25–50	75–150	1000–2500	1
Flexor carpi ulnaris	25–75	72–250	1500–5000	2–3
Flexor digitorum superficialis	25–50	75–200	1000–2500	2–4
Flexor digitorum profundus	20–50	75–150	750–2500	1–2
Flexor pollicis longus	10–20	30–60	500–1000	1
Thenar adductors and flexors of thumb	5–10	20–40	250–500	1
Upper limb extensors				
Triceps	50–100	100–250	250–750	2–3
Extensor carpi ulnaris	10–30	30–100	50–150	1–2
Extensor carp radialis	10–30	30–100	50–150	1–2
Extensor digitorum communis	10–20	30–60	50–100	1–2
Lower limb				
Iliopsoas	75–150	250–500	5000–7500	1–2
Adductor group: magnus, longus and brevis	100–300	500–1000	5000–7500	3–6
Quadriceps group: rectus femoris, vastus medialis, vastus lateralis, sartorius	100–300	500–1000	5000–7500	3–6
Hamstring group: biceps femoris long head and short head, semitendinosus, semimembranosus	100–300	500–1000	5000–7500	3–6
Triceps surae: medial and lateral gastrocnemius, soleus	100–200	250–1000	5000–7500	3–4
Tibialis posterior	50–100	150–250	2500–5000	1–2
Extensor hallucis longus	25–75	75–200	1000–2500	1
Tibialis anterior	25–75	75–200	1000–2500	1–2

[a] The majority of the dosing recommendations in this table were formed as a consensus among members of the WE MOVE Spasticity Study Group (2005a,b) and may be accessed online. These consensus recommendations have been supplemented with additional muscles and doses based on Pathak *et al.* (2006), Kaňovský *et al.* (2009) and Barnes *et al.* (2010).

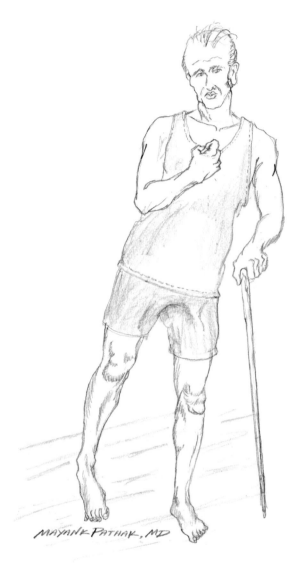

Fig. 14.1 Common pattern of spasticity in upper and lower limbs.

The most common pattern of spasticity in the lower limb involves extension at the knee, plantarflexion at the ankle and sometimes inversion of the foot (Mayer *et al.*, 2002) (Fig. 14.1). This pattern is seen unilaterally in stroke. It occurs bilaterally in cerebral palsy and some spinal cord lesions, producing a "toe-walking pattern." Other patterns of spasticity in the lower limbs include "scissoring" adduction at the hip joints, flexion or extension at the knees and spastic extension of the great toe (Mayer *et al.*, 2002).

It is important to distinguish plantarflexion posture caused by spastic contraction of the calf muscles from flaccid "drop foot" caused by paresis of the tibialis anterior and other dorsiflexor muscles. Drop foot

classically occurs with peroneal nerve palsy or lumbar radiculopathy and occasionally after stroke. Use of BoNT is not indicated in flaccid drop foot, and ankle–foot orthotic splints are usually sufficient to bring the foot and ankle to neutral position.

Extensor posturing at the knee also requires careful consideration before injection because quadriceps strength is important in maintaining weight-bearing stance during walking, and some degree of residual spasticity may be helpful. Additionally, the large powerful muscles of the proximal lower limb require high doses of BoNT approaching recommended maximums, and most patients will benefit more from the application of this dose elsewhere.

Treatment guide

Note that in Figs. 14.2 to 14.16 (below) target muscles are printed in bold and lines with arrowheads represent approximate injection vectors.

The upper limb

Flexion at the proximal interphalangeal joints

Inject flexor digitorum superficialis (Fig. 14.2).

The flexor digitorum superficialis muscle is involved in the clenched hand posture. The muscle is often treated in conjuction with the flexor digitorum profundus. The needle is inserted obliquely approximately one-third of the distance from the antecubital crease to the distal wrist crease. It is advanced toward the radius, passing through fasicles for each of the fingers as the bolus is injected. The muscle is activated by the patient flexing the fingers. Confirmation of needle placement can be performed using EMG or electrical stimulation.

Flexion at distal interphalangeal joints

Inject flexor digitorum profundus (Fig. 14.3).

The flexor digitorum profundus muscle is involved in the clenched hand. This muscle is often treated in conjunction with the flexor digitorum superficialis. Flexor digitorum profundus lies against the ventral surface of the ulna. The needle is inserted along the ulnar edge of the forearm one-third of the distance from the antecubital crease to the distal wrist crease and directed across the ventral surface of the ulnar shaft. After advancing through a thin section of the flexor carpi ulnaris, the first fibers of the flexor digitorum profundus entered will be those for the fifth and

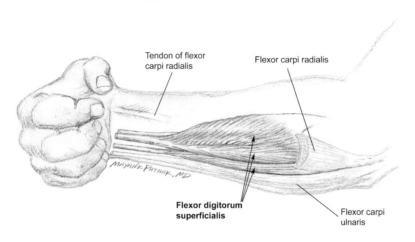

Fig. 14.2 Injection of flexor digitorum superficialis.

Tendon of flexor carpi radialis

Flexor carpi radialis

Flexor digitorum superficialis

Flexor carpi ulnaris

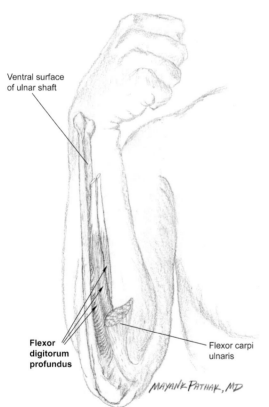
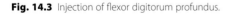

Ventral surface of ulnar shaft

Flexor digitorum profundus

Flexor carpi ulnaris

Fig. 14.3 Injection of flexor digitorum profundus.

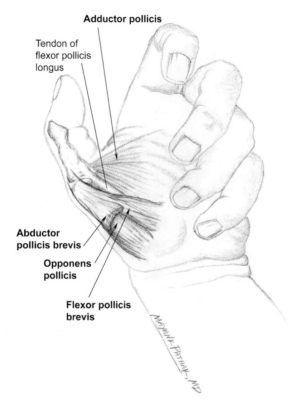

Adductor pollicis

Tendon of flexor pollicis longus

Abductor pollicis brevis

Opponens pollicis

Flexor pollicis brevis

Fig. 14.4 Injection of adductor pollicis and other thenar muscles.

fourth digits. The muscle fibers are activated by the patient flexing the distal phalanges of these fingers. Deeper fibers flex the distal phalanges of the third and second digits.

Thumb curling

Inject adductor pollicis and other thenar muscles (Fig. 14.4); *inject flexor pollicis longus* (Fig. 14.5).

Thumb curling may present with the clenched hand or alone. A curled thumb can prevent a patient from having an effective grasp and may also get caught during activities of daily living such as dressing.

Adductor pollicis spans the web between the first two metacarpals. It may be approached from the dorsal surface by going through the overlying first dorsal interosseus muscle or, more commonly, approached from the

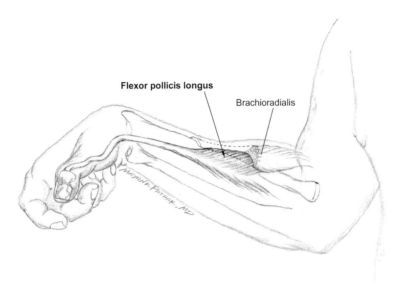

Fig. 14.5 Injection of flexor pollicis longus.

Flexor pollicis longus

Brachioradialis

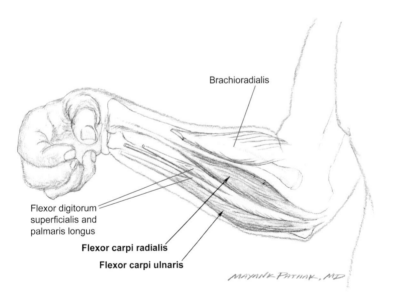

Fig. 14.6 Injection of wrist flexors.

Brachioradialis

Flexor digitorum superficialis and palmaris longus

Flexor carpi radialis

Flexor carpi ulnaris

palmar side. Three other thenar muscles can be injected with insertion in the palmar surface over the proximal half of the first metacarpal. The needle will first encounter abductor pollicis brevis, which may be injected if required, followed by the deeper opponens pollicis, activated by flexion of the first metacarpal in opposing the thumb against the fifth digit. Flexor pollicis brevis lies medial and adjacent to abductor pollicis brevis and may be reached by partially withdrawing the needle and directing it toward the base of the second digit; it is activated by flexion of the metacarpophalangeal joint.

Flexor pollicis longus is approached by inserting the needle in the middle third of the ventral forearm, adjacent to the medial border of the brachioradialis, and directing it toward the ventral surface of the radius. The radial pulse may be palpated and avoided. Once contact with bone is made, withdrawing the tip a few millimeters will place it in the muscle belly, which is activated by flexion of the interphalangeal joint.

Wrist flexion

Inject flexor carpi ulnaris and flexor carpi radialis (Fig. 14.6).

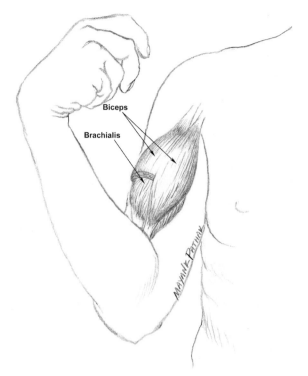

Fig. 14.7 Injection of biceps and brachialis muscles.

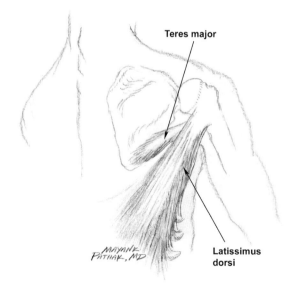

Fig. 14.9 Injection of latissimus dorsi and teres major.

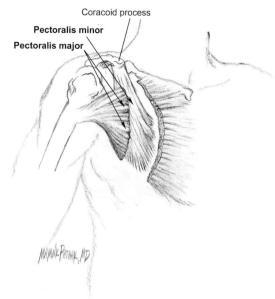

Fig. 14.8 Injection of pectoralis major and minor.

The flexed wrist may present with the flexed elbow and/or flexed hand, or alone. Persistent flexion of the wrist may cause pain and often interferes with a useful grasp regardless of involvement of the finger flexors.

Flexor carpi ulnaris is approached directly at the medial border of the forearm midway between the antecubital and distal wrist creases. This superficial muscle is activated by the patient flexing the wrist with slight ulnar deviation.

Flexor carpi radialis lies along the ventral surface of the forearm just medial to the midline. It is located by having the patient flex the wrist and then the line of the tendon can be followed from its insertion at the wrist toward the lateral edge of the biceps aponeurosis, where its fibers of origin may be palpable. The muscle is superficial, and injection is made four to five finger-breadths distal to the antecubital crease.

Elbow flexion

Inject biceps and brachialis muscles (Fig. 14.7).

The elbow may be flexed alone or in combination with the flexed hand and/or wrist. The flexed elbow may be exacerbated by walking and contribute to gait abnormalities, interfere with functional activities such as reaching and lifting and impair activities of daily living such as dressing and eating.

The biceps is approached from the ventral arm surface. The BoNT dose is divided between the short (medial) and long (lateral) heads. The brachialis lies lateral and deep to both heads of the biceps. It is injected by advancing the needle further toward the ventral

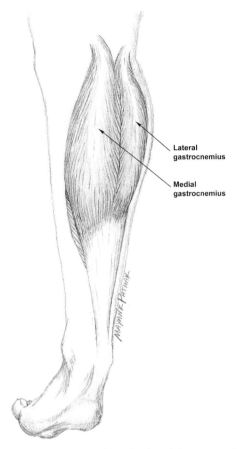

Fig. 14.10 Injection of lateral and medial gastrocnemii.

surface of the humerus. These muscles are activated by the patient flexing the elbow against resistance.

Adduction and internal rotation at the shoulder

Inject pectoralis major and minor (Fig. 14.8); *optional injection of latissimus dorsi and teres major* (Fig. 14.9).

Overactivity of the shoulder muscles may limit movements used in such routine activities as reaching, dressing and eating.

The pectoralis insertion fibers are palpated at the anterior axillary fold and the needle is inserted parallel to the chest wall to minimize the risk of pneumothorax. The muscles are activated by the patient pressing his or her palms together. Pectoralis major is superficial and the needle should advance through it to reach pectoralis minor. The dose is distributed among several sites. Latissimus dorsi and teres major may both also cause shoulder adduction. They are accessible below the posterior axillary fold.

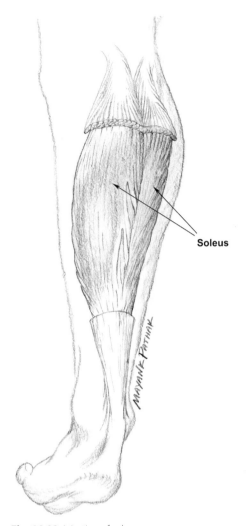

Fig. 14.11 Injection of soleus.

The lower limb

Plantarflexion spasm

Inject lateral gastrocnemius and medial gastrocnemius, plus soleus (Figs. 14.10 and 14.11, respectively); *optional injection of the tibialis posterior* (Fig. 14.12).

Plantarflexion is a typical posture of the spastic limb and interferes with fitting of splints and placement of the foot flat in activities such as walking and transfers. Care must be taken to distinguish this spastic posture from flaccid "drop foot," as discussed above.

The lateral and medial heads of the gastrocnemius lie superficially in the calf and should be injected separately. When the tip is inside the muscle belly,

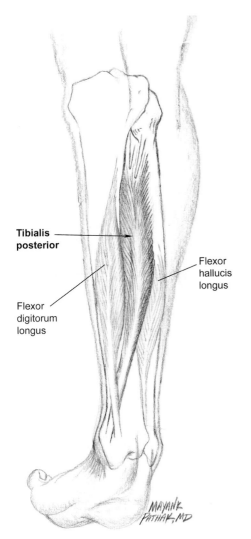

Fig. 14.12 Injection of tibialis posterior.

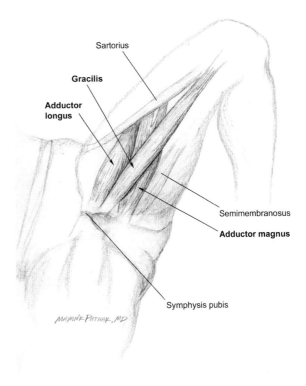

Fig. 14.13 Injection of the adductor group.

the syringe will wiggle back and forth as the muscle is stretched and relaxed by passively rocking the foot at the ankle with the knee extended. The soleus is best reached by advancing the needle through the medial gastrocnemius. The position of the needle tip is checked by the patient first flexing the knee to minimize movement of the gastrocnemii and then passively rocking the foot at the ankle until movement of the syringe is seen. All of these muscles are activated by the patient plantarflexing.

The tibialis posterior is an often overlooked contributor to foot plantarflexion and inversion, a posture noted in the spastic and dystonic foot. Those patients with the tibialis posterior involved may walk on the side of the foot or be unable to wear

shoes or orthotics. Because tibialis posterior lies deep and is difficult to localize, we recommend guidance by electrical stimulation or EMG and the use of a 50 mm injection needle. Approaching through the tibialis anterior can be painful for patients whose muscles are in involuntary spasm, and inadvertent injection into the tibialis anterior may cause foot drop, exacerbating the plantarflexion. We prefer a medial approach, slipping the needle behind the medial border of the tibia, advancing along its posterior surface through the smaller flexor digitorum longus and into the tibialis posterior. Injection into either of the two adjacent muscles, the flexor digitorum longus or flexor hallucis longus, will not be problematic and may also ameliorate plantarflexion posturing.

Adductor spasm

Inject the adductor group (Fig. 14.13).

Patients with overactive adductor muscles will present with difficulty with personal hygiene and dressing.

The adductor muscles are approached with the patient supine, thighs flexed and abducted at the hips,

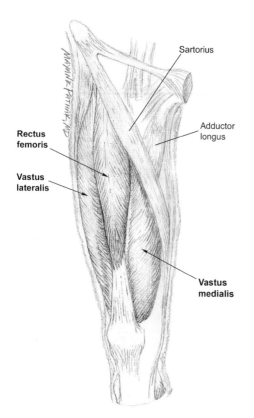

Fig. 14.14 Injection of the quadriceps group.

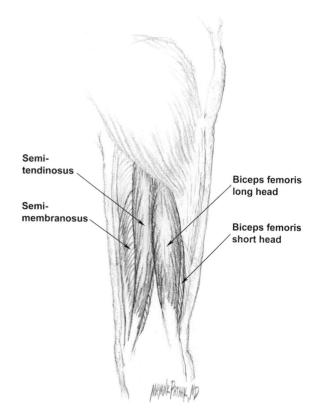

Fig. 14.15 Injection of hamstring muscles.

and knees flexed. The muscles are best found proximally in the anteromedial thigh approximately a handbreadth distal to the groin fold, where they are superficial and the separation (in anterior to medial progression) of the adductor longus and gracilis is palpable. The adductor brevis lies deep to adductor longus. Adductor magnus may be injected by advancing deep through the gracilis, or entered directly just posterior to the posterior edge of gracilis.

Extensor posturing at the knee

Inject the quadriceps group (Fig. 14.14).

Patients with involvement of the quadriceps group may have difficulty with relaxing the thigh, making it difficult to balance, walk or fit in a wheelchair. For patients in which a quadriceps injection is warranted, the rectus femoris, vastus lateralis and vastus medialis are readily approached in the anterior thigh. The rectus femoris and vastus lateralis are injected halfway between the patella and the groin fold. The vastus medialis is best found more distally.

Knee flexion spasm

Inject hamstring muscles (Fig. 14.15).

Patients with overactive hamstrings may present with pain. Spasticity in these muscles will make bending the knee difficult and may result in difficulty with sitting or walking. These large muscles are palpable in the posterior thigh of most patients and approaches are straightforward. The semitendinosus and semimembranosus muscles are medial in the posterior thigh, while the long and short heads of the biceps femoris are lateral.

Toe extension

Inject extensor hallucis longus (Fig. 14.16).

Patients with involvement of the great toe extensor may present with excessive wear to the top of the shoe or abrasions to the great toe. Patients or caregivers may have difficulty applying footwear or splints. This muscle is located by palpating its tendon just lateral to the tendon of the tibialis anterior and following it proximally about one-third of the way up the tibia.

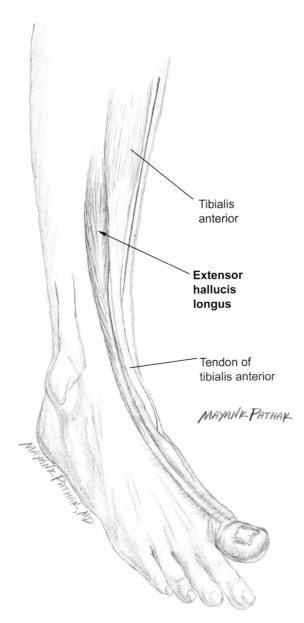

Tibialis anterior

Extensor hallucis longus

Tendon of tibialis anterior

MAYANK PATHAK

MAYANK PATHAK, MD

Fig. 14.16 Injection of extensor hallucis longus.

At this level, its muscular belly lies one fingerbreadth lateral to the tibia. It is activated by the patient extending the toe. Injection into the belly of the tibialis anterior should be avoided as this can result in foot drop.

References

Baricich A, Carda S, Bertoni M *et al.* (2008). A single-blinded, randomized pilot study of botulinum toxin type A combined with non-pharmacologica l treatment for spastic foot. *J Rehabil Med*, **40**, 870–2.

Barnes M, Schnitzler A, Medeiros L *et al.* (2010). Efficacy and safety of NT 201 for upper limb spasticity of various etiologies – a randomized parallel-group study. *Acta Neurol Scand*, **122**, 295–302.

Bergfeldt U, Borg K, Kullander K *et al.* (2006). Focal spasticity therapy with botulinum toxin: effects on function, activities of daily living, and pain in 100 adult patients. *J Rehabil Med*, **38**, 166–71.

Berweck S, Feldkamp A, Francke A *et al.* (2002). Sonography-guided injection of botulinum toxin A in children with cerebral palsy. *Neuropediatrics*, **33**, 221–3.

Bhakta BB, Cozens JA, Chamberlain M *et al.* (2000). Impact of botulinum toxin type A on disability and carer burden due to arm spasticity after stroke: a randomised double blind placebo controlled trial. *J Neurol Neurosurg Psychiatry*, **69**, 217–21.

Bleyenheuft C, Cockx S, Gilles C *et al.* (2009). The effect of botulinum toxin injections on gait control in spastic stroke patients presenting with a stiff-knee gait. *Gait Posture*, **30**, 168–72.

Brashear A, Gordon MF, Elovic E *et al.* (2002). Intramuscular injection of botulinum toxin for the treatment of wrist and finger spasticity after a stroke. *N Engl J Med*, **347**, 395–400.

Brashear A, Mcafee AL, Kuhn E *et al.* (2003). Treatment with botulinum toxin type B for upper-limb spasticity. *Arch Phys Med Rehabil*, **84**, 103–7.

Brashear A, Mcafee AL, Kuhn ER *et al.* (2004). Botulinum toxin type B in upper-limb poststroke spasticity: a double-blind, placebo-controlled trial. *Arch Phys Med Rehabil*, **85**, 705–9.

Childers MK (2003). The importance of electromyographic guidance and electrical stimulation for injection of botulinum toxin. *Phys Med Rehabil Clin N Am*, **14**, 781–92.

Childers MK, Brashear A, Jozefczyk P *et al.* (2004). Dose-dependent response to intramuscular botulinum toxin type A for upper-limb spasticity in patients after a stroke. *Arch Phys Med Rehabil*, **85**, 1063–9.

Chin T, Nattrass G, Selber P *et al.* (2005). Accuracy of intramuscular injection of botulinum toxin A in juvenile cerebral palsy: a comparison between manual needle placement and placement guided by electrical stimulation. *J Pediatr Orthop*, **25**, 286–91.

Dressler D, Benecke R (2003). Autonomic side effects of botulinum toxin type B treatment of cervical dystonia and hyperhidrosis. *Eur Neurol*, **49**, 34–8.

Dressler D, Adib Saberi F (2006). Safety aspects of high dose Xeomin therapy. *J Neurol*, **253**(Suppl 2), 141–2.

Dressler D, Mander G, Fink K (2012). Measuring the potency labelling of onabotulinumtoxinA (Botox®) and incobotulinumtoxinA (Xeomin®) in an LD50 assay. *J Neurol Transm*, **119**, 13–15.

Elia AE, Filippini G, Calandrella D et al. (2009), Botulinum neurotoxins for post-stroke spasticity in adults: a systematic review. *Mov Disord*, **24**, 801–12.

Francisco GE (2004). Botulinum toxin: dosing and dilution. *Am J Phys Med Rehabil*, **83**, S30–7.

Hesse S, Jahnke MT, Luecke D et al. (1995). Short-term electrical stimulation enhances the effectiveness of botulinum toxin in the treatment of lower limb spasticity in hemiparetic patients. *Neurosci Lett*, **201**, 37–40.

Hyman N, Barnes M, Bhakta B et al. (2000). Botulinum toxin (Dysport) treatment of hip adductor spasticity in multiple sclerosis: a prospective, randomised, double blind, placebo controlled, dose ranging study. *J Neurol Neurosurg Psychiatry*, **68**, 707–12.

Kaňovský P, Slawek J, Denes Z et al. (2009). Efficacy and safety of botulinum neurotoxin NT201 in poststroke upper limb spasticity. *Clin Neuropharm*, **32**, 259–65.

Lance JW (1981). Disordered muscle tone and movement. *Clin Exp Neurol*, **18**, 27–35.

Mayer NH, Esquenazie A, Childers MK (2002). Common patterns of clinical motor dysfunction. In Mayer NH, Simpson DM (eds.) *Spasticity: Etiology, Evaluation, Management and the Role of Botulinum Toxin*. New York, WE MOVE, pp. 1–11.

Monnier G, Parratte B, Tatu L et al. (2003) [EMG support in botulinum toxin treatment.] *Ann Readapt Med Phys*, **46**, 380–5.

O'Brien CF (1997). Injection techniques for botulinum toxin using electromyography and electrical stimulation. *Muscle Nerve*, **6**(Suppl), S176–80.

Pathak MS, Nguyen HT, Graham HK et al. (2006). Management of spasticity in adults: practical application of botulinum toxin. *Eur J Neurol*, **13**(Suppl 1), 42–50.

Raj PPE (2004). Treatment algorithm overview: BoNT therapy for pain, Appendix A. *Pain Pract*, **4**, S60–4.

Ryuji K, Osako Y, Suyama K et al. (2010a). Botulinum toxin type A in post-stroke upper limb spasticity. *Curr Med Res Opin*, **26**, 1983–92.

Ryuji K, Osako Y, Suyama K et al. (2010b). Botulinum toxin type A in post-stroke lower limb spasticity: a multicenter, double-blind, placebo-controlled trial. *J Neurol*, **257**, 1330–7.

Shaw L, Price CIM, VanWijk FMJ et al. on behalf of the BoTULS Investigators (2011). Botulinum toxin for the upper limb after stroke (BoTULS) Trial: effect on impairment, activity limitation, and pain. *Stroke* **42**, 1371–9.

Sheean GL (2001). Botulinum treatment of spasticity: why is it so difficult to show a functional benefit? *Curr Opin Neurol*, **14**, 771–6.

Simpson DM, Gracies JM, Graham HK et al. (2008). Assessment: botulinum neurotoxin for the treatment of spasticity (an evidence-based review): report of the Therapeutics and Technology Assessment Subcommittee of the American Academy of Neurology. *Neurology*, **70**, 1691–8.

Suputtitada A, Suwanwela NC (2005). The lowest effective dose of botulinum A toxin in adult patients with upper limb spasticity. *Disabil Rehabil*, **27**, 176–84.

Traba Lopez A, Esteban A (2001). Botulinum toxin in motor disorders: practical considerations with emphasis on interventional neurophysiology. *Neurophysiol Clin*, **31**, 220–9.

WE MOVE Spasticity Study Group (2005a). *BTX-A Adult Dosing Guidelines*. New York: WE MOVE (http://www.mdvu.org/classrooms/cme/CHEMD3/AdultSpastDosing.pdf, accessed 21 May 2013).

WE MOVE Spasticity Study Group (2005b). *BTX-B Adult Dosing Guidelines*. New York: WE MOVE (http://www.mdvu.org/classrooms/cme/CHEMD3/AdultSpastDosing.pdf, accessed 21 May 2013).

Westhoff B, Seller K, Wild et al. (2003). Ultrasound-guided botulinum toxin injection technique for the iliopsoas muscle. *Dev Med Child Neurol*, **45**, 829–32.

Wissel J, Ward A, Erztgaard P et al. (2009). European consensus table on the use of botulinum toxin type A in adult spasticity. *J Rehabil Med*, **41**, 13–25.

The use of botulinum neurotoxin in spastic infantile cerebral palsy

Ann Tilton and H. Kerr Graham

Introduction

Cerebral palsy is not a specific disease but a clinical syndrome caused by a non-progressive injury to the developing brain that results in a disorder of movement and posture that is permanent but not unchanging. It is the most common cause of physical disability affecting children in developed countries. The incidence is steady in most countries at approximately 2 per 1000 live births. The prevalence of cerebral palsy is much higher in children with birth weight under 1500 g and in those born earlier than 28 weeks of gestation. The location, timing and severity of the brain lesion are extremely variable, which results in many different clinical presentations. Despite the static nature of the brain injury, the majority of children with cerebral palsy develop progressive musculoskeletal problems such as posturing and muscle contractures (Koman *et al.*, 2004). Additionally, as pointed out in an expert consensus on cerebral palsy, it is important to recognize that there are also frequent yet inconsistent disturbances of sensation, cognition, communication and perception; abnormalities of behavior; and seizures (Bax *et al.*, 2005).

Classification

Cerebral palsy may be classified according to the cause of the brain lesion (when this is known), and the location of the brain lesion as noted on imaging such as MRI or CT. Clinically more useful classification schemes are based on the type of movement disorder, the distribution of the movement disorder (Box 15.1) and the gross motor function of the child.

It is important to correctly characterize the movement disorder because different movement disorders can be managed by different interventions.

Spasticity

Spasticity is the most common movement disorder, affecting between 60% and 80% of children with cerebral palsy (Fig. 15.1). Spasticity is defined as hypertonia in which one or both of the following signs are present:

- resistance to externally imposed movement increases with increasing speed of stretch and varies with the direction of joint movement
- resistance to externally imposed movement rises rapidly above a threshold speed or joint angle.

When focal, spasticity is often managed by injections of botulinum neurotoxin (BoNT). When severe or generalized, spasticity may be managed by selective dorsal rhizotomy or intrathecal baclofen.

Dystonia

Dystonia is characterized by involuntary sustained or intermittent muscle contractions that cause twisting and repetitive movements, abnormal postures, or both. Focal dystonia may also be treated with BoNT. In generalized dystonia, intrathecal baclofen may have a role. However, selective dorsal rhizotomy does not appear to offer improvement.

Athetosis

Athetosis, or intermittent writhing movement, is also very common. It is sometimes managed by oral medications and when severe by intrathecal baclofen pump, but never by selective dorsal rhizotomy.

Ataxia

Ataxia is less common in cerebral palsy and is difficult to treat successfully. In addition to the overactivity

Manual of Botulinum Toxin Therapy, 2nd edition, ed. Daniel Truong, Mark Hallett, Christopher Zachary and Dirk Dressler.
Published by Cambridge University Press. © Cambridge University Press 2013.

Box 15.1 Clinically based classification systems of cerebral palsy

Movement disorder
Spastic
Dystonic
Mixed
Athetoid
Ataxic

Topographical distribution
Unilateral: monoplegia, hemiplegia
Bilateral: diplegia, triplegia, quadriplegia

Gross Motor Function Classification System (GMFCS)
Level I: walk and run independently
Level II: walk independently
Level III: walk with assistance
Level IV: stand for transfers
Level V: absent head control and sitting balance

Source: classification system from Palisano *et al.* (1997).

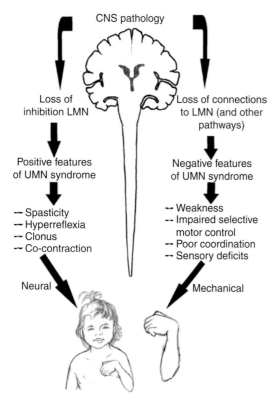

Fig. 15.1 Scheme of spasticity. LMN, lower motor neuron; UMN, upper motor neuron.

(positive) features of cerebral palsy such as spasticity and dystonia, there are also negative features – principally weakness and loss of selective motor control. In the long term, weakness and difficulty in controlling muscles have a much greater impact on gross motor function than the various forms of muscle overactivity. Nevertheless, spasticity has been implicated in the development of fixed deformities, which can further impair function and quality of life in the child or adolescent affected by cerebral palsy.

Topographical symptom distribution and anatomical approach to management

Understanding the topographical distribution of symptoms and recognizing the common clinical patterns of muscle overactivity form the basis for development of management strategies. These patterns are reviewed as the basis for intervention with BoNT and other therapies before turning to injection techniques.

As indicated in Box 15.1, involvement may be unilateral (monoplegic or hemiplegic) or bilateral (diplegic, paraplegic or quadriplegic). Spastic diplegia usually refers to individuals with minimal involvement of the upper limbs but bilateral lower limb involvement. Spastic quadriplegia refers to individuals with involvement of all four limbs, with the upper limbs sometimes more affected than the lower limbs. However, the differentiation between spastic diplegia and spastic quadriplegia is not clear cut and it is more clinically useful to classify bilateral cerebral palsy according to gross motor function, as noted above.

Unilateral cerebral palsy: spastic hemiplegia

In hemiplegia, motor pathway involvement on one side of the brain leads to contralateral motor symptoms (Fig. 15.2). The most common movement disorder is spastic but mixed spastic and dystonic types are also very common. Sometimes the upper limb has mainly a dystonic movement disorder and the lower limb a mainly spastic movement disorder.

Upper limb

Typical upper limb posturing includes adduction and internal rotation at the shoulder, pronation and flexion at the elbow/forearm, and flexion and ulnar

(a)   (b)

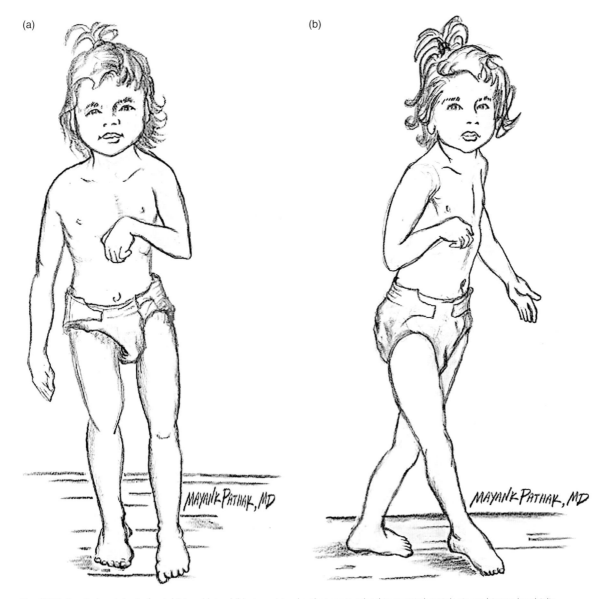

Fig. 15.2 Spastic hemiplegia, frontal (a) and lateral (b) views. Muscles that are involved in spastic hemiplegia are biceps, brachialis, adductor pollicis, flexor carpi ulnaris, flexor carpi radialis, pronator teres, gastrocnemius, soleus, tibialis posterior.

deviation at the wrist with flexed digits and "thumb in palm." The muscles typically involved in each pattern are indicated in Table 15.1, along with guidelines for injection of BoNT-A as onabotulinumtoxinA (Botox, Allergan, Irvine, CA, USA).

Without intervention, spastic posturing in the hemiplegic upper limb can progress to painful fixed contracture and deformities, which further impair function, and cosmesis. It is tempting to think that the spasticity or dystonia is the main functional limitation in the hemiplegic upper limb, and that relaxing the overactive muscles will necessarily restore function. On the contrary, the main barriers to function are impaired selective motor control and sensation. Muscle relaxation may set the stage for functional gains but may not be adequate by itself. Therefore, focal treatment with BoNT alone is rarely indicated and it should usually be combined with a program of splinting and occupational therapy or upper limb training.

Table 15.1 Muscle involvement and dosing guidelines

Clinical pattern	Potential muscles[a]	OnabotulinumtoxinA		AbobotulinumtoxinA	
		Dosing (U/kg)	No. injection sites	Dosing (U/kg)	No. injection sites
Upper extremity					
Internally rotated shoulder	Pectoralis complex	2	2–3	5–10	2–3
	Latissimus dorsi	2	2	5–10	2
	Teres major	2	1–2	5–10	1–2
	Subscapularis	1–2	1–2	5	1–2
Flexed elbow	Brachioradialis	1	1	5–10	1
	Biceps	2	2	5–10	2
	Brachialis	2	1–2	5–10	1–2
Pronation	Pronator quadrates	0.5–1	1	5	1
	Pronator teres	1	1	5–10	1
Wrist flexion	Flexor carpi ulnaris	1–2	1	5–10	1
	Flexor carpi radialis	1–2	1	5–10	1
Thumb in palm	Flexor pollicis longus	0.5–1	1	5	1
	Flexor pollicis brevis	0.5–1	1	5	1
	Adductor pollicis	0.5–1	1	5	1
Clenched fist	Flexor digitorum superficialis	1–2	1–2	5–10	1–2
	Flexor digitorum profundus	1–2	1–2	5–10	1–2
Intrinsic hand muscles	Lumbricals/interossei	0.5–1	1	5	1
Lower extremity					
Hip flexion	Iliacus	1–2	1	3–15/muscle group	1
	Rectus femoris	1–2	2	3–15/muscle group	1
	Psoas (with guidance)	2–3	2	3–15/muscle group	2
				3–15/muscle group	
Knee flexion	Medial hamstrings	3–6	3–4	3–15/muscle group	3–4
	Lateral hamstrings	2–3	2–3	3–15/muscle group	2–3
	Gastrocnemius	3–6	3–6	3–15/muscle group	3–6
				3–15/muscle group	
Scissoring adduction	Adductor group	3–6	1–2	3–15/muscle group	1–2
Extended knee	Quadriceps	3–6	3–4	3–15/muscle group	3–4
Equinovarus foot	Gastrocnemius medial/lateral	3–6	2–4	3–15/muscle group	2–4
		2–3	1–2	3–15/muscle group	1–2
	Soleus	1–2	1	3–15/muscle group	1
	Tibialis posterior	1–2	1	3–15/muscle group	1
	Flexor digitorum longus/brevis	1–2	1	3–15/muscle group	
	Flexor hallucis longus			3/muscle group	
				3/muscle group	
Striatal toe	Extensor hallucis longus	1–2	1	1–3	1

[a] See Chapters 10 and 14 for illustrations of the position of the muscles described in the table.

Sources: adapted from Russman *et al.* (2002) based on information in French Summary of Product Characteristics information; Fehlings *et al.*, 2010; Heinen *et al.*, 2010.

> **Box 15.2** Grading of lower limb involvement in spastic hemiplegia
>
> Type I: a drop foot in the swing phase of gait but no calf contracture
> Type II: spastic or contracted gastrocsoleus complex (gastrocnemius and soleus) resulting in equinus gait
> Type III: involvement extends to the knee with spasticity and co-contraction of the hamstrings and rectus femoris
> Type IV: involvement extends to the hip, which is typically flexed, adducted and internally rotated
>
> *Source*: Winters *et al.* (1987).

Lower limb

The involved lower limb is usually slightly shorter than that on the uninvolved side, with muscle atrophy particularly affecting the calf muscle. Typically, involvement is more pronounced distally than proximally (Box 15.2).

In younger children, the hemiplegic lower limb can be managed quite effectively using a combination of focal injections of BoNT, an ankle–foot orthosis and a physical therapy program. An ankle–foot orthosis is useful in all four grades of spasticity because it controls drop foot in swing. In type II, injection of BoNT once calf spasticity is noted can be very effective in improving gait and function. We usually start injection of the gastrocsoleus complex (gastrocnemius plus soleus) from the age of 18 months to 2 years and continue until age 6 years. By this time, either the spasticity is well controlled or a contracture has developed, which is more effectively treated by casting or an orthopedic muscle tendon-lengthening procedure. Types III and IV hemiplegia may be treated with multilevel injections of BoNT in the younger child and multilevel surgery in the older child. Multilevel injections typically are directed to the spastic gastrocsoleus; sometimes the tibialis posterior if the posturing is equinovarus; the hamstrings; the hip adductors and hip flexors; and occasionally the rectus femoris when there is a stiff knee gait.

Bilateral cerebral palsy: spastic diplegia

Children with spastic diplegia have usually been born prematurely and have generalized lower limb spasticity but often normal cognition and few medical comorbidities. Walking is typically delayed until age 2 to 5 years in children with spastic diplegia, and when they first walk, it is typically with a "tip toe" gait pattern. Spastic equinus is very common and may impair stability in stance and the ability to progress in standing and walking (Fig. 15.3). In the younger child, spastic equinus is safely and effectively managed by injection of BoNT into the gastrocsoleus muscle complex in the distribution shown and the provision of ankle–foot orthoses in the context of a physical therapy program. This allows many children to achieve flat foot and to progress in standing and walking at a faster rate than would be otherwise the case.

Older children with spastic diplegia frequently develop fixed contractures of the flexor muscles, including the iliopsoas at the hip, the hamstrings at the knee and the plantarflexors of the ankle. There are also frequently torsional abnormalities of the long bones, including medial femoral torsion and lateral tibial torsion. There may be instability of the hip joint and breakdown of the mid-foot. These more advanced musculoskeletal problems are best dealt with by multilevel orthopedic surgery, typically between the ages of 6 and 10 years. However, the use of spasticity management in the younger child is still an excellent option for these children. It avoids the need for early surgery, eliminates the need for repeated surgery and allows the orthopedic procedures to be performed at an age when an outcome is much more predictable. The sequence of early management by focal injections of BoNT followed by multilevel orthopedic surgery yields superior functional outcomes than have been achieved in the past by serial orthopedic procedures. A small number of children with spastic diplegia have such severe lower limb spasticity that it is not amenable to multilevel injections of BoNT. Such children are more effectively managed by intrathecal baclofen or in some cases by selective dorsal rhizotomy.

Bilateral cerebral palsy: spastic quadriplegia

Children with spastic quadriplegia have spasticity and/or dystonia in all four limbs and have much greater functional impairment than children with spastic diplegia. Some children can stand for transfers and walk short distances (GMFCS level IV). However some children lack head control and sitting balance and are unable to stand or transfer. These children are

(a)

(b)

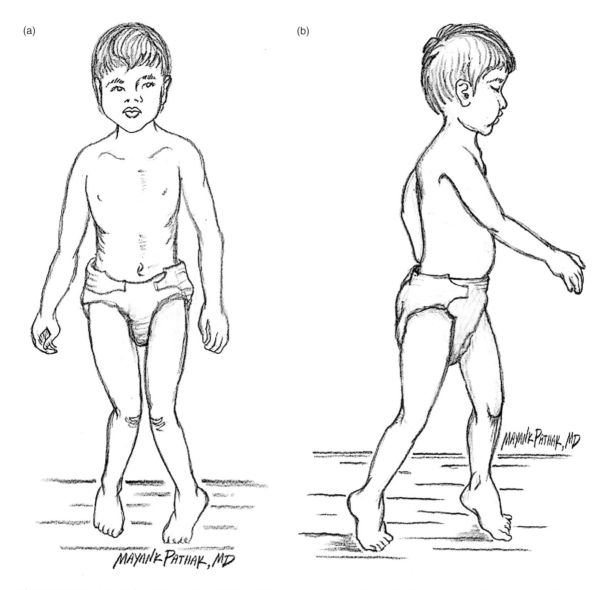

Fig. 15.3 Spastic diplegia, frontal (a) and lateral (b) views. Muscles that are involved in spastic diplegia are hamstrings, gastrocnemius and soleus.

transported in a wheelchair and are dependent for all aspects of their care (Fig. 15.4).

Functional walking is not a major goal for these children, but spasticity management can still be very useful to prevent postural deformities from becoming fixed and to make care and comfort easier for children and adolescents. Focal injections of BoNT are sometimes useful in the upper limb to permit easier use of wheelchair controls for children at GMFCS level IV. Injections of the hip adductors (see Fig. 14.13) and hamstrings (see Fig. 14.15) may aid sitting position

when standing and walking are not functional goals. Injections of the calf muscles may permit more comfortable sitting; allow the orthoses, shoes and socks to be worn; and keep the feet on a wheelchair foot plate.

Progression of spastic posturing to fixed contractures and joint instability is very common in these children. The majority will develop hip instability, which can be detected by serial radiographic examination of the hips. Injection of BoNT to the hip adductors may slow the progression of hip displacement, but the majority will eventually require preventative or

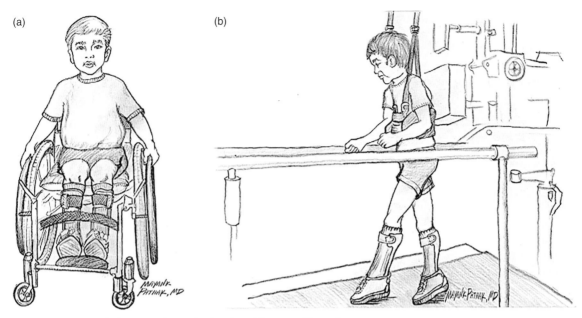

(a)　　　　(b)

Fig. 15.4 Spastic quadriplegia. Muscles involved are hip adductors and hamstrings.

reconstructive orthopedic surgery. If spastic dystonia is severe and causing discomfort or difficulties with care, the use of an intrathecal baclofen pump can be very effective.

Treatment techniques for botulinum neurotoxin

Following definition of treatment goals and a discussion of the risks and benefits of the medication, the patient is prepared for the BoNT treatment procedure. Patients often prefer some measure of local anesthesia. Topical lidocaine cream or ethyl chloride as a local coolant is helpful at the time of injection. Additionally, oral midazolam can be utilized as an anxiolytic. While most children and adults can tolerate the procedure well, combative patients, such as those with autism or extreme anxiety, may benefit from general anesthesia. Parents traditionally prefer to stay for the injections and provide reassurance (Russman *et al.*, 2002).

Assistance from technicians or medical personnel is important to stabilize and appropriately position the child. The patient is placed in a position to activate the muscle of interest (e.g. frog-legged for injection of the adductors). The skin is prepared with alcohol or povidone–iodine and universal precautions are utilized. While palpation is the most commonly and easily utilized method, electromyography or electrical stimulation guidance may be very helpful when surface

landmarks are not easily localized or when precise targeting of smaller muscles in the upper extremities is required. Ultrasonography is useful, particularly to accurately localize muscles and confirm the presence of the needle in muscles that are deeper and hard to reach.

Treatment guidelines

Dosing guidelines for BoNT type A (BoNT-A) have been developed by experienced injectors and reflect concern for avoidance of antibody-based resistance while delivering a clinically effective dose to the target muscles (Box 15.3) (Russman *et al.*, 2002). Because of the maximum dose limitation, not all muscles may be injected in one treatment session. Target muscles and dose ranges are shown in Table 15.1 (see also Chapter 14). The characteristics of BoNT, such as the mode of action, diffusion in muscle, and side effect profile, influence dosing. Additionally, because of the intrinsic molecular diversity and differences in manufacturing, units of the commercially available BoNT products are not equivalent. As a result, a standard conversion among the products is not possible.

Adverse effects

When used according to published guidelines, BoNT-A is safe for use in most children with cerebral palsy (Delgado *et al.*, 2010). There is insufficient evidence

---

Box 15.3 Guidelines for dosing of botulinum neurotoxin for children

OnabotulinumtoxinA
1. Maximum dosing per session: the lesser of 15 U/kg or 400 U; experienced injectors may use more
2. Dose range:

   - upper extremity, 0.5–2.0 U/kg
   - lower extremity smaller muscles, 1–3 U/kg and larger muscles 3–6 U/kg
   - no more than 50 U per injection site

3. Reinjection interval 3 months or greater
4. Dilution 1–2 ml of non-bacteriostatic saline per 100 U vial
5. Spread of the neurotoxin is 4–5 cm in the muscle; therefore muscles may need more than one injection site based on size, fascial planes and dose

AbobotulinumtoxinA
1. Maximum dosing per session: the lesser of 10–20 U/kg or 1000 U; experienced injectors may use more
2. Dose range:

   - upper extremity, 1–10 U/kg
   - lower extremity smaller muscles, 3–10 U/kg and larger muscles 3–15 U/kg
   - no more than 250 U per injection site

3. Reinjection interval 3 months or greater
4. Dilution 1–5 ml of non-bacteriostatic saline per 500 U vial
5. Spread of the neurotoxin is 4–5 cm in the muscle; therefore, muscles may need more than one injection site based on size, fascial planes and dose

---

for BoNT-B. The most common side effects are at the site of the injection and include muscle soreness and bruising. These complications are minor and self-limiting. There are no reports of deep infection after intramuscular injection or permanent neurovascular injury. Remote side effects, including incontinence and dysphagia, have occasionally been reported. Incontinence is of great concern to parents but usually resolves quickly. Dysphagia, which may lead to aspiration and chest infection, is the most serious complication. Children with spastic quadriplegia with pseudobulbar palsy seem to be much more sensitive to systemic spread after focal injection of BoNT, and treatment may be relatively contraindicated in this group for this reason. For the current US Food and Drug Administration recommendations refer to website (http://www.fda.gov/Drugs/DrugSafety/Postmark etDrugSafetyInformationforPatientsandProviders/Dr ugSafetyInformationforHeathcareProfessionals/ucm1 74959.htm).

Treatment planning and considerations

Botulinum neurotoxin is approved for use in cerebral palsy in some countries (including Canada) but not others (including the USA), and the age threshold also varies by country. Off-label use is common, but ideally should be in the context of approved clinical trials. There is reasonable clinical evidence to suggest that younger children respond more fully and for longer periods of time than do older children. This may simply be because of the progression from dynamic posturing to fixed contracture in the older child.

Children with spastic hemiplegia and spastic diplegia can be safely injected from age 18 to 24 months. Treatment seems to be most effective between the ages of 2 and 6 years, and should be in the context of a global tone management program, including the use of orthoses, serial casting and physical therapy. By age 6–10 years, children will have plateaued in terms of physical functioning and many no longer require injection therapy. Some will have developed fixed contractures and are more effectively managed by orthopedic surgical procedures.

References

Bax M, Goldstein M, Rosenbaum P *et al.* (2005). Proposed definition and classification of cerebral palsy, *Dev Med Child Neurol*, **47**, 571–6.

Delgado MR, Hirtz D, Aisen M *et al.* (2010). Practice parameter: pharmacologic treatment of spasticity in children and adolescents with cerebral palsy (an evidence-based review). *Neurology*, **74**, 336–43.

Fehlings D, Novak I, Berweck S (2010). Botulinum toxin assessment, intervention and follow-up for paediatric upper limb hypertonicity: international consensus statement. *Eur J Paediatr Neurol*, **17**, 36–56.

Heinen F, Desloovere K, Schroeder AS *et al.* (2010). The updated European Consensus 2009 on the use of botulinum toxin for children with cerebral palsy. *Eur J Paediatr Neurol*, **14**, 45–66.

Koman LA, Smith BP, Shilt JS (2004). Cerebral palsy. *Lancet*, **363**, 1619–31.

Palisano RJ, Rosenbaum P, Walter S *et al.* (1997). Development and reliability of a system to classify gross motor function in children with cerebral palsy. *Dev Med Child Neurol*, **45**,113–20.

Russman BS, Tilton AH, Gormley ME Jr. (2002). Cerebral palsy: a rational approach to a treatment protocol, and the role of botulinum toxin in treatment. In Mayer NH, Simpson DM (eds.) *Spasticity: Etiology, Evaluation, Management, and the Role of Botulinum Toxin*. New York, WE MOVE, pp. 134–43.

Winters TF Jr., Gage JR, Hicks R (1987). Gait patterns in spastic hemiplegia in children and young adults. *J Bone Joint Surg*, **69**, 437–41.

The role of ultrasound for botulinum neurotoxin injection in childhood spasticity

Bettina Westhoff

Introduction

Botulinum neurotoxin type A (BoNT-A) injections are established as a standard procedure for the treatment of functional shortening of different muscles in spastic or dystonic children. Preconditions for beneficial effects are:

- a functional problem resulting from dynamic hyperactive muscle shortening without major structural changes
- a focal problem caused by hyperactivity of a few muscles
- application of the BoNT in the target muscle close to the neuromuscular junctions
- a sufficient dose
- no antibodies to BoNT-A.

Muscles that are superficial and palpable are easy to inject. In contrast, exact placement of the needle is more difficult and less controllable in muscles that are not palpable and deeply situated (e.g. iliopsoas) or are small and difficult to selectively identify (such as forearm muscles). Exact needle placement is, however, essential for optimal functional result, avoidance of side effects and evaluation of therapeutic failures.

To localize the target muscle and to control the placement of the injection needle several techniques are available:

- orientation at anatomical landmarks and palpation supported by moving the distal joint to observe the motion of the needle placed in the target muscle (Buchthal technique)
- electromyography
- electrical stimulation
- real-time ultrasound
- CT.

Clinical application of BoNT has been shown to be inaccurate except for the gastrocsoleus complex (Chin *et al.*, 2005). Electromyography is good, but many muscles may be simultaneously active. Control by electrical stimulation is quite uncomfortable and painful and often requires anesthesia. Guidance under CT is not appropriate for routine use because of the exposure to radiation and high costs. By comparison, the advantages of the ultrasound-guided technique are clear:

- real-time observation of the injection
- readily available
- easily applicable after a manageable learning period
- cost effective
- no serious side effects.

Technical prerequisites

For muscle sonography, a linear-array transducer is used. This provides a considerable contact area and, therefore, good coupling, as well as a geometrically exact image. Depending on the depth of the target muscle, different ultrasound frequencies are indicated: superficial muscles are best assessed by probes working at high frequencies (frequency band 7.5–12 MHz), and deep muscles best at lower frequencies (5–7.5 MHz). The penetration depth of a 12 MHz transducer is about 4 cm and of a 7.5 MHz transducer about 8 cm. Ideally, a multifrequency transducer is used.

Ultrasound morphology of muscles

The anatomy of a skeletal muscle is shown in Fig. 16.1. The echotexture of normal skeletal muscles has a hypoechoic background, which corresponds to the muscle fascicles, and multiple hyperechoic structures consistent with fibroadipose septa (perimysium).

Manual of Botulinum Toxin Therapy, 2nd edition, ed. Daniel Truong, Mark Hallett, Christopher Zachary and Dirk Dressler. Published by Cambridge University Press. © Cambridge University Press 2013.

Within the muscle, there might be a hyperechoic band where the fascicles converge, which is the aponeurosis. The muscle itself is surrounded by a hyperechoic fascia (epimysium). The ratio between the hypoechoic and the hyperechoic components gives information about the proportion of connective tissue and muscle fascicles, which is variable and differs among muscles. On longitudinal scans, the fibroadipose septa appear as straight, almost parallel, hyperechoic lines (Fig. 16.2a). On transverse scans, the fibroadipose septa appear as small dot-like reflectors (Fig. 16.2b) (Zamorani and Valle, 2007).

Patient preparation

The patient should be placed as comfortable as possible and in a way that the target muscle can be reached without major difficulties. Standard disinfectant fluid can be used as the contact medium. Alternatively, before performing the ultrasound, standard skin disinfection can be performed and the injection carried out through the standard bacteriostatic gel (Berweck and Heinen, 2005).

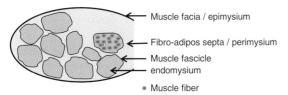

Fig. 16.1 Cross-section of muscle.

Ultrasound-guided injection technique

The target muscle is identified and scanned by ultrasound in the longitudinal and transverse planes. The optimum injection area is located where most of the motor endplates are assumed to be (Campenhout and Molenaers, 2011).

There are two ways to place the needle with ultrasound guidance.

Indirect technique. The puncture site is marked by ultrasound and the depth of the target region is measured. The needle is then placed blindly perpendicular to the skin surface and as deep as measured before. There is no real-time control of the injection itself.

Real-time technique. The target region is shown by ultrasound and the needle is advanced under direct ultrasound control. This technique is preferred.

The muscle can be viewed in a longitudinal or transverse plane. The transverse projection allows the differentiation of structures in the neighborhood and the identification of the muscles based on their characteristic pattern. This is especially helpful when injecting smaller muscles such as those of the upper extremity. For iliopsoas injection, the longitudinal view is favored.

For the injection, two basically different approaches are described: needle parallel to the long axis of the probe and needle perpendicular to the long axis of the probe.

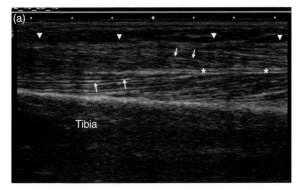

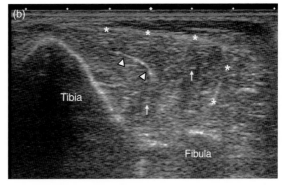

▽ Margin of the m. tibialis anterior to the subcutanous tissue

* hyperechoic band corresponding to the intramuscular aponeurosis

↑ hyperechoic fibroadipose septa converging to the aponeurosis

* Margin of the m. tibialis anterior to the subcutanous tissue

▽ hyperechoic band corresponding to the intramuscular aponeurosis

↑ hyperechoic fibroadipose septa

Fig. 16.2 Ultrasound of skeletal muscle. Longitudinal (a) and transverse (b) scans.

(a)

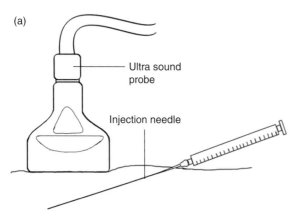

- Ultra sound probe

- Injection needle

(b)

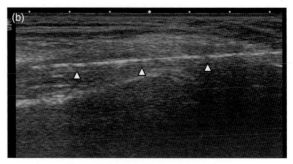

△ Injection needle

Fig. 16.3 Injection technique with the needle parallel to the long axis of the probe. (a) The relationship of the probe to the needle. Illustrated by Mayank Pathak. (b) Ultrasound view with the arrowheads indicating the position of the needle.

Needle parallel to the long axis of the probe

The needle is inserted approximately 1 to 2 cm distal to the probe and advanced under real-time control in the longitudinal axis of the probe (Fig. 16.3); the advancement of the needle can be followed as a hyperechoic line. The higher the injection angle relative to the ultrasound beam, the better the visualization of the needle. If the needle advancement cannot be followed directly, the position can be estimated indirectly by imaging the movements of the surrounding soft tissues during real-time observation. After correct placement and control aspiration, BoNT is injected under real-time observation mode. The solution of BoNT in saline presents mostly as a hyperechoic area within the muscle, sometimes with a dorsal echo-extinction. By changing the position of the needle, the BoNT can be well distributed in the muscle belly.

Needle perpendicular to the long axis of the probe

The target region should be focused in the middle of the screen. In this way, it is possible to place the injection needle in the middle of the probe and, from that point, inject into the muscle. By swaying the probe around its longitudinal axis, the advancement of the needle may be followed as a hyperechoic dot; the tip of the needle can also be identified as a hyperechoic dot which appears on the screen while advancing the needle and holding the probe position stable. In that moment, the target region is reached and the needle should not be advanced further. The distribution of the BoNT can be followed on the screen.

The problem of this technique is that the tip cannot always be identified with certainty, as the echoic reflection of the tip and the shaft looks the same (Fig. 16.4b,c).

The needle length required depends on the anatomic location of the target region and the injection technique: if the needle is inserted parallel to the probe it has to be longer.

As an example, the injection of the iliopsoas muscle from the distal approach is described in detail (Westhoff *et al.*, 2003). The patient lies in supine position and standard disinfectant fluid is used as contact medium. The iliopsoas muscle is examined in the groin by a 5.0 or 7.5 MHz linear transducer in the longitudinal plane. The femoral head serves as a bony landmark and is identified in the groin in the standard longitudinal sectional plane (Fig. 16.5a). The relationship between the iliopsoas muscle and the femoral vessels is demonstrated in the transverse sectional plane (Fig. 16.5b). The iliopsoas muscle is in direct contact with the capsule over the femoral head. For an optimum placement of the BoNT injection, the transducer is moved cranially following the iliopsoas muscle. The injection needle is introduced distal to the inguinal ligament and approximately 1 to 2 cm distal to the transducer (Fig. 16.5c); it is advanced cranially and placed into the iliopsoas muscle under real-time ultrasound control (Fig. 16.5d). We use a TSK-Supra 0.8-gauge, 12 cm length injection needle (TSK, Tochigi/Japan). The needle is located either directly as the typical hyperechoic structure or indirectly by imaging the movements of the surrounding soft tissues during real-time observation. After correct placement and control aspiration, the BoNT is injected under real-time observation mode. By changing the position of the needle, the BoNT can

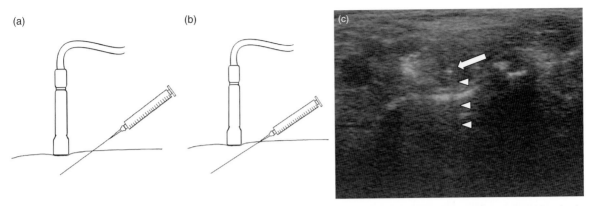

Fig. 16.4 Injection technique with the needle perpendicular to the long axis of the probe. (a) The tip of the needle is positioned under the probe in the target region; in this position the injection should be made. (b) The tip of the needle should be advanced further and is no longer located in the target region; the shaft of the needle will be visualized by the ultrasound image. Illustrated by Mayank Pathak. (c) In the ultrasound image, the hyperechoic dot (arrow) corresponds to the needle. There is no difference in the image whether it shows the tip or the shaft. A wave-extinction can be identified (triangles) with ultrasound waves completely reflected at the "changeover" between soft tissue and needle; consequently behind the needle no echo can be seen.

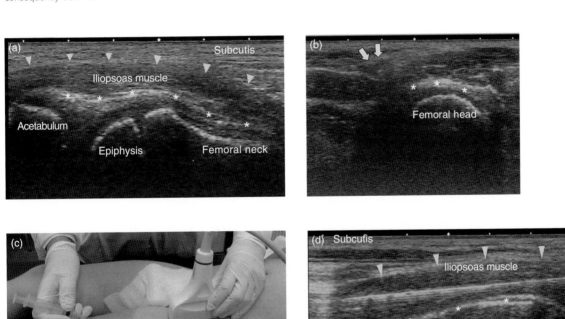

Fig. 16.5 Injection of the iliopsoas muscle (a) Longitudinal ultrasound view of the hip joint; the iliopsoas muscle lies directly on the joint capsule (*); the triangles mark the border to the subcutis. (b) Transverse ultrasound view of the iliopsoas at the level of the femoral head; the arrows marks the femoral vessels. During real-time imaging, pulsation can be followed. (c) Clinical picture showing needle and probe during injection. (d) Ultrasound showing the needle placed in the iliopsoas muscle; the triangles mark the border of the iliopsoas muscle; the injection needle is identified as a hyperechoic white line; in this case an artifact is visible as there are further white lines behind the needle itself (repeating echos); * correspondings to the OS ilium.

be distributed safely in the muscle belly. The needle is introduced up to 12 cm depending on the patient's stature.

This technique for the iliopsoas injection is well suited to children. In adults, the motor endplate zone might be too far proximal and, therefore, cannot be reached from the groin. It is located at about 30% and 70% of the distance between T12 and the passing of the psoas under the inguinal ligament (Campenhout *et al.*, 2010).

References

Berweck S, Heinen F (2005). *Blue Book. Treatment of Cerebral Palsy with Botulinum Toxin. Principles, Clinical Practice, Atlas*, 2nd edn. Berlin: Child & Brain.

Campenhout A, Molenaers G (2011). Localization of the motor endplate zone in human skeletal muscles of the lower limb: anatomical guidelines for injection with botulinum toxin. *Dev Med Child Neurol*, **53**, 108–19.

Campenhout A, Hubens G, Fagard K, Molenaers G (2010). Localization of motor nerve branches of the human psoas muscle. *Muscle Nerve*, **42**, 202–7.

Chin T, Nattrass G, Selber P *et al.* (2005). Accuracy of intramuscular injection of botulinum toxin A in juvenile cerebral palsy: a comparison between manual needle placement and placement guided by electrical stimulation. *J Pediatr Orthop*, **25**, 286–91.

Westhoff B, Seller K, Wild A, Jäger M, Krauspe R (2003). Ultrasound-guided botulinum toxin injection technique for the iliopsoas muscle. *Dev Med Child Neurol*, **45**, 829–32.

Zamorani MP, Valle M (2007). Muscle and tendon. In Bianchi S, Martinoli C (eds.) *Ultrasound of the Musculoskeletal System*. Berlin: Springer, pp. 46–50.

The use of botulinum neurotoxin in spasticity using ultrasound guidance

Andrea Santamato, Franco Molteni and Pietro Fiore

Introduction

One important factor influencing the effectiveness of botulinum neurotoxin (BoNT) injection in the treatment of upper and lower limb spasticity is the accuracy of administration into the target muscle. Indeed, incorrect needle placement can result in complete failure of treatment. Neurotoxin diffusion outside of target muscles can cause weakness or paresis, particularly for small muscles of the hand and forearm. The use of various guidance techniques may improve both effectiveness and safety, decreasing the occurrence of side effects.

A wide range of injection techniques has been described, such as manual needle placement using surface anatomy landmarks or palpation, electromyographic guidance, electrical stimulation of the muscle and ultrasound guidance (Childers 2003; Berweck et al., 2004). Generally, manual needle placement is considered to be an acceptable technique for delivering the BoNT to large, superficial muscles, but not for small, slender, deep muscles. Therefore, guidance is recommended where the goal of treatment is the modulation of muscle hypertonicity to improve the dexterity of spastic muscles (particularly for hand spasticity), as well as for deep and small muscles of the limbs, whereas it is considered optional for larger easily palpated muscles.

In recent years, the availability of portable ultrasound devices has facilitated the application of ultrasound technology for guidance in BoNT injection procedures. It is easy, quick, painless and available in most hospitals. Ultrasonography has been used to guide BoNT administration in the urinary system and salivary glands and is being assessed for skeletal muscles (Westhoff et al., 2003; Berweck et al., 2004).

Skeletal muscle ultrasound

First characterized in the early 1950s, ultrasound has become an innovative technique in medical practice to visualize several living tissues by combining non-invasive, high-frequency ultrasonic waves with real-time display (Wild and Neal, 1951). Currently, ultrasound is widely available, with muscle tissue resolutions up to 0.1 mm (Cosgrove, 1992). This resolution permits the identification of several muscles from near structures such as bone, nerves, blood vessels, fibrosis and fat (Fig. 17.1). Additionally, Heckmatt and colleagues (1980) discovered that muscles affected by certain disorders show a different appearance to healthy muscles when viewed on ultrasound.

Echogenicity may vary somewhat with different ultrasound probe frequencies and machine set-up. Usually, the main ultrasound technique to observe

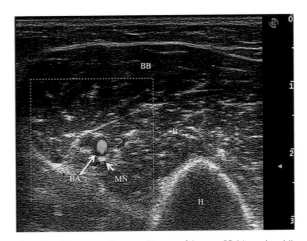

Fig. 17.1 Transverse ultrasound image of the arm. BB, biceps brachii muscle; B, brachial muscle; H, humerus; MN, median nerve; BA, brachial artery.

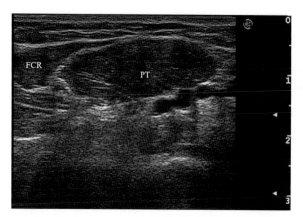

Fig. 17.2 Transverse ultrasound image of pronator teres (PT) and flexor carpi radialis (FCR) muscles in the left forearm.

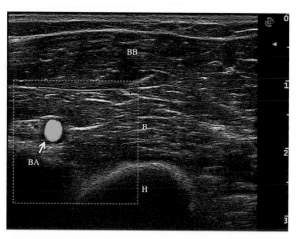

Fig. 17.3 Power-Doppler imaging of brachial artery (BA) with surrounding biceps brachii (BB) and brachialis (B) muscles in transverse ultrasound image of the left arm. H, humerus.

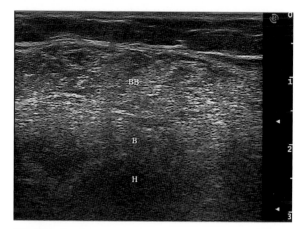

Fig. 17.4 Fibrotic area into transverse ultrasound image of biceps brachii (BB) muscle. Boundaries of the muscles are not clearly visible. B, brachialis muscle; H, humerus.

skeletal muscles is the brightness mode (B-mode), which provides a two-dimensional image with different brightness points in a gray scale. Surrounding tissue also influences echogenicity through beam attenuation. Normal muscle is relatively black with hypoechoic intensity; between muscle fibers, some hyperechoic interfaces may be seen (reflections of perimysial connective tissue). Hyperechoic fascia surrounds each muscle belly, delineating the muscle groups. The boundaries of the muscle are clearly visible, as the epimysium surrounding the muscle is a highly reflective structure (Fig. 17.2).

The acoustical impedance is very different between muscles and bones, causing a strong reflection with hardly any sound passing through. In normal subjects, the echo from the bone and periosteum forms a highly reflective hyperechoic linear or curvilinear line with a characteristic anechoic bone shadow underneath (Fig. 17.1). The hyperechoic tendon consists of parallel fibers running in the long axis of the tendon. The tendon sheath is hyperechoic and separated from the tendon by a thin hypoechoic area (Bradley and O'Donnell, 2002). Nerves are relatively hyperechoic, linear nerve bundles being separated by hyperechoic interfaces, whereas blood vessels are hypo- or anechoic circles or lines depending on the direction of the ultrasound beam. To correctly identify blood vessels in muscle sections, power Doppler imaging is used as it shows blood flow (Fig. 17.3).

In neuromuscular disorders such as spasticity, when the muscle tissue is replaced by fat and by infiltration of intramuscular connective tissue (fibrosis), the ultrasound beam encounters tissues with different acoustic impedance and much reflection. This explains why the muscle ultrasound image appears white (Fig. 17.4).

Subcutaneous fat is hypoechoic, but the echogenicity varies in different anatomies and pathologies, and several echogenic septa of connective tissue may be visible within this tissue. Other fatty areas may vary in echogenicity depending on their structure and surrounding tissue.

Skeletal muscle ultrasound examination can be performed by a transverse or longitudinal evaluation. In the transverse plane, perpendicular to the long axis of the muscle, the muscle has a speckled appearance, whereas in the longitudinal plane (along the long axis of the muscle) the fascicular architecture of the muscle becomes visible (Pillen, 2010). Usually, a probe with a resolution of 7.5–12 MHz is adequate to observe all superficial muscles, but it is not useful for the identification of individual small muscles. For small muscles, a high frequency (18 MHz) with a corresponding higher resolution transducer must be used. In the case of deeper muscles, it is possible to use lower frequencies (5–7.5 MHz) or a convex transducer.

Ultrasound guidance for botulinum neurotoxin injection in spastic muscles

Why use ultrasound guidance?

Ultrasonography is well established as a reliable and reproducible imaging method in muscle anatomy (Bradley and O'Donnell, 2002) and several studies have shown applicability of the procedure for visually controlled BoNT injections as an alternative to electrophysiological techniques (Willenborg *et al.*, 2002; Westhoff *et al.*, 2003; Berweck *et al.*, 2004). Kwon and colleagues (2010) compared the clinical outcomes of two different BoNT injection guidance techniques, electric stimulation and ultrasound, into both gastrocnemius muscles in 30 children with cerebral palsy. Gait pattern and hindfoot position–maximum foot/floor contact during stance significantly improved in the ultrasound-guided group while no statistical differences were noted in the Modified Ashworth Scale, Modified Tardieu Scale or Selective Motor Control. These authors concluded that visual feedback by ultrasonography could improve the accuracy of selective neuromuscular blocking of the gastrocnemius muscles.

Yang and colleagues (2009) investigated the accuracy of manual needle placement for BoNT injection into the gastrocnemius muscle in 39 children with spastic cerebral palsy. These authors showed that the needle was accurately inserted into gastrocnemius muscles in 78.7% of cases. Accuracy was 92.6% into gastrocnemius medialis and 64.7% into gastrocnemius lateralis. Muscle thickness at the needle insertion site was significantly thinner in gastrocnemius lateralis than gastrocnemius medialis, so injection of the BoNT into gastrocnemius muscles through the use of an anatomical landmark was acceptable in gastrocnemius medialis but not in gastrocnemius lateralis. Finally, Py and colleagues (2009) showed that ultrasonically guided BoNT injections into the lower limbs of children with cerebral palsy led to greater functional improvement than seen in those performed with manual needle placement. Therefore, reasons to use ultrasound guidance for BoNT administration include the accuracy of muscle identification, correct needle placement into the

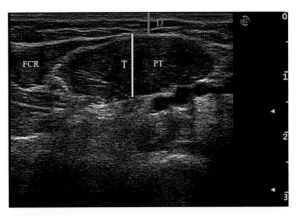

Fig. 17.5 Transverse ultrasound image of pronator teres (PT) muscle. D, depth; FCR, flexor carpi radialis; T, thickness.

muscle mass and reduced likelihood of inserting the needle into tissues surrounding the target muscle.

An additional advantage of ultrasound guidance may also be a reduction in the time required for muscle identification. Berweck and colleagues (2004) assessed more than 6000 ultrasound-guided BoNT injections and demonstrated that the average time to identify and inject the targeted muscle ranged from 5 seconds in superficial muscles such as the gastrocnemius muscle to 30 seconds in deep-seated muscles such as the tibialis posterior or the iliopsoas muscle.

Moreover, ultrasound guidance permits the identification of a muscle's depth and thickness. Depth is defined as the distance from the skin to the superficial aponeurosis of each muscle. Thickness is defined as the distance from the superficial to the deep aponeurosis of each muscle (Fig. 17.5).

It is known that immobilization and spasticity lead to changes in muscle morphology over time, represented by atrophy, fibrosis and fat replacing sarcomeres. Therefore, a risk of BoNT administration is the needle's insertion over the thickness of target muscle, particularly in cases of atrophy and for small and superficial muscles. The advanced ultrasound machines show the exact muscle depth measured in centimeters, allowing the choice of a specific sized needle for injection. For example, to inject gastrocnemius muscle, it is sufficient to use a 25-gauge (0.5 mm × 16 mm) needle. The injection of soleus muscle with the same needle may be difficult in adult patients considering its depth (Fig. 17.6).

In obese patients, the needle needs to pass through the fat between skin and superficial aponeurosis of each muscle. Immobilization and spasticity of the arm disrupts the normal muscle architecture through the infiltration of fat and the development of fibrosis.

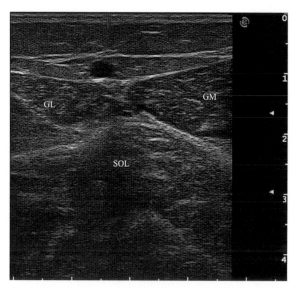

Fig. 17.6 Transverse ultrasound image of the left calf. Depth of single muscles is indicated by green arrows. GM, gastrocnemius medialis; GL, gastrocnemius lateralis; SOL, soleus.

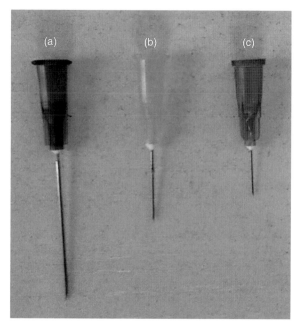

Fig. 17.7 Needles: (a) 0.7 mm × 30 mm; (b) 0.5 mm × 16 mm; (c) 0.45 mm × 10 mm.

Box 17.1 Characteristics of ultrasound guidance for botulinum neurotoxin injections

- Accuracy of muscle identification
- Correct needle placement into the muscle tissue
- Awareness of muscle's depth and thickness
- Assessment of atrophy, fibrosis and fat in muscle tissue
- Differentiation of muscle tissue from surrounding structures (vessel, nerves, bone)
- Independent of patient cooperation
- Painless evaluation
- Option of documenting the injections

Ultrasound guidance avoids administration of BoNT into fibrotic or fatty areas and increases its accuracy.

Ultrasound guidance for BoNT administration can also facilitate the identification of nerves and vessels, thereby avoiding unwanted bleeding and enhancing the accuracy of BoNT placement (Fig. 17.1). It also allows estimation of muscle volumes so that the amount of BoNT needed for specific muscles can be calculated. However, ultrasound technology is unable to register muscular hyperactivity or to localize neuromuscular junctions. There is evidence from animal models and clinical studies that distance to neuromuscular junctions influences efficiency of BoNT treatment.

Box 17.1 lists the advantages of using ultrasound guidance for BoNT injections.

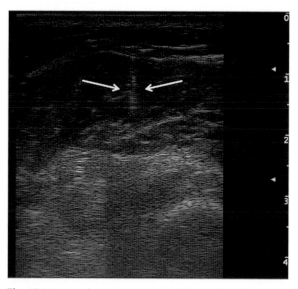

Fig. 17.8 Hyperechogenic appearance of the needle in the muscle.

Technique for ultrasound-guided botulinum neurotoxin injection

Transverse as opposed to longitudinal scans permit "panoramic" images, which make it possible to visualize several muscles in one plane. In this mode, the injector can move the probe laterally or medially along the target muscle's areas, facilitating the identification of muscles that are to be treated with BoNT. Moreover, the injector can activate the muscle identified, consider their motor function biomechanically and can observe this activation with the probe.

Before proceeding to the injection, it is better to prepare several needles of various sizes for the different muscle depths (Fig. 17.7). To observe the correct placement into target muscles, it is important to introduce the needle tip under ultrasound beam at an angle of 30 degrees with the axis of the probe. The needle is identified directly as an echogenic line or indirectly by imaging the movements of the surrounding soft tissues during real-time observation (Fig. 17.8).

After correct placement, BoNT is injected under real-time observation mode, and by changing the position of the needle, the BoNT can be well distributed in the muscle belly. The appropriate number of injection sites usually depends on the size of the muscle. Injecting a small volume at several sites is preferred over a large volume at a single site.

Ultrasound-guided botulinum neurotoxin injections for common patterns of upper and lower limb spasticity

In the following paragraphs, the common muscles involved in spasticity are shown with their position in upper or lower limb and their transverse ultrasound image.

Upper limb spasticity

The most common patterns of spasticity in the upper limb involve flexion of the fingers, wrist and elbow; adduction with internal rotation at the shoulder; and flinched fist with thumb in palm (Mayer *et al.*, 2002). Wrist or elbow extension is less common.

Shoulder: adduction and internal rotation

Inject pectoralis major and minor (Fig. 17.9); *optional injection of latissimus dorsi and teres major* (Fig. 17.10).

It is useful to identify the coracobrachialis muscle at the proximal and anterior surface of the arm.

From there, moving the probe medially to the axillary fold, it is possible to palpate the pectoralis major muscle insertion fibers at the anterior axillary fold. The pectoralis major muscle is superficial (Fig. 17.9); advance through it to reach pectoralis minor muscle. Latissimus dorsi is approached at the posterior chest wall, looking for its origin, spinous processes of lower thoracic vertebrae, lumbodorsal fascia and posterior crest of ilium (Fig. 17.10).

Arm: elbow flexion

Inject biceps brachii, brachialis and/or brachioradialis muscles (Figs. 17.11 and 17.12).

Biceps brachii muscle is approached at the third medium of the anterior arm surface, superficially, with brachialis muscle separating it from humerus (Fig. 17.11). Brachioradialis muscle is approached at the third proximal of dorsal surface of the forearm (Fig. 17.12).

Forearm

For the forearm, ultrasound evaluation is carried out while the patient lies in a supine position with a forceful fully supinated forearm. In this mode, transverse ultrasound image allows visualization of several flexor muscles in one plane. At the proximal third of the ventral surface of the forearm, the pronator teres muscle can be easily observed because of its size and hypoechogenicity with respect to other surrounding muscles. By first identifying this muscle, it is possible to observe the other muscles from lateral to medial: pronator teres, flexor carpi radialis, palmaris longus, flexor digitorum superficialis, flexor carpi ulnaris muscles, flexor digitorum profundus (Fig. 17.13).

Pronated forearm

Inject pronator teres muscle (Fig. 17.14).

Inject pronator teres muscle at the proximal third of the ventral surface of forearm (Fig. 17.14).

Wrist flexion

Inject flexor carpi radialis and/or flexor carpi ulnaris (Figs. 17.14 and 17.15).

Flexor carpi ulnaris is approached directly at the medial border of the forearm midway between

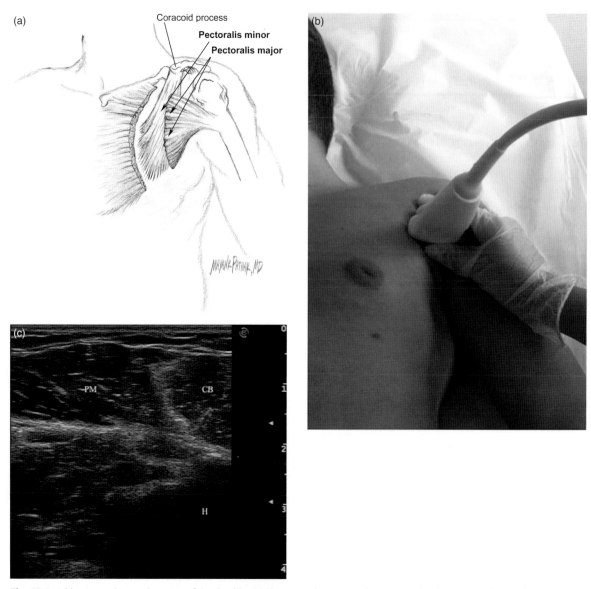

Fig. 17.9 Adduction and internal rotation of the shoulder. (a) The pectoralis major and minor muscles. (b) Position of probe for a transverse ultrasound image. (c) The left pectoralis major (PM) muscle, coracobrachialis (CB) muscle and humerus (H).

the antecubital and distal wrist creases (evaluation can be facilitated with forearm flexion). Flexor carpi radialis lies along the ventral surface of the forearm just medial to the midline.

Hand: clenched fist

Inject flexor digitorum superficialis and flexor digitorum profundus (Fig. 17.16).

The flexor digitorum superficialis muscle is injected for flexion at the proximal interphalangeal joints and the flexor digitorum profundus muscle to reduce flexion at distal interphalangeal joints.

Flexor digitorum superficialis lies between flexor carpi radialis and flexor carpi ulnaris, while flexor digitorum profundus is approached between flexor digitorum superficialis and flexor carpi ulnaris (Fig. 17.16).

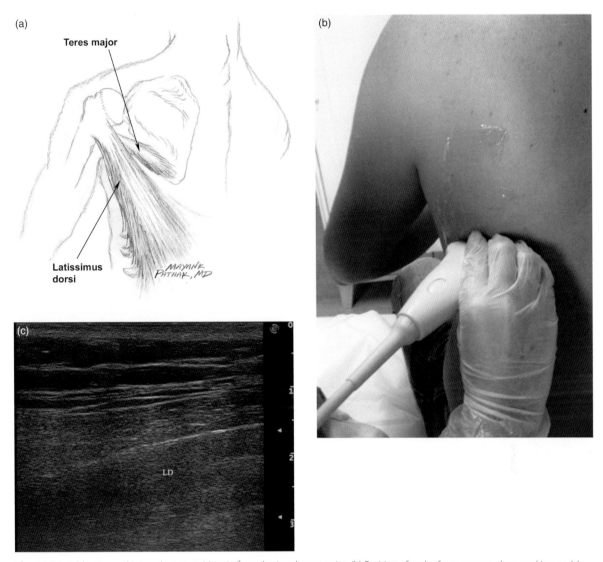

(a)

Teres major

Latissimus dorsi

MAYANK PATHAK, MD

(b)

(c)

LD

Fig. 17.10 Adduction and internal rotation. (a) Latissimus dorsi and teres major. (b) Position of probe for transverse ultrasound image. (c) Latissimus dorsi (LD) muscle.

Hand: thumb in palm

Inject flexor pollicis longus, adductor pollicis and other thenar muscles (Figs. 17.17 and 17.18).

Flexor pollicis longus muscle is approached from the middle to the distal third of the ventral forearm, adjacent to the medial border of the brachioradialis muscle (Fig. 17.17). Adductor pollicis muscle may be approached from the dorsal surface by going through the overlying first dorsal interosseus muscle, or, more commonly, from the palmar side. The other thenar muscles that may be injected include opponens pollicis, flexor pollicis brevis and abductor pollicis brevis. Into the palmar side, flexor pollicis brevis muscle lies medial and adjacent to abductor pollicis brevis muscle (Fig. 17.18).

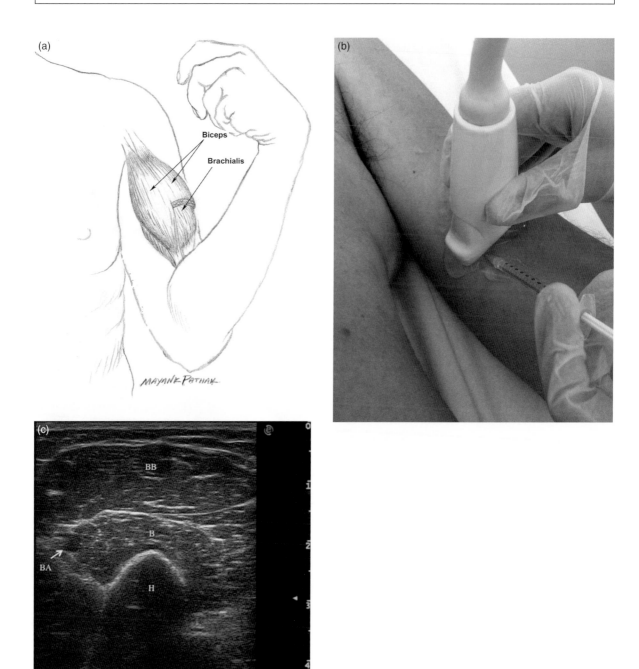

Fig. 17.11 Elbow flexion. (a) Biceps and brachialis. (b) Position of probe for a transverse ultrasound image. (c) The biceps brachii (BB) and brachialis (B) muscles and brachial artery (BA). H, humerus.

(a)

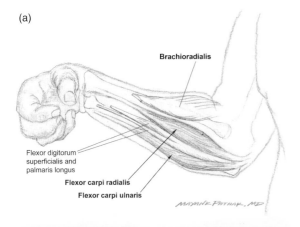

Brachioradialis

Flexor digitorum
superficialis and
palmaris longus

Flexor carpi radialis

Flexor carpi ulnaris

MAYANK PATHAK, MD

(b)

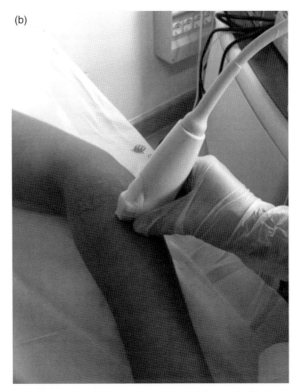

Fig. 17.12 Elbow flexion. (a) The brachioradialis muscle. (b) The probe approachs the muscle at the third proximal dorsal surface of the forearm. (c) Transverse ultrasound image of left brachioradialis (BR), extensor carpi radialis longus (ECRL) and supinator (S) muscles in the left forearm. R, radius.

(c)

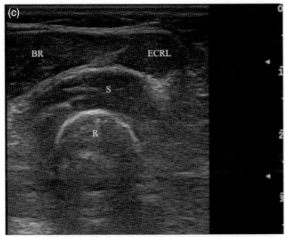

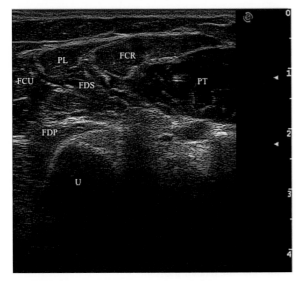

Fig. 17.13 Transverse ultrasound image of left forearm. PT, pronator teres; FCR, flexor carpi radialis; PL, palmaris longus; FDS, flexor digitorum superficialis; FCU, flexor carpi ulnaris; FDP, flexor digitorum profundus; U, ulna.

Other upper limb muscles

Elbow extension

Inject triceps brachii (Fig. 17.19).

The triceps brachii muscle is injected in cases of elbow extension or to reduce co-contraction with biceps brachii and brachialis muscles. Triceps brachii is approached behind the posterior surface of humerus at the third medium (Fig. 17.19).

Wrist extension

Inject extensor carpi radialis longus, extensor carpi radialis brevis or extensor carpi ulnaris (Figs. 17.20 and 17.21).

In case of upper limb spasticity, it's possible to inject extensor carpi radialis longus, brevis or extensor carpi ulnaris muscles. Extensor carpi radialis longus and extensor carpi ulnaris muscles are approached at the third proximal of dorsal surface of the forearm (Figs. 17.20 and 17.21).

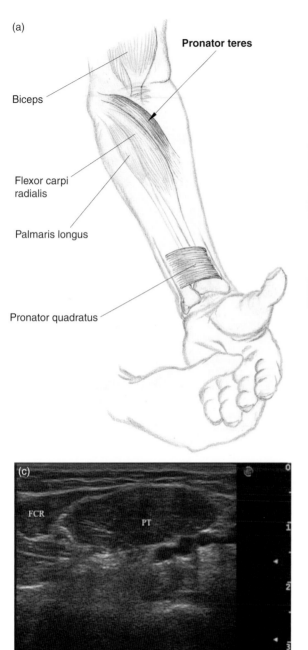

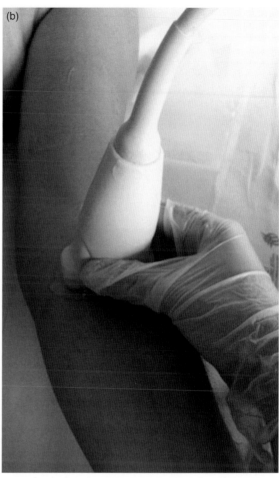

Fig. 17.14 Pronated forearm. (a) The muscles of the forearm. (b) Position of probe for a transverse ultrasound image. (c) Ultrasound image of left pronator teres (PT) and flexor carpi radialis (FCR) muscles in the left forearm.

Lower limb spasticity

The most common pattern of spasticity in the lower limb involves extension at the knee, plantar-flexion at the ankle and inversion of the foot (Mayer *et al.*, 2002). Other patterns of spasticity in the lower limbs include "scissoring" adduction at the hip joints, along with flexion or extension at the knees and spastic extension of the great toe.

Ankle: plantar-flexion position

Inject lateral gastrocnemius, medial gastrocnemius and soleus (Fig. 17.22); optional injection of the tibialis posterior.

(a)

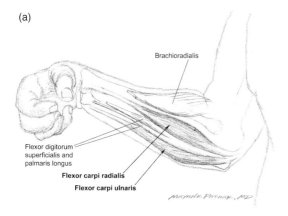

Brachioradialis

Flexor digitorum superficialis and palmaris longus

Flexor carpi radialis

Flexor carpi ulnaris

(b)

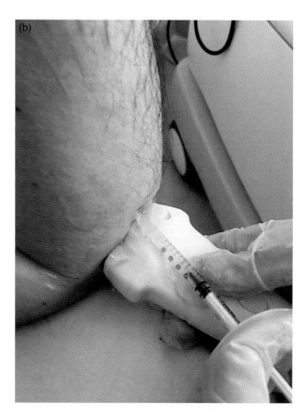

(c)

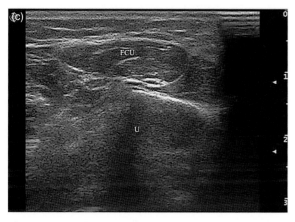

FCU

U

Fig. 17.15 Wrist flexion. (a) Muscles of flexion. (b) Position of probe for a transverse ultrasound image. (c) Ultrasound image of left flexor carpi ulnaris (FCU) and ulna (U) in the left forearm.

The lateral and medial heads of the gastrocnemius muscle lie superficially, while the tibialis posterior muscle (injected in cases of foot inversion) lies deep in the calf. Because of the great depth of the tibialis posterior muscle, it is better to put the probe on the middle third of the anterior and medial surface of the leg to facilitate its identification (Fig. 17.23).

Foot: extension of the great toe

Inject extensor hallucis longus (Fig. 17.24).

The extensor hallucis longus is located by palpating its tendon just lateral to the tendon of the tibialis anterior and following it about to the proximal third of the tibia. At this level, its muscular belly lies one fingerbreadth lateral to the tibia (Fig. 17.24).

Flexion of the great toe and other toes

Inject flexor hallucis longus and flexor digitorum longus (Fig. 17.25).

Both flexor hallucis longus and flexor digitorum longus are below the soleus muscle in the calf, between the tibia and fibula. Flexor hallucis longus is approached adjacent to the posterior distal fibula, while flexor digitorum longus is adjacent to the medial posterior tibia (Fig. 17.25).

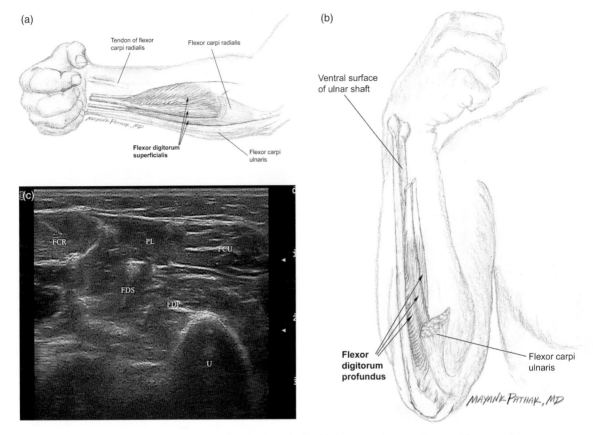

Fig. 17.16 Clenching the fist. (a,b) Muscles utilized in clenching the fist. (c) Transverse ultrasound image of flexor muscles in the left forearm. FCR, flexor carpi radialis; PL, palmaris longus; FDS, flexor digitorum superficialis; FCU, flexor carpi ulnaris; FDP, flexor digitorum profundus; U, ulna.

Other lower limb muscles sometimes injected

Thigh: hip adduction

Inject adductor muscles: longus, brevis and magnus (Fig. 17.26).

We prefer that the patient lies in the supine position with thighs flexed, abducted at the hips and the knees flexed. The adductor muscles (longus, brevis and magnus) are found proximally in the anteromedial thigh approximately a handbreadth distal to the groin fold, where they are superficial and the separation (in anterior to medial progression) of the adductor longus and gracilis muscles are palpable. The magnus adductor muscle lies deep in the medial part of the thigh; the longus adductor muscle is approached superficially while the brevis adductor muscle is between magnus and longus adductor muscles (Fig. 17.26). In this mode, it is possible to treat all adductor muscles with only one BoNT administration by varying the depth of needle insertion into the muscle tissue.

Leg: knee flexion

Inject hamstring muscles (Fig. 17.27).

The hamstring muscles are biceps femoris, semimembranonus and semitendinosus muscles. The semitendinosus and semimembranosus muscles are medial in the posterior surface of the thigh, while the long and short heads of biceps femoris are lateral.

Leg: knee extension

Inject extensor muscles (Fig. 17.28).

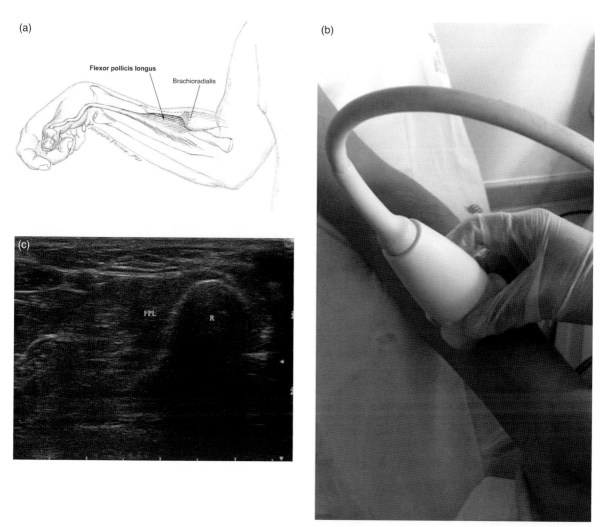

Fig. 17.17 (a) Flexor pollicis longus muscle. (b) Position of probe for a transverse ultrasound image. (c) The flexor pollicis longus (FPL) muscle in the left forearm. R, radius.

It is sometimes useful to inject the extensor muscles of the leg to improve gait and balance. The rectus femoris, vastus lateralis and vastus medialis muscles are readily approached in the anterior thigh (Fig. 17.28).

Foot: eversion position

Inject peroneus muscles (Fig. 17.29).

Peroneus longus and brevis are approached from the proximal one-third of the fibula. The peroneus tertius is approached at the distal one-third of the fibula.

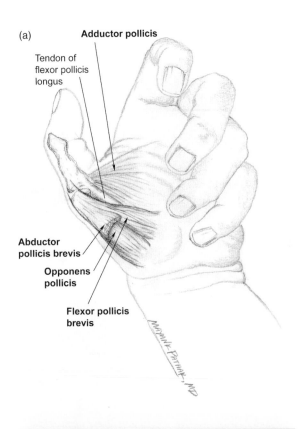

(a)

Adductor pollicis

Tendon of
flexor pollicis
longus

Abductor
pollicis brevis

Opponens
pollicis

Flexor pollicis
brevis

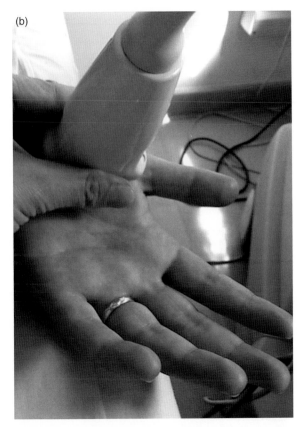

(b)

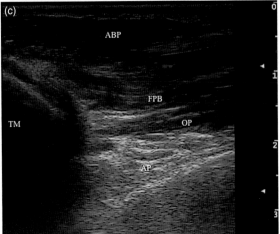

(c)

ABP

FPB

TM

OP

AP

Fig. 17.18 (a) The thenar muscles. (b) Position of probe for a transverse image. (c) Ultrasound image showing the abductor brevis pollicis (ABP), flexor pollicis brevis (FPB), opponens pollicis (OP) and adductor pollicis (AP) muscles. TM, thumb metacarpal.

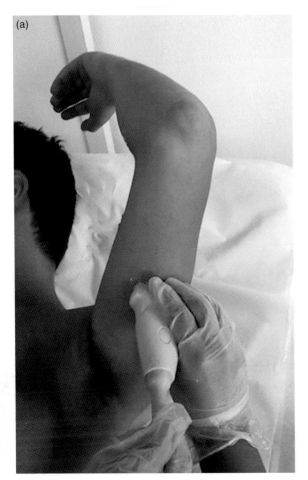

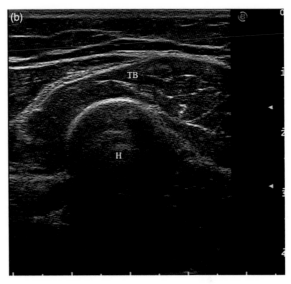

Fig. 17.19 Elbow extension. (a) Probe position for the triceps brachii muscle. (b) Transverse ultrasound image of triceps brachii (TB) muscle in the left arm. H, humerus.

(a)

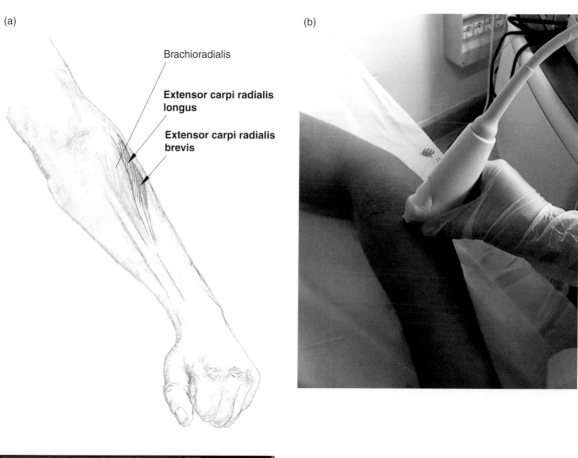

Brachioradialis

Extensor carpi radialis longus

Extensor carpi radialis brevis

(b)

(c)

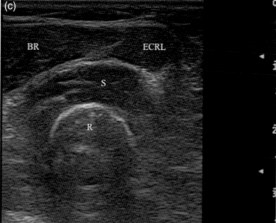

BR   ECRL

S

R

Fig. 17.20 Wrist extension. (a) Muscles of the forearm. (b) Probe position for a transverse ultrasound image. (c) The extensor carpi radialis longus (ECRL), brachioradialis (BR) and supinator (S) muscles in the left forearm. R, radius.

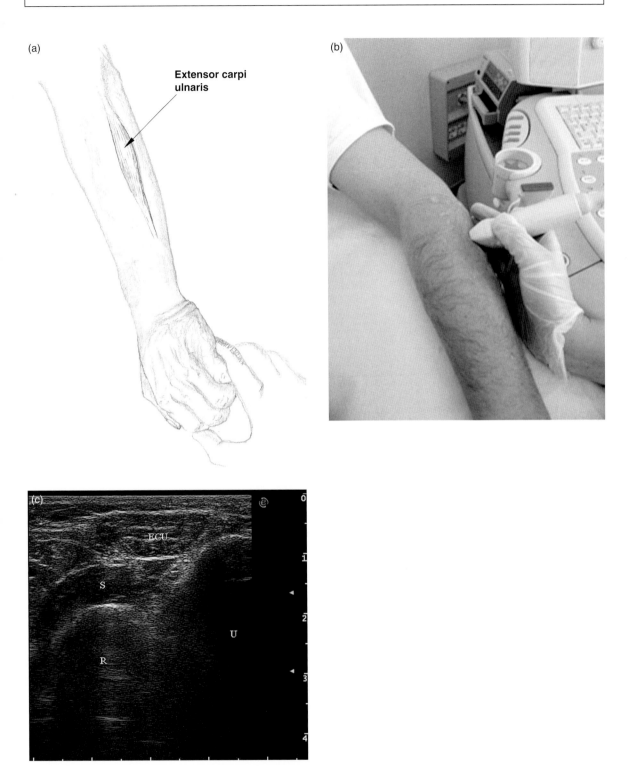

Fig. 17.21 Wrist extension. (a) The extensor carpi ulnaris. (b) Probe position for a transverse ultrasound image. (c) The extensor carpi ulnaris (ECU) and supinator (S) muscles in the left forearm. R, radius, U, ulna.

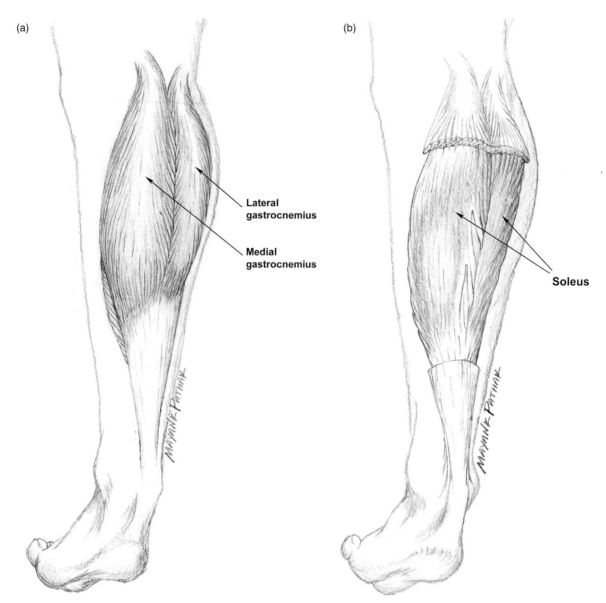

Fig. 17.22 Plantar-flexion position of the ankle. (a,b) The plantar flexor muscles of the left calf. (c) Transverse ultrasound image of the gastrocnemius medialis (GM), gastrocnemius lateralis (GL) and soleus (SOL) muscles. (d) Probe and injection for gastrocnemius medialis muscle. (e) Probe and injection for soleus muscle.

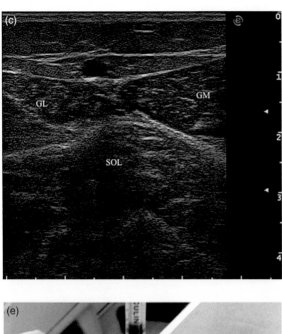

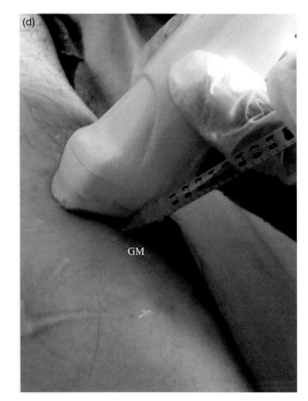

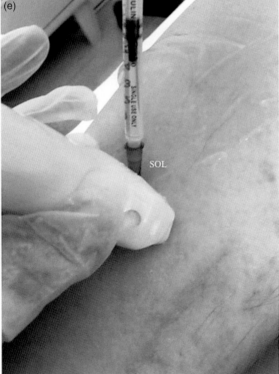

Fig. 17.22 (cont.)

(a)

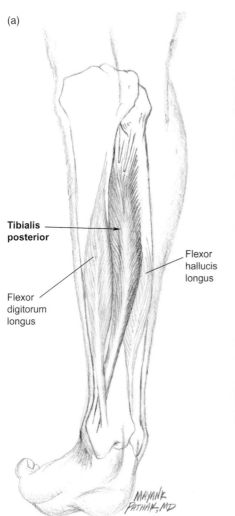

Tibialis posterior

Flexor hallucis longus

Flexor digitorum longus

MAYANK PATHAK, MD

(b)

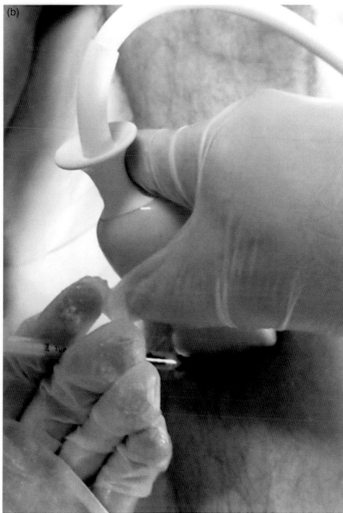

(c)

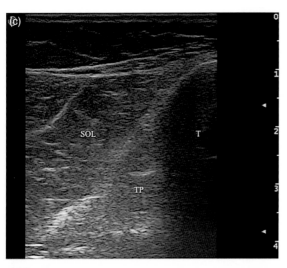

SOL

T

TP

Fig. 17.23 The anterior and medial surface of the left leg. (a) The tibialis posterior muscle. (b) Probe on the middle third of the anterior and medial surface of the leg. (c) Ultrasound image of the soleus (SOL) and tibialis posterior (TP) muscles. T, tibia.

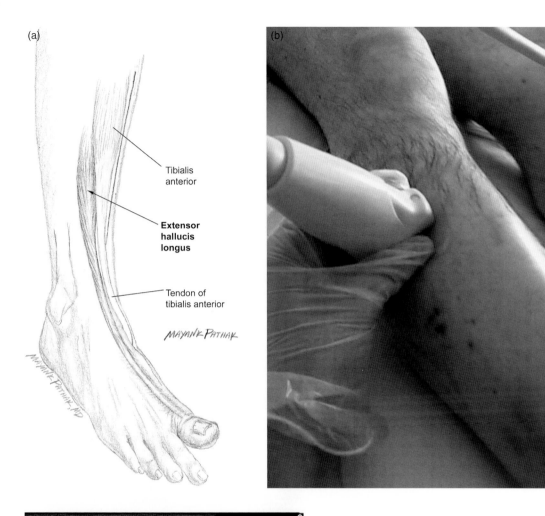

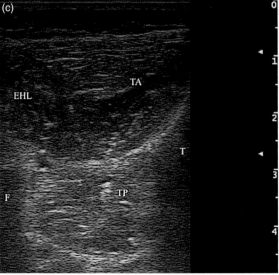

Fig. 17.24 Extension of the great toe. (a,b) Muscles involved in the movement of the great toe. (c) Transverse ultrasound image of the anterior surface of the right leg. EHL, extensor hallucis longus muscle; TP, tibialis posterior muscle; TA, tibialis anterior muscle; T, tibia; F, fibula.

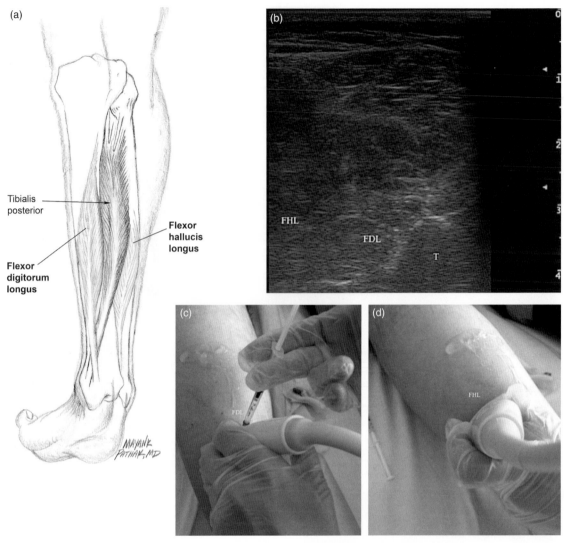

Fig. 17.25 Flexion of the toes. (a) The flexor hallucis longus and flexor digitorum longus muscles. (b) Transverse ultrasound image of the left calf showing the flexor digitorum longus (FDL) and flexor hallucis longus (FHL) muscles and the tibia (T). (c) Probe and injection for the flexor digitorum longus muscle. (d) Probe and injection for the flexor hallucis longus muscle.

(a)

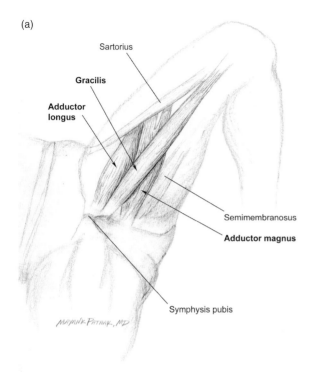

Sartorius

Gracilis

Adductor longus

Semimembranosus

Adductor magnus

Symphysis pubis

MAYANK PATHAK, MD

(b)

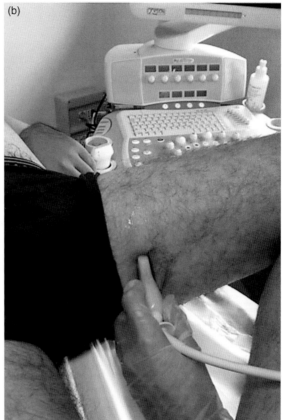

(c)

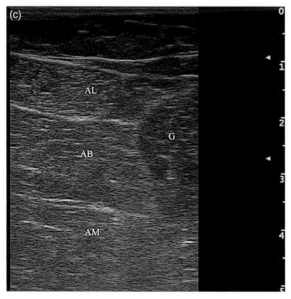

Fig. 17.26 Hip adduction. (a) The adductor muscles. (b) Position of probe for transverse ultrasound image of the anterior and medial surface of the left thigh. (c) Ultrasound image showing the adductor longus (AL), adductor brevis (AB), adductor magnus (AM) and gracilis (G) muscles.

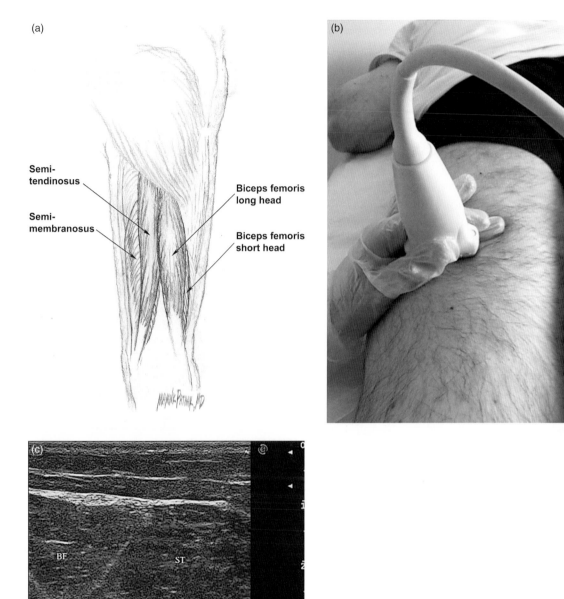

Fig. 17.27 Leg flexor muscles. (a) The hamstring muscles. (b) Position of probe for transverse image of posterior surface of the left thigh. (c) Ultrasound image showing biceps femoris (BF) and semitendinosus (ST) muscles.

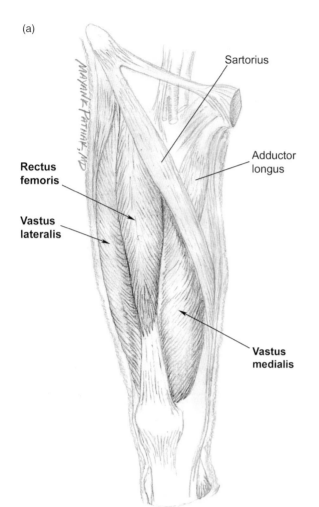

(a)

Sartorius

Rectus
femoris

Vastus
lateralis

Adductor
longus

Vastus
medialis

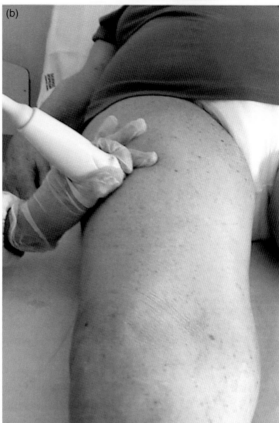

(b)

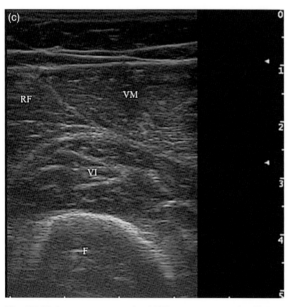

(c)

RF

VM

VI

F

Fig. 17.28 Leg extensor muscles. (a) The extensor muscles. (b) Position of probe for transverse image of the anterior surface of the right thigh. (c) Ultrasound image showing the vastus medialis (VM), rectus femoris (RF) and vastus intermedius (VI) muscles. F, femur.

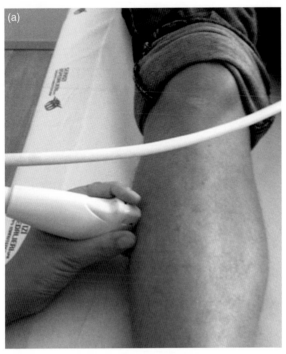

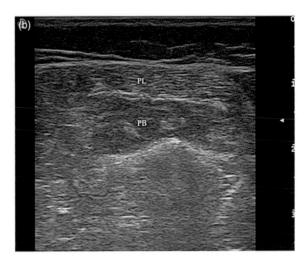

Fig. 17.29 Foot eversion position. (a) Probe position on the proximal one-third of the fibula of the right leg. (b) Transverse ultrasound image showing the peroneus longus (PL) and peroneus brevis (PB) muscles.

References

Bradley M, O'Donnell P (2002). *Atlas of Musculoskeletal Ultrasound Anatomy*. Cambridge, UK: Cambridge University Press.

Berweck S, Schroeder AS, Fietzek UM, Heinen F (2004). Sonography-guided injection of botulinum toxin in children with cerebral palsy. *Lancet*, **17**, 249–50.

Childers MK (2003). The importance of electromyographic guidance and electrical stimulation for injection of botulinum toxin. *Phys Med Rehabil Clin N Am*, **14**, 781–92.

Cosgrove D (1992). Ultrasound: general principles. In Grainger RG, Allison DJ (eds.) *Diagnostic Radiology*. Edinburgh: Churchill Livingstone, pp. 65–77.

Heckmatt JZ, Dubowitz V, Leeman S (1980). Detection of pathological change in dystrophic muscle with B-scan ultrasound imaging. *Lancet*, **i**, 1389–90.

Kwon JY, Hwang JH, Kim JS (2010). Botulinum toxin A injection into calf muscles for treatment of spastic equinus in cerebral palsy: A controlled trial comparing sonography and electric stimulation-guided injection techniques: A preliminary report. *Am J Phys Med Rehabil*, **89**, 279–86.

Mayer NH, Esquenazi A, Childers MK (2002). Common patterns of clinical motor dysfunction. In Mayer NH, Simpson DM (eds.) *Spasticity: Etiology, Evaluation, Management and the Role of Botulinum Toxin*. New York: WE MOVE, pp. 16–26.

Pillen S (2010). Skeletal muscle ultrasound. *Eur J Transl Myol*, **1**, 145–55.

Py AG, Zein Addeen G, Perrier Y, Carlier RY, Picard A (2009). Evaluation of the effectiveness of botulinum toxin injections in the lower limb muscles of children with cerebral palsy. Preliminary prospective study of the advantages of ultrasound guidance. *Ann Phys Rehabil Med*, **52**, 215–23.

Westhoff B, Seller K, Wild A, Jaeger M, Krauspe R (2003). Ultrasound-guided botulinum toxin injection technique for the iliopsoas muscle. *Dev Med Child Neurol*, **45**, 829–32.

Wild JJ, Neal D (1951). Use of high-frequency ultrasonic waves for detecting changes of texture in living tissues. *Lancet*, **i**, 655–7.

Willenborg MJ, Shilt JS, Smith BP *et al.* (2002). Technique for iliopsoas ultrasound-guided active electromyography-directed botulinum a toxin injection in cerebral palsy. *J Pediatr Orthop*, **22**, 165–8.

Yang EJ, Rha DW, Yoo JK, Park ES (2009). Accuracy of manual needle placement for gastrocnemius muscle in children with cerebral palsy checked against ultrasonography. *Arch Phys Med Rehabil*, **90**, 741–4.

Chapter 18

The use of botulinum neurotoxin in tic disorders and essential hand and head tremor

Joseph Jankovic

Introduction

This chapter describes aspects of tics and tremors including clinical features, oral medication treatment and the utility of botulinum neurotoxin (BoNT) injections as a therapeutic modality.

Tics

Tics are brief, sudden, movements (motor tics) or sounds (phonic tics) that are intermittent but may be repetitive and stereotypic (Jankovic and Kurlan, 2011). When motor tics and phonic tics coexist without other neurological abnormalities, the diagnosis of Tourette's syndrome should be considered. Most patients with Tourette's syndrome have also a variety of comorbid disorders such as attention deficit disorder, obsessive compulsive disorder and impulse control disorders. Tourette's syndrome is considered a genetic neuro-developmental disorder but its pathogenesis is not well understood (Jankovic and Kurlan, 2011). Although Tourette's syndrome is the most common cause of childhood-onset tics, there are many other causes of tics, including autistic disorder and various insults to the brain and basal ganglia (infection, stroke, head trauma, drugs and neurodegenerative disorders).

Clinical features of tics

Motor and phonic tics consist of either simple or complex movements, which may be seemingly goal directed. Motor tics may be rapid (clonic) or more prolonged (tonic or dystonic). Many patients exhibit suggestibility and temporary suppressibility; they may also have a compulsive component, sometimes perceived as an irresistible need to perform the movement or sound repetitively until it feels "just right." One feature that is particularly helpful in differentiating tics from other jerk-like movements is a premonitory sensation in the region of the tic or more generalized "urge." Some patients repeat other's gestures (echopraxia) or sounds (echolalia).

Treatment options for tics

The most commonly used effective anti-tic medications, the so-called neuroleptics, act by blocking dopamine receptors or by depleting dopamine but they can be associated with troublesome side effects (Jankovic and Kurlan, 2011; Pringsheim et al., 2012). These include drowsiness, weight gain, school phobia, parkinsonism and tardive dyskinesia. Tardive dyskinesia, however, has not been reported with tetrabenazine, a depleter of dopamine, approved for the treatment of chorea associated with Huntington's disease (Jankovic and Clarence-Smith, 2011). Although not yet approved for Tourette's syndrome, this drug has been found to be safe and effective in the treatment of Tourette's syndrome, even though it may be potentially associated with adverse effects, such as parkinsonism, depression, drowsiness and akathisia.

Use of botulinum neurotoxin

When oral medications fail to provide relief of tics, local chemodenervation with BoNT offers the possibility of relaxing the muscles involved in focal tics without causing undesirable systemic side effects. Focal tics that are repetitively performed are more effectively treated with BoNT than tics with complex movements, as the latter would require injections in multiple muscles. In a pilot study, onabotulinumtoxinA (BoNT-A; Botox) injections demonstrated marked reduction in the frequency and intensity of dystonic tics in 10 patients with Tourette's syndrome (Jankovic 1994). An important

Manual of Botulinum Toxin Therapy, 2nd edition, ed. Daniel Truong, Mark Hallett, Christopher Zachary and Dirk Dressler.
Published by Cambridge University Press. © Cambridge University Press 2013.

observation was that premonitory sensory symptoms were reduced. Kwak *et al.* (2000), in a second open-label study of 35 patients (34 with Tourette's syndrome), demonstrated a peak effect of 2.8 on a self-rating scale (range 0–4, with 0 for no effect and 4 for marked relief in both severity and function). The effect lasted a mean of 14.4 weeks. The mean dose per session was 57.4 U in the upper face, 79.3 U in the lower face, 149.6 U in the cervical muscles and 121.7 U in other muscles of the shoulder, forearm and scalp. Four patients received 17.8 U in the vocal cords. In the 25 patients in the study with premonitory sensory symptoms, 21 (84%) had notable reduction in these symptoms. Complications, which were all mild and transient, included neck weakness (four), dysphagia (two), ptosis (two), nausea (one), hypophonia (one), fatigue (one) and generalized weakness (one).

A randomized, placebo-controlled, double-blind, crossover study of onabotulinumtoxinA for motor tics was conducted with 18 patients (Marras *et al.*, 2001). There was a 37% reduction in the number of tics per minute within 2 weeks compared to that seen with vehicle. The premonitory urge was reduced, with an average change in urge scores of –0.46 in the treatment phase and +0.49 in the placebo phase (score range 0–4, with 0 for none and 4 for severe). Although 50% of patients noted motor weakness in the injected muscles, the weakness was not functionally disabling. Two patients noted motor restlessness that paralleled the weakness induced by the onabotulinumtoxinA during the active treatments. Problems with the study included insufficient power to demonstrate significant differences in measured variables such as severity, global impression and pain. In addition, the patients were only assessed at 2 weeks after injection and the full effect of the treatment may not have been realized. Finally, the patients did not rate their tics as significantly compromising at baseline, indicating that their Tourette's syndrome was rather mild.

In an open-label study of 30 patients with phonic tics treated with 2.5 U onabotulinumtoxinA in both vocal cords (Porta *et al.*, 2004), patient assessments occurred after 15 days and then four times over a 12-month period. Phonic tics improved after treatment in 93% patients, with 50% being tic free. The percentage of subjects stating their condition severely impacted their social life reduced from 50% to 13% after injection and those with tics causing a severe effect on work or school activities reduced from 47% to 10%. In the 16 subjects (53%) experiencing

premonitory symptoms, only 6 (20%) continued to have these sensations after injection. Hypophonia, which was mild, was the only side effect of note (in 80% of patients).

In 1996 we described two patients with Tourette's syndrome who had compressive cervical myelopathy as a result of severe motor tics involving the neck (so-called "whiplash tics") (Krauss and Jankovic, 1996). The first patient, a 21-year-old man, had complex tics consisting of violent twisting and extending movements of the neck preceded by an irresistible urge to produce the abnormal postures. Two years after onset of these tics, he developed paresthesia, sensory deficits up to the level of C4 and a gait disturbance. Despite initial neuroimaging evidence of compressive myelopathy, the symptoms gradually improved with onabotulinumtoxinA injections into the posterior cervical muscles. The second patient, a 42-year-old man, had had violent "whiplash" tics since the age of 10 years. At age 23, he developed progressive weakness of all four extremities and bladder and sexual dysfunction. Myelography demonstrated cervical spinal canal stenosis; after cervical decompression by C3–C5 laminectomies, his spinal cord symptoms improved temporarily. The tics, however, continued, and the neurologic deficits of cervical myelopathy progressed again after age 34. He did not benefit from a second operation but his symptoms of myelopathy recovered completely with repeat BoNT injections into the posterior neck muscles. Subsequently, another patient with Tourette's syndrome was reported with violent dystonic tics resulting in cervical myelopathy and quadriparesis and who had not responded to high doses of neuroleptic drug. His tics completely resolved after two injections of onabotulinumtoxinA (50 U injected bilaterally to the sternocleidomastoid muscle and 100 U to the splenius capitis) at follow-up at 12 months. These reports draw attention to the possibility that some tics can produce disabling compressive myelopathy and, therefore, need to be treated early and aggressively (Cheung *et al.*, 2007).

Long-term experience with a large number of patients has confirmed the beneficial effects of BoNT injections in the treatment of motor and phonic tics (Vincent, 2008), including severe coprolalia (Scott *et al.*, 1996) (Table 18.1).

Our experience with botulinum neurotoxin

Our long-term experience with BoNT in well over 1000 patients with tics provides further evidence that

Table 18.1 Selected studies of botulinum neurotoxin injection for tics

Reference	Design	Size	Treatment (technique, dose)	Brand	Follow-up	Outcome	Adverse events
Kwak et al. (2000)	Open-label, case series with unblinded assessments	35	57.4 U in the upper face, 79.3 U in the lower face, 149.6 U in the cervical muscles and 121.7 U in other muscles of the shoulder, forearm and scalp. 4 patients received 17.8 U in the vocal cords	OnabotulinumtoxinA	Mean duration of follow-up was 21.2 months (range, 1.5–84); mean peak effect over 115 sessions was 2.8 weeks (range, 0–4); the mean duration of benefit was 14.4 weeks (maximum, 45 weeks); mean latency to onset of benefit was 3.8 days (maximum, 10 days)	Clinical effect on 4 point self-rating scale	Mild and transient, including neck weakness (4), dysphagia (2), ptosis (2), nausea (1), hypophonia (1), fatigue (1) and generalized weakness (1)
Marras et al. (2001)	Double-blinded, crossover, placebo-controlled	20 randomized, 18 completed (2 lost to follow-up)	Variable doses based on clinical judgment	OnabotulinumtoxinA	All outcomes compared week 2 to baseline measurement; patients reassessed at weeks 6 and 12 and every 4 weeks until patient and examiners agreed tic disorder had reached baseline and then the patient crossed over to the second phase of the trial	Primary measure: number of treated tics per minute on a videotape segment. Secondary measures: number of untreated tics per minute, the Shapiro Tourette Syndrome Severity Scale score, a numerical assessment of the urge to perform the treated tic (0 to 4), the premonitory sensation associated with the treated tic (0 to 4) and the patient's global impression of change	50% of patients noted weakness not functionally disabling of the injected muscles; 2 patients noted a significant motor restlessness during the active treatment; 2 patients felt the inability to perform the treated tic led to a new tic to replace it
Porta et al. (2004)	Open-label, case series with unblinded assessments	30	2.5 IU in both vocal cords; mean number injections were 1.9 per patient with a mean interval 4.2 months apart	OnabotulinumtoxinA	Assessed after 15 days and then 4 times over a 12-month period	Phenomenology of tics, global impression of changes by physician and patient, number of BoNT-A injections given, interval between injections	Mild hypophonia was the only side effect of note (80% of patients).

BoNT, botulinum neurotoxin.

BoNT is a safe and effective treatment modality, particularly in patients with focal tics, such as blinking, facial grimacing, jaw clenching, neck extensions ("whiplash tics") and shoulder shrugging.

Dosages and muscles injected

The exact muscles and location of injections are determined by considering which movements are of particular concern to the patient, by observing the predominant movement (including severity) of the tic being performed and by determining whether or not there is a significant localized premonitory sensation or urge associated with the tic. Dosing varies depending on the intensity of the premonitory sensation, force of the contraction and size of the muscle, but the average starting dose is 25–50 U onabotulinumtoxinA/incobotulinumtoxinA (onabotulinumtoxinA/incobotulinumtoxinA), 75–150 U abobotulinumtoxinA (Dysport) or 1500–2500 U rimabotulinumtoxinB (MyoBloc/NeuroBloc) into the splenius muscle (see Adult Dosing Guidelines and dosage recommendations of the WE MOVE Spasticity Study Group (2005)). The dosages of BoNT injected into vocal folds for phonic tics are, of course, substantially smaller, about 1–2 U onabotulinumtoxinA/incobotulinumtoxinA and 3–5 U abobotulinumtoxinA on each side. On occasion, as patients experience improvement of their treated tic, they may have a worsening of tics in other areas, but this is quite rare.

Tremors

Tremor is one of the most common movement disorders and essential tremor is the most common reason for referral to a movement disorders clinic for evaluation and treatment of tremor.

Clinical features

Essential tremor consists of involuntary, rhythmic or oscillatory movements, usually involving the hands, head and voice, and may be associated with other movement disorders such as dystonia and parkinsonism (Elble and Deuschl, 2011).

Treatment options for tremors

A recent review and practice parameter report by the American Academy of Neurology recommended propranolol, long-acting propranolol and primidone as the only first-line, class A medication therapies for essential tremor (Zesiewicz et al., 2011). Primidone is associated, however, with moderate to high frequency of acute adverse events and a decline in efficacy with long-term treatment in the majority of patients. Drugs such as topiramate, pregabalin and other anticonvulsants may also be useful in the treatment of essential tremor (Elble and Deuschl, 2011).

Use of botulinum neurotoxin

When oral medications for tremor have poor efficacy or intolerable side effects, BoNT injections may be used as an adjunctive treatment. There have been more than a dozen studies in which BoNT has been evaluated for efficacy and safety in treating hand tremor. The majority of these have focused on patients with essential tremor, but some have included subjects with Parkinson's disease or parkinsonian rest tremor. There have been two randomized, double-blind, controlled studies to evaluate the efficacy of BoNT-A in treating essential hand tremor. In the first study by Jankovic et al. (1996), 25 patients were injected in both the wrist flexors and extensors with 50 U onabotulinumtoxinA and with an additional 100 U after 4 weeks if they failed to respond. Some of the patients had rest tremors, but all clinically met the criteria for essential tremor. Rest, postural and kinetic tremors were evaluated at intervals of 2 to 4 weeks for 16 weeks using tremor severity rating scales, accelerometry and assessments of tremor improvement and functional disability. A significant ($p < 0.05$) improvement on the tremor severity rating scale 4 weeks after injection was seen in the onabotulinumtoxinA-treated group compared with placebo. Additionally, at 4 weeks after injection, 75% of onabotulinumtoxinA-treated patients compared with 27% of placebo-treated patients ($p < 0.05$) demonstrated mild to moderate (peak effect of ≥ 2) subjective improvement in their tremor on a 0 to 4 rating scale. There were no significant improvements in the functional rating scales. Postural accelerometry measurements showed a $\geq 30\%$ reduction in amplitude in 9 of 12 onabotulinumtoxinA-treated subjects and in 1 of 9 placebo-treated subjects. All patients treated with onabotulinumtoxinA reported some mild, transient degree of finger weakness.

In a randomized, multicenter, double-masked clinical trial by Brin et al. (2001), 133 patients with essential tremor were randomized to treatment with either low-dose (50 U) or high-dose (100 U) onabotulinum-toxinA or placebo. Injections were made into the wrist flexors and extensors and patients were followed for 16 weeks. Tremor severity was assessed with the hand at rest and in postural and kinetic positions. The effect of treatment was assessed by clinical rating scales, measures of motor tasks and functional disability, and global assessment of treatment. All assessments were scored on a scale of 0–4 measuring severity or disability (0, none; 1, mild; 2, moderate; 3, marked; 4, severe). Hand strength was evaluated by clinical rating and a dynamometer. The assessment of tremor severity based on rating scale evaluation indicated a significant difference ($p < 0.05$) from baseline for the low- and high-dose groups for postural tremor at 6, 12 and 16 weeks, and for kinetic tremor only at the 6-week evaluation, compared with placebo. Measures of motor tasks and functional disability were not consistently improved, but drawing a spiral and a straight line at 6 and at 16 weeks improved. The results of treatment on assessment using functional rating scales indicated that low-dose onabotulinumtoxinA significantly ($p < 0.05$) improved feeding, dressing and drinking at 6 weeks and writing at 16 weeks compared with placebo. In the high-dose group, onabotulinumtoxinA significantly ($p < 0.05$) improved feeding at 6 weeks; drinking at 6, 12 and 16 weeks; hygiene at 6 weeks; writing at 16 weeks; and fine movements at 6, 12 and 16 weeks. The Sickness Impact Profile scores and ratings on speaking, working, embarrassment and anxiety state were not significantly improved. The subjects had dose-dependent, finger or wrist weakness in flexion and extension, with a tendency for greater weakness in wrist and finger extension.

In both placebo-controlled studies, patients had statistically significant finger or wrist weakness in flexion and extension, with a tendency for greater weakness in wrist and finger extensors.

In an open-label study of BoNT treatment, 20 patients with disabling essential tremor not responding to conventional pharmacological therapy were enrolled (Pacchetti et al., 2000). Activities of daily living self-questionnaire, Severity Tremor Scale, accelerometry and surface electromyography were used to assess the severity of the tremor and identify the arm muscles involved in generating the tremor during certain positions. Treatment with BoNT was associated with a significant reduction in both severity and functional rating scales scores (activities of daily living self-questionnaire, Severity Tremor Scale) and of tremor amplitude as measured with accelerometry and electromyography (Table 18.2). The most common adverse effect, which occurred in 15% of patients,

was a slight, transient, weakness of the third finger extension.

Essential head tremor was initially reported to improve with onabotulinumtoxinA injections into the cervical muscles in 1991 (Jankovic and Schwartz, 1991). This observation was subsequently confirmed by a double-blind, placebo-controlled study (Pahwa et al., 1995). In the study by Jankovic and Schwartz (1991), both splenius capitus muscles were injected if patients had a lateral oscillation ("no–no" tremor) of the head and one or both sternocleidomastoid muscles if they had an anterior–posterior ("yes–yes" tremor) oscillation. The average dose of onabotulinumtoxinA was 107 U (± 38). There was a 3.0 (± 1.1) improvement on a 0–4 scale with 4 indicating complete resolution of tremor. A few patients had mild transient neck weakness (9.5%) or dysphagia (28.6%). In the study by Pahwa et al. (1995), 10 patients received 40 and 60 U onabotulinumtoxinA injected into the sternocleidomastoid and splenius muscles, respectively. Each subject received placebo or onabotulinumtoxinA on separate injection visits 3 months apart. Examiner and subject ratings showed 50% versus 10% and 50 versus 30%, respectively, in improvement in tremor between onabotulinumtoxinA and placebo. Accelerometry measurements failed to demonstrate a significant difference. Side effects were also mild and transient and included neck weakness and dysphagia.

Use of BoNT has been also found to be effective in patients with voice tremor. In one study involving 27 patients with adductor spasmodic dysphonia and vocal tremor and in four patients with severe vocal tremor alone, a significant improvement in various acoustic measures was observed after thyroarytenoid and interarytenoid BoNT injections and less tremor was demonstrated in 73% of the paired comparisons (Kendall and Leonard, 2011).

Our experience with botulinum neurotoxin

As a result of long-term experience with hundreds of patients treated with BoNT for various tremors, we have modified our protocol and have markedly decreased the dosage in the forearm extensor muscles (to less than 15 U), or completely omit injections into these muscles altogether. With this modification (i.e. injecting mainly into the forearm flexor muscles), we now obtain similar benefits in terms of reduction in the amplitude of the tremor without the undesirable extensor weakness. Patients with essential tremor of the head are poorly treated with oral medications and

Table 18.2 Class I studies in botulinum neurotoxin injection for treatment of essential hand tremor

Reference	Design	Cohort size	Treatment (technique, dose)	Brand	Follow-up	Outcome (1-primary 2-secondary)	Drop outs	Adverse events
Jankovic et al. (1996)	Double-blinded, parallel, placebo controlled	25; 13 treated and 12 placebo	50 U, if no response, 100 U at 4 weeks	OnabotulinumtoxinA	16 weeks	Tremor rating physician/patient subjective rating, Sickness Impact Profile, accelerometry	1 in placebo due to pregnancy	Finger weakness, mild in 50%, moderate in 42%
Brin et al. (2001)	Double-blinded, parallel, placebo controlled	133; 43 (50 U) 45 (100 U) 45 (placebo)	Electromyography-guided into forearm muscles	OnabotulinumtoxinA	16 weeks	Tremor rating physician/patient subjective rating, Sickness Impact Profile	None	Weakness in 30% of 50 U and 70% of 100 U groups

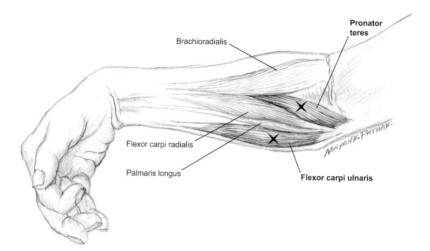

Fig. 18.1 Injection sites in the forearm.

may also benefit from BoNT injections. If the tremor is primarily a "no–no" tremor of the head, injections into the sternocleidomastoid muscles as well as the splenius capitis muscles should be considered, as opposed to the splenius capitis muscles only in a "yes–yes" tremor.

Dosages and muscles injected

We usually inject the forearm flexor muscles predominantly involved, but the flexor carpi radialis and ulnaris muscles are the muscles most frequently injected in patients with essential tremor (Fig. 18.1). The average starting dose is 25–50 U onabotulinumtoxinA/incobotulinumtoxinA, 75–150 U abobotulinumtoxinA and 1500–2500 U rimabotulinumB equally divided between the two muscles. Patients with resting hand tremor in Parkinson disease have, and patients with severe essential hand tremor may have, pronation–supination of the forearm. If present, this component of tremor may require an additional injection into the biceps brachii muscle to decrease it by weakening supination. The initial dose injected is based on the severity, but we usually start at the lower end of the range of recommended dosages.

References

Brin MF, Lyons KE, Doucette J et al. (2001). A randomized, double masked, controlled trial of botulinum toxin type A in essential hand tremor. *Neurology*, **56**, 1523–8.

Cheung MY, Shahed J, Jankovic J (2007). Malignant Tourette syndrome. *Mov Disord*, **22**, 1743–50.

Elble R, Deuschl G (2011). Milestones in tremor research. *Mov Disord*, **26**, 1096–105.

Jankovic J (1994). Botulinum toxin in the treatment of dystonic tics. *Mov Disord*, **9**, 347–9.

Jankovic J, Clarence-Smith K (2011). Tetrabenazine for the treatment of chorea and other hyperkinetic movement disorders. *Expert Rev Neurotherapeut*, **11**, 1509–23.

Jankovic J, Kurlan R (2011). Tourette syndrome: Evolving concepts. *Mov Disord*, **26**, 1149–56.

Jankovic J, Schwartz K (1991). Botulinum toxin treatment of tremors. *Neurology*, **41**, 1185–8.

Jankovic J, Schwartz K, Clemence W, Aswad A, Mordaunt JA (1996). Randomized, double-blind, placebo-controlled study to evaluate botulinum toxin type A in essential hand tremor. *Mov Disord*, **3**, 250–6.

Kendall KA, Leonard RJ (2011). Interarytenoid muscle botox injection for treatment of adductor spasmodic dysphonia with vocal tremor. *J Voice* **25**, 114–19.

Krauss JK, Jankovic J (1996). Severe motor tics causing cervical myelopathy in Tourette's syndrome. *Mov Disord*, **11**, 563–6.

Kwak C H, Hanna PA, Jankovic J (2000). Botulinum toxin in the treatment of tics. *Arch Neurol*, **57**, 1190–3.

Marras C, Andrews D, Sime E, Lang AE (2001). Botulinum toxin for simple motor tics: a randomized, double-blind, controlled clinical trial. *Neurology*, **56**, 605–10.

Pacchetti C, Mancini F, Bulgheroni M et al. (2000). Botulinum toxin treatment for functional disability induced by essential tremor. *Neurol Sci*, **21**, 349–53.

Pahwa R, Busenbark K, Swanson-Hyland EF et al. (1995). Botulinum toxin treatment of essential head tremor. *Neurology*, **45**, 822–4.

Porta M, Maggioni G, Ottaviani F, Schindler A (2004). Treatment of phonic tics in patients with Tourette's syndrome using botulinum toxin type A. *Neurol Sci*, **24**, 420–3.

Pringsheim T, Doja A, Gorman D *et al.* (2012). Canadian guidelines for the evidence-based treatment of tic disorders: pharmacotherapy. *Can J Psychiatry*, **57**, 133–43.

Scott BL, Jankovic J, Donovan DT (1996). Botulinum toxin into vocal cord in the treatment of malignant coprolalia associated with Tourette's syndrome. *Mov Disord*, **11**, 431–3.

Vincent DA Jr. (2008). Botulinum toxin in the management of laryngeal tics. *J Voice* **22**, 251–6.

WE MOVE Spasticity Study Group (2005). *BTX-A Adult Dosing Guidelines*. New York: WE MOVE (http://www.mdvu.org/classrooms/cme/CHEMD3/AdultSpastDosing.pdf, accessed 21 May 2013).

Zesiewicz TA, Elble RJ, Louis ED *et al.* (2011). Evidence-based guideline update: treatment of essential tremor: report of the Quality Standards Subcommittee of the American Academy of Neurology. *Neurology*, **77**, 1752–5.

Treatment of stiff-person syndrome with botulinum neurotoxin

Diana Richardson and Bahman Jabbari

Introduction

Stiff-person syndrome (SPS) is characterized by muscular rigidity and episodic spasms that principally involve the trunk and lower limbs. The muscle spasms are typically symmetric, more proximal in distribution and associated with an increased sensitivity to external stimuli.

The syndrome was first described by Frederick Moersch and Henry Woltman in the *Proceedings of the Staff Meeting of the Mayo Clinic* in 1956 (Moersch and Woltman, 1956). These astute clinicians eventually described a total of 14 afflicted patients who were observed over a 32-year period. Because of the magnitude of this finding and such meticulous records, the condition was also coined Moersch–Woltman syndrome, but this term is not used any more.

In the 1980s, increased levels of antibodies against glutamic acid decarboxylase (GAD; catalyzing production of gamma-aminobutyric acid from glutamic acid in the central nervous system) were isolated in patients with SPS. Since then, an association with other autoimmune diseases such as type 2 diabetes mellitus, pernicious anemia and thyroiditis has been well established. Symptoms usually begin during adult life and affect both sexes, with a slight preference towards women. Stiff person syndrome can easily be misdiagnosed, especially in the early stages. If untreated, the symptoms can become disabling (Dalakas *et al.*, 2000). Electromyography demonstrates continuous and spontaneous firing of motor units in the rigid muscles.

Clinical features

Grimaldi *et al.* (1993) described several variants of SPS. The autoimmune variant (classic) is characterized by progressive axial rigidity, predominantly involving the paraspinal and abdominal muscles; hyperlordosis of the lumbar spine; and spontaneous or stimulus-sensitive disabling muscle spasms of the abdominal wall, lower extremities and other proximal muscles. Muscle rigidity in typical SPS is attributed to dysfunction of the inhibitory interneurons of the spinal cord. These patients have a high incidence of anti-GAD and anti-islet cell antibodies (ICA) (96% with antibodies to the isoform GAD-65 and 89% with anti-islet cell antibodies in Mayo clinic series) (Walikonis and Lennon, 1998). Anti-GAD titers usually exceed 20 nmol/L. The muscle rigidity partially responds to high doses of diazepam and/or baclofen.

The paraneoplastic and idiopathic variants typically have rigidity that mainly involve the limbs. Patients have other central nervous system symptoms, and their response to diazepam and baclofen is less favorable. Elevations in anti-GAD titers in the serum or cerebrospinal fluid are less common or absent. The presence of other autoantibodies such as for amphiphysin may be found.

About 35% of patients with SPS have the idiopathic variant. These patients have no evidence of antibodies and SPS is not associated with other identifiable diseases. Subgroups of atypical SPS (SPS-Plus) have also been reported by Brown and Marsden (1999). At least three variants of SPS-Plus have been identified:

Progressive encephalomyelitis with rigidity. These patients demonstrate additional brainstem and long tract signs, cognitive changes and cerebrospinal fluid pleocytosis. Rigidity and dystonic posturing involves one or more limbs, and some patients have myoclonus. The pathology is an encephalomyelitis that primarily involves the gray matter. The muscle rigidity seems to be related to the release of inhibitory influence of interneurons on alpha motor neurons (alpha rigidity).

Manual of Botulinum Toxin Therapy, 2nd edition, ed. Daniel Truong, Mark Hallett, Christopher Zachary and Dirk Dressler. Published by Cambridge University Press. © Cambridge University Press 2013.

Jerky stiff-man syndrome. This variant is characterized by prominent brainstem signs and florid brainstem myoclonus in addition to symptoms of SPS. Muscle spasms can compromise respiration and prove fatal. Encephalomyelitis or paraneoplastic syndromes are pathological conditions associated with this variant.

Stiff-limb syndrome. Rigidity and painful spasms of the limbs are typical for this variant. Anti-GAD antibodies are positive in only 15% of patients but there is a high incidence of rheumatoid factor and autoantibodies (Barker *et al.*, 1998). Patients with carcinoma of the breast or lung (oat cell) may develop stiff-limb syndrome with high titers of anti-amphiphysin (Saiz *et al.*, 1999).

Paraneoplastic SPS tends to involve the upper limbs, neck and cranial nerves (Espay and Chen, 2006). Coexistence of other paraneoplastic conditions such as myelitis has been reported (Chamard *et al.*, 2011). Electromyography usually shows abnormally synchronous discharge of motor units both in low (6–12 Hz) and higher frequencies, a finding which is not seen in typical SPS.

Conventional treatment

In typical SPS, diazepam 5–200 mg daily, clonazepam 2.5–10 mg daily and baclofen 5–60 mg daily (alone or in combination) offer some relief of rigidity and muscle spasms (Gordon *et al.*, 1967; Barker *et al.*, 1998). Patients with high anti-GAD antibodies, rigidity and muscles spasms may respond to intravenous immunoglobulin treatment (Dalakas *et al.*, 2001). Anecdotal reports claim response to plasmaphoresis or steroid and other immunomodulator therapy.

Botulinum neurotoxin treatment

Treatment of the rigidity of SPS with botulinum neurotoxins (BoNTs) is based on several factors:

- BoNTs block the release of acetylcholine from presynaptic vesicles, which directly leads to muscle relaxation and reduction of spasms
- BoNTs decrease discharge of muscle spindles, the main reporters of muscle stretch to the central nervous system; this reduction can reduce spinal cord excitability
- BoNTs reduce exocytosis of substance P and glutamate, substances with potential for enhancing muscle spasms.

Anatomy of low-back paraspinal muscles

Because typical SPS often involves axial and paraspinal muscles usually in the thoracolumbar area, it is essential to understand the anatomy of these muscles for a successful treatment response. In the low-back area, the paraspinal muscles are arranged at different levels. The most superficial muscles, erectors of the spine, are long powerful muscles that receive innervation from multiple segments of the spinal cord. These muscles can be felt under the skin and contribute to the board-like appearance of the back area in SPS. The three components of spinal erectors, spinalis (medial), longissimus (middle) and iliocostalis (lateral) with attachments to cervical and thoracic vertebrae fuse and make a large single muscle mass (erector spinae) at the level of the upper lumbar region. This single mass of three muscles in the lumbar area ends in a strong tendon that attaches to the sacrum and to the medial surface of the iliac bone (Fig. 19.1).

On the lower end, some of the fibers of erector spinae are continuous with those of the multifidus

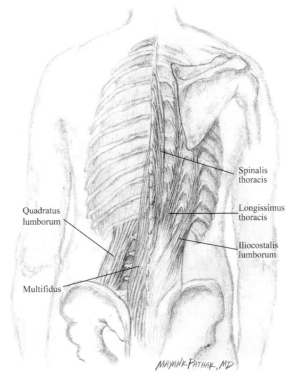

Fig. 19.1 Anatomy of low-back muscles based on *Gray's Anatomy*. As shown in the figure, the superficial erector spinae make a single mass in the lumbar region (right side).

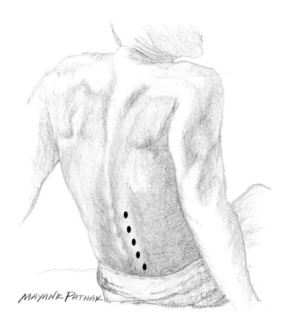

Fig. 19.2 In most individuals, the erector spinae are easily visible and palpable in the lumbar area. The figure shows the site of injections in one side (40–50 U/site). Patients with stiff-person syndrome usually require bilateral treatment.

and gluteus maximus muscles (Williams *et al.*, 1995). The multifidus muscle (Fig. 19.1) lies deep and medially to erector spinae and is made up of muscle bands (multifidii) that cross obliquely upward and attach to the whole length of the spine of each vertebrae. The lowest multifidus band is attached to sacral vertebra 4. Multifidus bands stabilize and to some degree rotate the spine. Deeper muscles such as rotatores (cervicis, thoracis and lumborum) mainly rotate the spine. Short interspinales and intertransversalis muscles are stabilizers and rotators and play an important role in maintaining posture.

Early treatment reports

Davis and Jabbari (1993) first reported significant improvement of "muscle stiffness" and painful muscle "spasms" with onabotulinumtoxinA (Botox) in a 36-year-old man who developed clinical features of typical SPS over a period of 18 months. The rigidity and painful muscle spasms involved mainly the paraspinal muscles at the T12 to L5 level. His anti-GAD antibody titers (Mayo Clinic laboratory) were 1/122 000 in serum (normal <1/120) and 1/128 (normal <1/2) in cerebrospinal fluid. Treatment with baclofen

and high-dose diazepam (100mg daily) provided only partial relief. OnabotulinumtoxinA was injected at five levels (L1–L5) into the paraspinal muscles bilaterally, 40–50 U/level for a total of 560 U. Within a week, the patient reported marked reduction in muscle spasms along with improvement of sleep and ambulation. On examination, a reduction in the board-like rigidity of paraspinal muscles was noted. Over a follow-up period of 3 years, four additional treatments of 400 U (200 U per side) maintained relief.

In a blinded study by Liguori *et al.* (1997), two patients who received onabotulinumtoxinA showed improvement of muscle rigidity and muscle spasm. The patients were 58 and 59 years of age with probable stiff-limb variant of SPS and raised anti-GAD antibodies. In one patient, a number of lower limb muscles (adductors magnus and longus, biceps femoris, tibialis posterior, gastrocnemius and soleus) were injected with doses ranging from 50 to 100 U/muscle. The second patient was injected in the trapezius, deltoid and biceps with doses of 50–300 U/muscle. Both muscle rigidity and muscle spasm showed significant improvement. The authors reported continued responsiveness with smaller doses over a 2-year follow-up period.

The Yale treatment protocol

Thoracolumbar paraspinal muscles in typical stiff-person syndrome

In typical SPS with board-like rigidity of back muscles, the superficial paraspinal muscles (erectors of the spine) in the thoracolumbar region are the main focus of treatment. Since some fibers of the erector spinae are continuous with the multifidii and glutei in the lumbosacral region, treatment of the erector spinae at this level with a sufficient dose can theoretically also affect at least a part of the deeper muscles.

OnabotulinumtoxinA is prepared with preservative-free saline to the strength 100 U/ml. For injection, the solution is drawn into a 1 ml syringe, using a 37.5 mm (1.5 inch), 27-gauge needle. It is our view that treatment of low-back spasms and rigidity in SPS should include injections at multiple sites/levels (at least five) because of the length of the erector muscles (Fig. 19.2). Furthermore, an adequate dosage at each level is needed in order to ensure sufficient lateral, longitudinal and depth spread of the solution. While there is experience

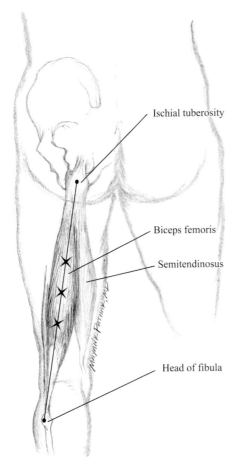

Ischial tuberosity

Biceps femoris

Semitendinosus

Head of fibula

Fig. 19.3 For hamstring spasticity, injections into biceps femoris may be made in three or more sites with a dose of 30–50 U/site.

only with onabotulinumtoxinA for SPS, there is no reason to think that other forms of toxin would not be similarly effective.

After careful inspection and palpation of the back, the silhouette of erector muscles (medial and lateral borders) can be identified in most patients without difficulty (Fig. 19.2). Injection into erector muscles is made perpendicular to the surface with the patient either in the sitting position or lying down on the stomach or side. In a thin individual, an injection to the depth of 1.9–2.5 cm (0.75–1 inch) is sufficient. In larger individuals the depth of injection varies from 2.5 cm (1 inch) to 3.75 cm (1.5 inches). Five paraspinal levels are injected on each side: 40–50 U/site (total dose per session 400–500 U). In typical SPS, the injected area usually includes L1 to L5 or T12 to L4.

Injections are performed under electromyographic guidance.

Limb muscles in stiff-limb syndrome or typical stiff-person syndrome with proximal limb rigidity

Solution preparation, syringe and needle length are the same as that described above for rigid axial/paraspinal muscles. The method of injection is similar to that currently widely used for treatment of spasticity: two to four injections in the affected muscles (Figs. 19.3 and 19.4). Some physicians use larger volumes of 2 ml (50 U/ml) or 4 ml (25 U/ml) dilution in an attempt to achieve better diffusion into the muscle with larger volumes. Comparative studies are needed to prove the merits of larger volumes. Injections are performed under electromyographic guidance.

Dosage recommendations

Table 19.1 gives dosages for treatment of the proximal rigid muscles often involved in SPS.

Side effects

Because serious side effects may happen rarely with BoNT treatment, it is prudent to obtain patient acknowledgment of the side effect list before commencing treatment. Transient muscle weakness, pain in the site of injection, focal infection and a transient low-grade flu-like syndrome may occur. We have not seen any serious side effects in treatment of a dozen patients with SPS and over 300 patients with low-back pain and spasms. Lack of weakness or gait impairment most likely reflects protection of the spine by a number of powerful deep muscles and ligaments. Furthermore, spinal erectors may not yield to weakness easily because of their exceptional long length and the multiplicity of their attachments. Nevertheless, long-term follow-up data are not available and the clinician should enquire about weakness and examine the patient carefully at each visit. Finally, repeated treatments with large doses of BoNT subject the patients to the potential to develop antibodies and non-responsiveness. In clinical practice, however, the development of non-responsiveness to onabotulinumtoxinA became rare after 1997 because of the reduced protein content of the preparation in the vial (from 25 ng to 5 ng).

Table 19.1 Dosage of onabotulinumtoxinA (Botox) used for treatment of the proximal rigid muscles often involved in stiff-person syndrome[a]

Upper limb	Dose (U)	Lower limb	Dose (U)
Biceps	50–150	Hamstring	100–200
Triceps	50–150	Rectus femoris	100–200
Brachioradialis	50–100	Gastrocnemius	100–200
Deltoid	50–100	Soleus	50–100
Trapezius	150–200	Tibialis posterior	50–150
Levator scapulae	50–100	Tibialis anterior	50–150

[a] The recommended doses are slightly higher than those commonly used for spasticity.

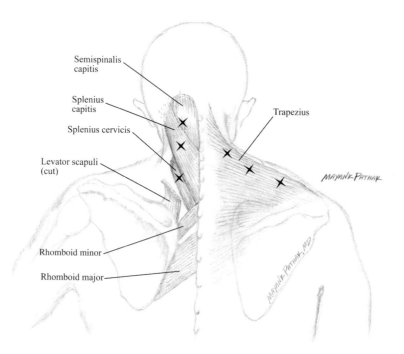

Fig. 19.4 Sites of injection in the neck and shoulder for the rigidity of stiff-person syndrome (20–30 U/site). The sites cover the trapezius muscle as well as splenius capitis and cervicis. Additional sites may be injected around the scapula if necessary to cover the levator scapula and rhomboids.

References

Barker RA, Revesz T, Thom M *et al.* (1998). A review of 23 patients with stiff man syndrome: clinical subdivision into stiff trunk (man) syndrome, stiff limb syndrome and progressive encephalomyelitis with rigidity. *J Neurol Neurosurg Psychiatry*, **65**, 633–40.

Brown P, Marsden CD (1999). The stiff man and stiff man plus syndromes. *J Neurol*, **246**, 648–52.

Chamard L, Magnin E, Berger E *et al.* (2011). Stiff leg syndrome and myelitis with anti-amphiphysin antibodies: a common physiopathology? *Eur Neurol*, **66**, 253–5.

Dalakas MC, Fuji, IM, Li M *et al.* (2000). The clinical spectrum of anti-GAD antibody-positive patients with stiff-person syndrome. *J Neurol*, **55**, 1531–5.

Dalakas MC, Fujii M, Li M *et al.* (2001). High-dose intravenous immune globulin for stiff-person syndrome. *N Engl J Med*, **345**, 1870–6.

Davis D, Jabbari B (1993). Significant improvement of stiff-person syndrome after paraspinal injections of Botulinum toxin A. *Mov Disord*, **8**, 371–3.

Espay AJ, Chen R (2006). Rigidity and spasms from autoimmune encephalomyelopathies: stiff-person. *Muscle Nerve*, **34**, 677–90.

Gordon EE, Januszko DM, Kaufman KL (1967). A critical review of stiff-man syndrome. *Am J Med*, **42**, 582–99.

Grimaldi LM, Martino G, Braghi S *et al.* (1993). Heterogeneity of autoantibodies in stiff-man syndrome. *Ann Neurol*, **34**, 57–64.

Liguori R, Cordivari C, Lugaresi E *et al.* (1997). Botulinum toxin A improves muscle spasms and rigidity in stiff-person syndrome. *Mov Disord*, **12**, 1060–3.

Moersch FP, Woltman HW (1956). Progressive fluctuating muscular rigidity and spasm ("stiff-man" syndrome); report of a case and some observations in 13 other cases. *Proc Staff Meet Mayo Clin*, **31**, 421–7.

Saiz A, Dalmau J, Butler MH *et al.* (1999). Anti-amphiphysin I antibodies in patient with paraneoplastic neurological disorders associated with small cell lung carcinoma. *J Neurol Neurosurg Psychiatry*, **66**, 214–17.

Walikonis JE, Lennon VA (1998). Radioimmunoassay for glutamic acid decarboxylase (GAD65) autoantibodies as a diagnostic aid for stiff-man syndrome and a correlate of susceptibility to type 1 diabetes mellitus. *Mayo Clin Proc*, **73**, 1161–6.

Williams PL, Bannister LH, Berry MM (eds) (1995). Muscles and fasciae of the trunk. *Gray's Anatomy*, 38th edn. Edinburgh: Churchill Livingstone, pp. 809–12.

Chapter 20

Botulinum neurotoxin applications in ophthalmology

Peter Roggenkamper and Alan Scott

Introduction

Justinus Kerner, a German medical doctor and poet, was the first to describe botulism in detail in the nineteenth century (see Chapter 1). However, it took another 150 years until botulinum neurotoxin (BoNT) was first used for therapeutic measures. This was done by Alan Scott, a co-author of this chapter, who examined a number of chemical substances in order to find one that could lengthen an extrinsic eye muscle in order to have an alternative to surgery for squint. In animal tests, BoNT proved to be the only substance that showed the desired paralytic effect and was locally and systemically well tolerated in a very low dose (Scott et al., 1973). The first patients were treated in 1978. It

is evident that this method is safe but cannot replace surgery for most patients with strabismus because the long-term effect is often not stable (Fig. 20.1).

This book illustrates that strabismus has been joined by a wide range of disorders for which BoNT has emerged as an important or even first-line treatment, in addition to cosmetic indications. Around the eye/orbit, a number of diseases can be treated with BoNT: predominantly essential blepharospasm and hemifacial spasm (Chapters 8 and 13; for both BoNT is the first choice treatment) but also to lengthen retracted lids and to overcome double vision in Graves' disease, to reduce oscillopsia and improve vision in nystagmus, to produce protective ptosis in lagophthalmos or corneal diseases, to reduce tearing through injections into the lacrimal gland, and to treat special cases of spastic entropion.

Treatment of strabismus with botulinum neurotoxin

Physical realignment of the eyes is often needed in strabismus treatment to remove diplopia and to align the eyes to allow development of binocular function, and also for cosmesis. Use of BoNT was developed as an alternative to surgery to treat small angles (Fig. 20.2), to treat infantile esotropia, to reduce antagonist contracture in acquired paralytic strabismus and

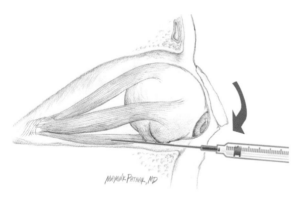

Fig. 20.1 Extraocular muscle injection.

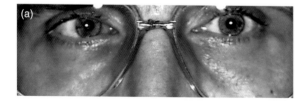
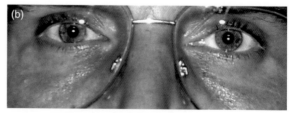

Fig. 20.2 Small angle esotropia. (a) Before treatment; (b) 3 months after botulinum neurotoxin injection of the medial rectus muscle.

Manual of Botulinum Toxin Therapy, 2ⁿᵈ edition, ed. Daniel Truong, Mark Hallett, Christopher Zachary and Dirk Dressler. Published by Cambridge University Press. © Cambridge University Press 2013.

for patients who decline surgery. In the eye muscle system, an interval of 3–4 months of reduced abnormal activity is not the goal as it is in blepharospasm and many other disorders. Instead, the induced paralysis acts to alter eye position and hence alters eye muscle lengths for a period of 2–3 months. The muscles respond to this change by sarcomeric adaptation, actual lengthening of the injected muscle and shortening of the antagonist, just as do skeletal muscles (Scott, 1994). In general, about 40% of patients are corrected to within 10 prism diopters at 1 year with one injection and about 65% corrected with an average of 1.6 injections.

Indications

Injections of BoNT in extraocular muscles are useful for both normal and restrictive strabismus.

Sixth nerve paralysis is a frequent indication: the medial rectus is injected to reduce contracture. There is often a good effect on double vision. In patients who have a good prognosis (e.g. a diabetic or hypertensive origin of the paresis), BoNT can provide earlier rehabilitation. In patients with more severe paresis where a long recovery time is anticipated, the contracture of the medial rectus and the increase of esotropia can be prevented. Functional as well as cosmetic results are available compared with those who do not receive BoNT injections. An operation such as a transposition procedure is necessary in patients with permanent paralysis, but BoNT can improve contracture of the medial rectus and thereby avoid surgical recession and its concomitant reduction of range of motion. In addition, the anterior ciliary artery supply is left intact, reducing or eliminating the problem of anterior segment ischemia.

Certain patients with third and fourth nerve paresis are also helped by BoNT injection (Mc Neer et al., 1999).

A number of strabismus specialists are treating children with infantile esotropia, acquired esotropia, intermittent exotropia and strabismus in cerebral palsy. Results approach those of surgery and the need for only brief general anesthesia is an added advantage.

In adult strabismus, BoNT injection is particularly valuable in patients who have had frequent surgery and who fear further operation without adequate long-term success. There are often rewarding results for strabismus after retinal detachment or cataract, particularly with smaller strabismic angle and normal binocular vision. Injection of BoNT is also useful as a

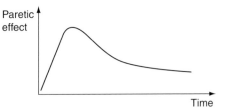

Fig. 20.3 Paretic effect of extraocular muscle injection over time. The maximum effect occurs 10–14 days after injection.

postoperative adjustment for those patients with squint when the intended goal of surgery has not been achieved or for whom further surgical procedure may threaten the vascularity of the anterior segment. Diplopia from strabismus in chronic myasthenia and in progressive external ophthalmoplegia is an additional indication. For a discussion of the place of BoNT in these specific strabismus cases, see McNeer et al. (1999).

In addition to the well-documented indications mentioned above, the authors use BoNT injection in adults who desire strabismus correction but who respond with diplopia to preoperative prism adaptation or forced duction tests. The eye position to be achieved by an operation can be temporarily tested with respect to double vision during the period of overcorrection, around 1 week after BoNT injection (Fig. 20.3). It has been shown that there is adaptation of suppression or habitation to double vision in 80% of patients (Nuessgens and Roggenkamper, 1993).

Electromyography guidance for injection

Teflon-insulated injection needles that record only from the tip localize the site of injection in active muscle. These and an electromyography (EMG) amplifier are important tools for use in eye muscle injection. Practiced injectors do well without EMG for previously unoperated medial rectus, but EMG guidance is very helpful for vertical muscles, for unusual muscle involvement (e.g. in Graves' disease) and for those who have had previous surgery. The sharp sound of individual motor units indicates correct penetration of the muscle; this is easily appreciated and differentiated from the general hum of nearby muscle. Injection under direct vision after a small conjunctival opening is also good practice. Occasionally, EMG is of use to locate muscles that have been displaced and to determine if a weak muscle is partly or wholly denervated (Figs. 20.4–20.6).

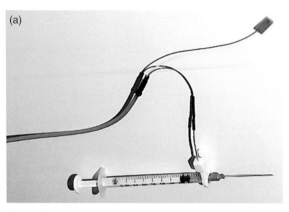

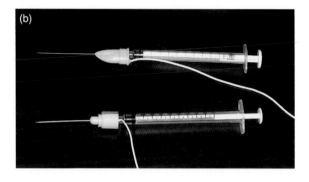

Fig. 20.4 Electromyography. (a) Bipolar wire for recording. One pole is connected to the special injection needle. (b) There are also fixed connections between the electric wire and needle that are commercially available.

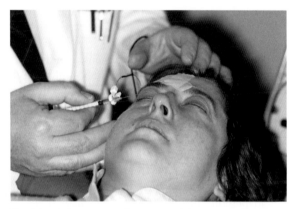

Fig. 20.5 Before injection, functioning of the equipment is tested by recording the electric activity of the orbicularis muscle.

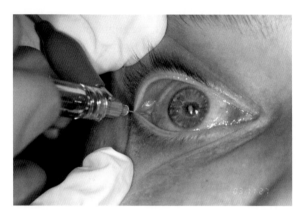

Fig. 20.6 Injection of the right lateral rectus muscle.

Dosage

For comitant strabismus of 15–30 prism diopters, the initial dose is 2.5 U onabotulinumtoxinA (Botox); for larger deviations 5.0 U onabotulinumtoxinA is used. (Other BoNT formulations could also be used, but we have less experience with them; all subsequent dosing in this chapter will also refer to onabotulinumtoxinA.) Based on the experience with other indications, a 1:1:3 relationship for onabotulinumtoxinA:incobotulinumtoxinA:abobotulinumtoxinA could be estimated but physicians should base the dose to use on personal experience. While most muscles respond well to this dosage scheme, occasionally individuals will require much more BoNT for treatment to be effective. We increase the dose by about 50% if an initial dose was inadequate as measured by the degree of induced paralysis and the resulting correction. For medial rectus injection in partial lateral rectus paresis, a dose of 1.0–1.5 U is appropriate.

The intended volume with some extra should be loaded into a 1.0 ml tuberculin syringe; the electrode needle is firmly attached and the excess fluid is ejected to assure patency of the needle and absence of leak at the needle/hub. For multiple muscles, multiple syringes are good, as it is often impossible to view the gradations on the syringe for partial volume injection. The EMG amplitude diminishes as the bolus of fluid pushes the muscle fibers away from the injection site, a sign of a good insertion. The needle is left in place 30–60 seconds after injection to allow the injection bolus to dissipate in the muscle – otherwise it can run back out the needle tract, as shown with dyed solution in animals.

Anesthesia

Proparacaine 1% drops are followed 30 seconds later by an alpha-agonist such as brimonidine tartrate ophthalmic solution (Alphagan) or epinephrine 0.1%.

Three additional proparacaine drops are placed at intervals of 1 minute. Where there is scar tissue from prior muscle surgery, injection of 100–200 μl lidocaine 2% beneath the conjunctiva is helpful.

Targeted muscles

Medial rectus

The patient gazes at a target slightly into abduction with the fellow eye. The electrode tip is inserted 8–10 mm from the limbus, avoiding blood vessels, and advanced straight back to a position behind the equator of the eye. Gaze is then slowly brought to moderate adduction to activate the muscle. The needle and syringe is rotated to keep the electrode tip in position relative to the muscle. Some muscle activity is usually heard at this point, but the needle should be advanced until a sharp motor unit sound is produced. Botulinum neurotoxin diffuses about 15 mm from the point of injection and so does not need to be placed far back in the muscle.

Lateral rectus

This is treated similarly to medial rectus, recognizing that the needle must be first directed backward behind the equator of the eye, then angled medially 40 degrees or so.

Inferior rectus

This is injected very much as for horizontal muscles. Keeping on the orbital side of the muscle to avoid penetrating the globe, the needle will often penetrate the inferior oblique. The path should be continued on through the inferior oblique, slanting medially about 23 degrees along the line of the inferior rectus. There is a step up in the orbital floor 15 mm from the orbital apex and the electrode will often hit against that – angling superiorly will put it directly in the inferior rectus. Injection through the lower lid is easier in thyroid eye disease. The electrode is inserted at the midpoint of the lid, about 8 mm from the lid margin. Penetration through the inferior oblique is usual.

Inferior oblique

The inferior oblique is injected through the conjunctiva, aiming for a point slightly temporal to the lateral border of the inferior rectus at about the equator of the eye. With the eye in far up-gaze, the inferior oblique is highly innervated and its insertion is moved forward, making the muscle accessible.

Superior rectus and superior oblique

These are seldom injected as prolonged and severe ptosis always results from diffusion of BoNT from the target muscle.

Complications and adverse outcomes

Overflow from diffusion of BoNT causes transient vertical deviation and ptosis, particularly after medial rectus injection in 5–10% of patients; in 1–2% these persist over 6 months. Undercorrection is the most frequent adverse outcome. If an earlier injection was not fully paralytic, reinjection at a higher dose can be considered. Progressive correction of large deviations is possible by multiple injections.

Bupivacaine and botulinum neurotoxin

The ability of bupivacaine to enlarge and strengthen eye muscles, used either alone or in conjunction with BoNT, with effects lasting years rather than a few months characteristic of BoNT treatment alone, has further enlarged the role of injection as a valuable treatment approach for strabismus (Scott *et al.*, 2009)

Endocrine disorders: endocrine myopathy

Although only 15% of the authors' patients achieved a permanent result, BoNT injection into the involved (thickened) eye muscles is very useful to diminish double vision and anomalous head position in patients where the angle of squint is yet not stable. After injection, the passive motility restriction becomes better and patients feel less tension around the eye. This disease is suitable for the beginner in eye muscle injection techniques because the eye muscles are thickened and easier to hit. In a number of patients, it has not been possible to get appropriate EMG signals, but even without these the injections were effective. Injection of the inferior rectus can also easily be performed transcutaneously, as mentioned above (Figs. 20.7 and 20.8).

Lid retraction in endocrine myopathy

The injection of BoNT (initially 5 or 7.5 U onabotulinumtoxinA) into the anterior part of the levator muscle and Mueller muscle is a valuable method for treatment of lid retraction in a mild or unstable situation as an alternative to the lid-lengthening operation. The transcutaneous injection

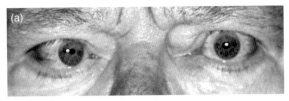

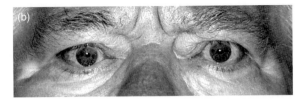

Fig. 20.7 Endocrine myopathy of the right medial rectus muscle. (a) Before treatment; (b) 3 weeks after botulinum neurotoxin injection into the affected muscle.

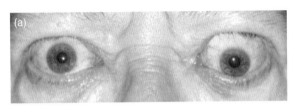

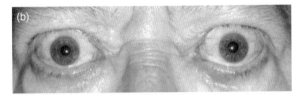

Fig. 20.8 Endocrine myopathy of the left inferior rectus muscle. (a) Before treatment; (b) 4 weeks after injection of the muscle.

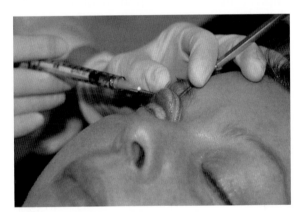

Fig. 20.9 Technique of lengthening levator and Mueller muscles in upper eyelid retraction (Graves' disease).

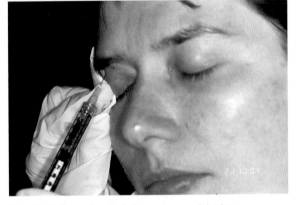

Fig. 20.10 Protective ptosis: transcutaneous injection.

technique used initially, with injection under the orbital roof similar to the technique used for protective ptosis, often gives an overeffect with ptosis. Therefore, we have proposed the following subconjunctival technique used by Uddin and Davies (2002), which gives an effect lasting around 3 months, with rare ptosis or double vision. After topical anesthesic drops, the upper lid is everted on a Desmarre retractor and an injection is made into the center of the levator aponeurosis above the upper tarsal rim; a second injection is made into the lateral third of the levator (Fig. 20.9).

Protective ptosis

Injection of BoNT into the levator palpebrae will last several months in closing the eye in order to protect the cornea or to promote corneal healing. Injection can be done through the upper lid, keeping to the

orbital roof and then angling downward until the sound of the levator is heard on the EMG, or by turning the upper lid and injecting the insertion of the levator. Paresis of the superior rectus from diffusion is variable; it is probably dose related and may be less with injection into the levator above the tarsus, as described above (Adams *et al.*, 1987; Naik *et al.*, 2008).

We always use the high amount of 20 U onabotulinumtoxinA because of some failures with less: 10 U is distributed into three sites with a 30-gauge needle transcutaneously and 10 U transconjunctively by lifting the upper lid with a Desmarre hook but not turning the lid (Figs. 20.10 and 20.11). For this application, EMG is not necessary, the effect is relatively sure to be achieved. Diplopia has not been a problem, probably because in injecting the anterior part of the levator the superior rectus was not reached or the superior rectus was only affected when the ptosis was present.

Temporary lagophthalmos

Another useful indication for BoNT injection of the levator is temporary lagophthalmos from seventh cranial nerve paresis, for example after neurosurgical intervention in the cerebellopontine angle for an acoustic neurinoma. Reinjection may be required until the facial nerve has recovered (Fig. 20.12).

Nystagmus in immobile patients

For chair- or bed-bound patients with vision of 20/80, or less the recovered ability to recognize persons, read and see TV after orbital BoNT injection can be very dramatic. It is only realistic to treat one (the better) eye because it is impossible to have both sides paralyzed symmetrically without incurring double vision. Ambulation is severely compromised by the spatial

distortion of the induced paralysis so this is not practical for mild nystagmus. The syringe is loaded with 20–25 U onabotulinumtoxinA. Without EMG, the needle is inserted through the lower lid to a point behind the eye as for retrobulbar anesthesia. The injection is placed slightly low in the orbit to reduce the chance of diffusion to the levator with consequent ptosis. Injection of the horizontal muscles for apparent horizontal nystagmus will often reveal a significant residual vertical or torsional component, so orbital injection is preferred. Unlike eye muscle injections that are expected to have a long duration, orbital injection for nystagmus will require repetition at intervals of 4–6 months.

Abnormal lacrimation

Injection of the lacrimal gland with BoNT is the first choice of treatment for the abnormal lacrimation in so-called crocodile tears (i.e. excess tearing during eating) caused after proximal facial nerve injury that misroutes to the lacrimal gland the autonomic nerve fibers that originally supplied the salivary gland. Suppression of lachrimal function with BoNT is useful also in other situations with excessive tearing, such as a blocked tear duct.

At first injections were done transcutaneously. However, it has been shown that the incidence of the side effects of ptosis and incomplete lid closure is reduced by injection through the conjunctiva. The following injection technique is recommended (Meyer 1995; Riemann et al., 1999). First, topical anesthetic eye drops are applied several times; the patient gazes in the direction away from the eye to be injected and the temporal part of the upper lid is lifted by a finger so that the palpebral part of the lacrimal gland is

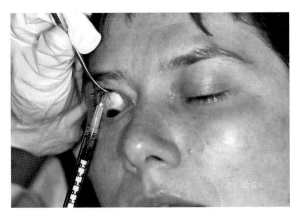

Fig. 20.11 Protective ptosis: transconjunctival injection.

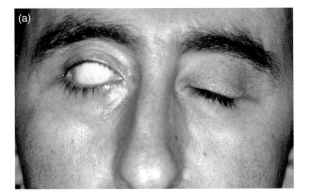
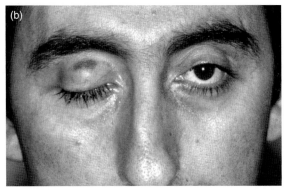

Fig. 20.12 Patient with transient lagophthalmos after surgery in the cerebellopontine angle for an acoustic neurinoma. (a) Intense Bell's phenomenon during attempt to close the eyes. (b) The patient after injection of the levator muscle.

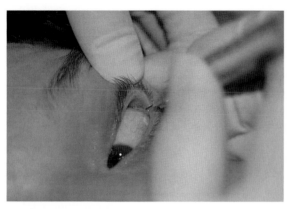

Fig. 20.13 Injection of the lacrimal gland.

visible. An injection of 2.0–2.5 U onabotulinumtoxinA is made using a 30-gauge needle directed temporarily between the secretory orifices (Fig. 20.13). The effect of this procedure lasts 4–6 months; reinjection in the same way is possible. Interestingly, the reduction of lacrimal function did not produce symptoms of dryness or corneal irritation in our patients; perhaps the accessory tear gland function is sufficient to prevent that.

Entropion

Injections of BoNT can be valuable in involutional (senile) and spastic entropion (not in cicatricial or congenital entropion). The involutional form, the most common type of entropion, results from the subcutaneous tissues and overlying skin of the lid becoming atonic and less adherent to the orbicularis muscle with age. As a result, a part of the orbicularis can override the upper end of the tarsus during lid closure and thus move the eyelashes against the cornea.

Long-term good results in this condition can be achieved by an operation. In some cases (e.g. if it is not clear if the disease will be permanent or the patient is confined long term to bed at home or in care), BoNT injections can free patients from their severe discomfort caused by the rubbing of the eyelashes on the cornea.

We follow a technique similar to that of Clarke *et al.* (1988). onabotulinumtoxinA 10–12.5 U is injected subcutaneously 3 mm in from the border of the eyelid using a very fine needle and spreading the injections over the full length of the lower lid. The beneficial effect will last around 3 months and then the easily performed procedure can be repeated again and again.

References

Adams GG, Kirkness CM, Lee JP (1987). Botulinum toxin A induced protective ptosis. *Eye*, **1**, 603–8.

Clarke JR, Spalton DJ (1988). Treatment of senile entropion with botulinum toxin. *Br J Ophthalmol*, **72**, 361–2.

McNeer KW, Magoon EH, Scott AB (1999). Chemodenervation therapy. In Rosenbaum AL, Santiago AP (eds.) *Clinical Strabismus Management*. Philadelphia, PA: Saunders, pp. 423–32.

Meyer M (1995). Krokodilstraenen und gustatorisches Schwitzen. *In Botulinum-Toxin-Forum 1995*. Hamburg: Wissenschaftsverlag Wellingsbuettel.

Naik MN, Gangopadhyay N, Fernandes M, Murthy R, Honavar SG (2008). Anterior chemodenervation of levator palpebrae superioris with botulinum toxin type-A (Botox) to induce temporary ptosis for corneal protection. *Eye*, **22**, 1132–6.

Nuessgens Z, Roggenkamper P (1993). Botulinum toxin as a tool for testing the risk of postoperative diplopia. *Strabismus*, **1**, 181–6.

Riemann R, Pfennigsdorf S, Riemann E, Naumann M (1999). Successful treatment of crocodile tears by injection of botulinum toxin into the lacrimal gland: a case report. *Ophthalmology*, **106**, 2322–4.

Scott AB (1994). Change of eye muscle sarcomeres according to eye position. *J Pediatr Ophthalmol Strabismus*, **31**, 85–8.

Scott AB, Rosenbaum AL, Collins C. C (1973). Pharmacologic weakening of extraocular muscles. *Invest Ophthalmol*, **112**, 924–7.

Scott AB, Miller JM, Shieh KR (2009). Treating strabismus by injecting the agonist muscle with bupivacaine and the antagonist with botulinum toxin. *Trans Am Ophthalmol Soc*, **107**, 104–9.

Uddin JM, Davies PD (2002). Treatment of upper eyelid retraction associated with thyroid eye disease with subconjunctival botulinum toxin injection. *Ophthalmology*, **109**, 1183–7.

Chapter 21

Cosmetic uses of botulinum neurotoxins

Joshua Spanogle, Dee Anna Glaser and Christopher Zachary

The injection of botulinum neurotoxin (BoNT) for cosmetic purposes is the most commonly performed cosmetic procedure in the USA, with 4 million such procedures performed in 2011 alone (American Society for Aesthetic Plastic Surgery, 2011).

With time, overlying skin loses both its elasticity and thickness. This, coupled with repeated pleating and contraction of the skin over many years, will result in wrinkles. Cosmetically, the primary function of BoNT is to paralyze the muscles of facial expression. By relaxing the relevant underlying muscles of facial expression, BoNT will eliminate the so-called "dynamic" rhytids (wrinkles). Over time, even the appearance of static rhytids may be improved. In a 2007 study, patients reported looking 3 years' younger than baseline 4 weeks after receiving BoNT to the upper face (Carruthers and Carruthers, 2007)

Currently (2012), there are three BoNT type A (BoNT-A) formulations with a cosmetic indication available in the USA: onabotulinumtoxinA (Botox, Allergan. Irvine, CA, USA), abobotulinumtoxinA (Dysport, Ipsen, Slough, UK) and incobotulinumtoxinA (Xeomin, Merz, Frankfurt/M, Germany). All are approved for the treatment of glabellar lines.

There is no agreed upon conversion ratio for the different formulations of BoNT-A. Ratios of 2.5:1 to 5:1 for abobotulinumtoxinA:onabotulinumtoxinA (Rzany et al., 2007; Talarico-Filho et al., 2007) have been suggested, although ratios of greater than 3:1 are probably too high (Wohlfarth et al., 2008). A ratio of 1:1 for onabotulinumtoxinA:incobotulinumtoxinA (Jost et al., 2005, 2007; Oliveira de Morais et al., 2012) has been suggested. In this chapter, all dosing will be given in onabotulinumtoxinA/incobotulinumtoxinA units. Dose of abobotulinumtoxinA is given separately.

Anatomy

The primary cosmetic use of BoNT-A relies on the relaxation of various muscles of facial expression (Fig. 21.1). Many of these muscles have soft tissue attachments, investing in the dermis itself (e.g. the platysma), other muscles of facial expression (e.g. orbicularis oris to the risorius) or the superficial muscular aponeurotic system. The interconnectedness and the soft tissue attachments of many of these muscles differentiate them from the skeletal muscles, which, by definition, have bony attachments. Broadly, the action of these muscles on the overlying skin contracts the tissue for functional purposes (speaking, eating) and/or for telegraphing emotion. Rhytids generally will be perpendicular to the contraction of the muscle, although the complexity of muscle attachment will alter the contours of the wrinkles.

Treatment techniques

Botulinum neurotoxin can be reconstituted using non-preserved normal saline (per the manufacturer's recommendations) or preserved normal saline. The benzyl alcohol preservative has no negative effects on the efficacy of the BoNT and, as a benefit, provides some anesthesia to the patient upon injection (Alam et al., 2002).

The dilution of BoNT varies between injectors but is generally in the 1–5 ml range per 100 U (onabotulinumtoxinA/incobotulinumtoxinA) or 300 U (abobotulinumtoxinA). At our institution, we dilute 100 U onabotulinumtoxinA/incobotulinumtoxinA or 300 U abobotulinumtoxinA with 2.5 ml of preserved normal saline. This yields 4 U/0.1 ml onabotulinumtoxinA/incobotulinumtoxinA and 12 U/ 0.1 ml abobotulinumtoxinA, effectively standardizing

Manual of Botulinum Toxin Therapy, 2nd edition, ed. Daniel Truong, Mark Hallett, Christopher Zachary and Dirk Dressler.
Published by Cambridge University Press. © Cambridge University Press 2013.

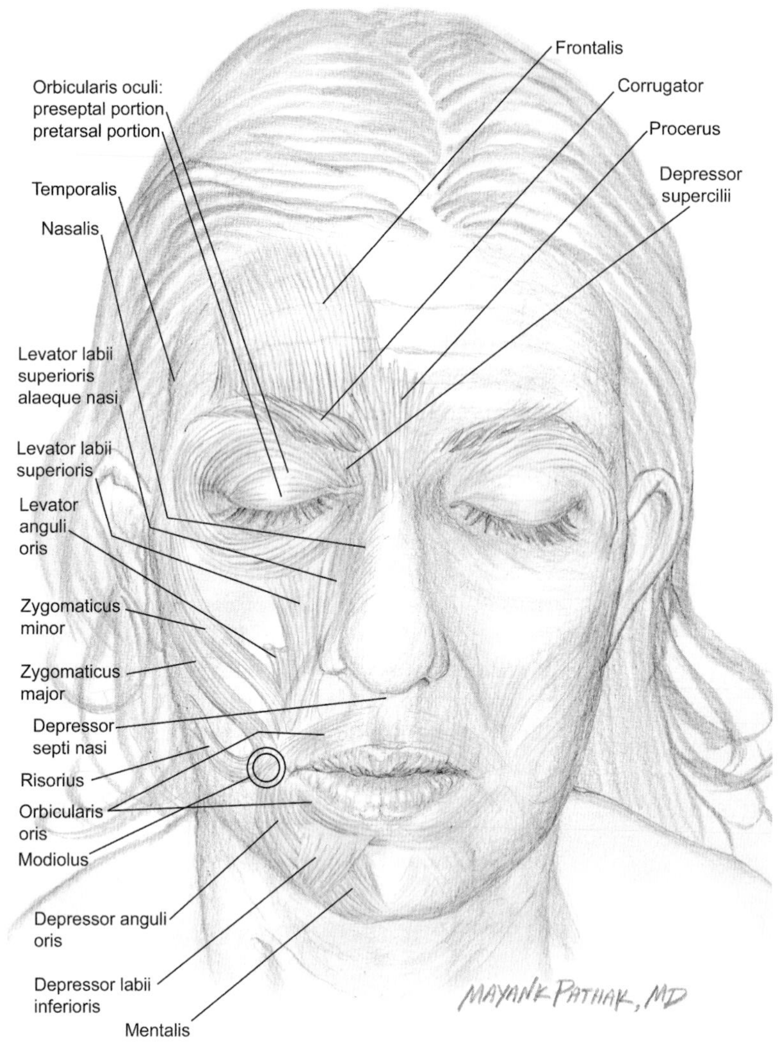

Fig. 21.1 Muscular anatomy of the face.

Frontalis

Orbicularis oculi:
preseptal portion,
pretarsal portion

Corrugator

Procerus

Depressor
supercilii

Temporalis

Nasalis

Levator labii
superioris
alaeque nasi

Levator labii
superioris

Levator
anguli
oris

Zygomaticus
minor

Zygomaticus
major

Depressor
septi nasi

Risorius

Orbicularis
oris

Modiolus

Depressor anguli
oris

Depressor labii
inferioris

Mentalis

MAYANK PATHAK, MD

the volume injected across BoNT products. This ensures an appropriate level of dosing irrespective of which BoNT product is chosen.

For a syringe, most injectors chose either a 1 ml tuberculin syringe or an insulin syringe. The 1 ml tuberculin syringe offers flexibility in needle selection for drawing up the product (e.g. an 18- or 25-gauge for a more rapid draw) and for injection (generally a 30- or 32-gauge needle). An insulin syringe offers very good injection control, a fine needle and no product left in the hub.

Ideally, to mitigate bruising, a patient would not be taking any medication to thin the blood: aspirin or other non-steroidal anti-inflammatory drug, fish oil, gingko biloba, warfarin, vitamin E, garlic. In practice,

however, it is often inconvenient or medically unwise to discontinue the medications.

In preparation for injection, the patient should be upright on the examination table or chair. The skin is cleansed with alcohol. Although topical anesthetics and ice packs are unnecessary, they can be used pre-operatively for patients who experience excessive discomfort.

Many physicians recommend the following after injection:

- contract the treated muscles periodically for 2–3 hours following injection
- *do not* bend over for 2–3 hours, for example to tie shoes or pick an object off the floor

- *do not* massage the treated area for 2–3 hours following injection
- *do not* lie down for 2–4 hours following injection
- limit heavy activity for 2–4 hours.

In practice, there is little evidence to support such recommendations.

Cosmetic uses of botulinum neurotoxin

The first step to achieving desirable results (and pleasing the patient) is a clear understanding of the patient's reason for presentation, followed by a thorough analysis of the patient's facial expression and appearance. The primary use of BoNT is to soften or eliminate dynamic rhytids – those wrinkles that deepen with movement – and, less often, for facial sculpting.

A careful analysis of the patient's face – often conducted with the patient looking into the mirror – is critical. Many, if not most, humans have facial asymmetry. This often goes unnoticed by the patient and is important to identify and to discuss with the patient. The size and strength of the target muscles needs to be assessed since this will have significant bearing on the amount of product needed. Once the patient's concerns are noted, and the facial analysis completed, a treatment strategy can be discussed.

Dynamic rhytids

Glabella

The glabellar wrinkles – those wrinkles between the eyebrows – are perhaps the most common area for injection of BoNT. The so-called "glabellar complex" or "depressor complex" comprises four muscles that pull the central brow down and in: procerus, orbicularis oculi, corrugator supercilliaris and depressor supercillii. The primary targets for BoNT are procerus and corrugator supercilliaris, but the entire depressor complex will be affected.

Prior to injection, the patient should be asked to frown, which will delineate the target muscles (Fig. 21.2). Procerus is a relatively easily identifiable muscle, the belly becoming more obvious with contraction. The bulk of the muscle generally lies between the brows, just over the nasal root. Landmarks can be of help in identifying the procerus injection site: an "X" is drawn connecting the medial eyebrows and the contralateral medial canthi (Fig. 21.3).

The corrugators extend superolaterally from the procerus, and their lateral insertion sites can usually be seen as subtle dimples above the brow in the vicinity of the mid-pupillary line. The belly of the muscle generally lies above the medial canthus. The tail (which is often treated) is located approximately 1cm above the supraorbital notch in the midpupillary line. Since the insertion of the corrugators can vary, it is important to identify the muscles themselves, and not just target a region. Furthermore, the injection site

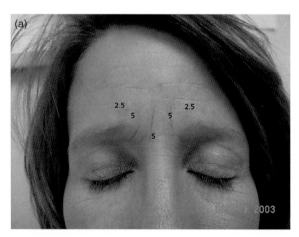

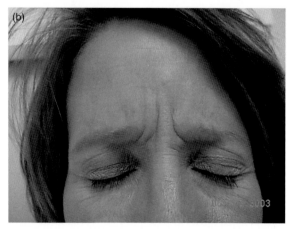

Fig. 21.2 Treatment of the glabellar complex. (a) The glabellar lines at rest. The numbers indicate the approximate units of onabotulinumtoxinA/incobotulinumtoxinA recommended; 20 U onabotulinumtoxinA/incobotulinumtoxinA (60 U abobotulinumtoxinA) were used. (b) Accentuation of the lines with frowning. (c,d) Post-treatment, the lines are diminished and the eyebrows elevated both at rest (c) and with activation (d).

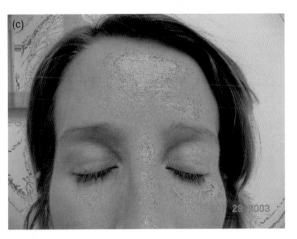
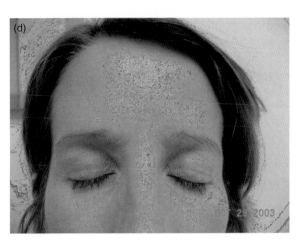

Fig. 21.2 (cont.)

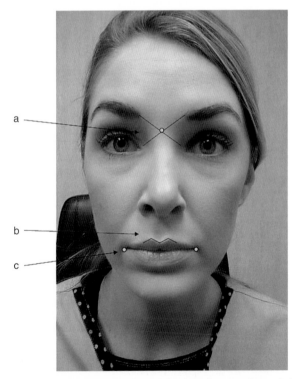

Fig. 21.3 Cosmetic landmarks. An "X" is drawn between the medial border of the eyebrow and the contralateral medial canthus (arrow a). The center of the "X" denotes the procerus muscle. The cupid's bow of the mouth is normally not injected (arrow b). The oral commissure is a landmark for locating the depressor anguli oris muscle (arrow c).

should generally be at least 1 cm above the orbital rim in order to avoid blepharoptosis.

Five injections are commonly used to treat the area: belly of procerus, right and left medial corrugator (in the belly), and right and left lateral corrugator (the tail). Altogether 30–40 U onabotulinumtoxinA/incobotulinumtoxinA (90–120 U abobotulinumtoxinA) should be used for this area. Some injectors grip procerus between the thumb and forefinger of the non-dominant hand to stabilize the muscle, distract the patient and improve accuracy. Injections of 5–10 U onabotulinumtoxinA/incobotulinumtoxinA (15–30 U abobotulinumtoxinA) are often used here. Likewise, many injectors will grab the belly of corrugator between non-dominant thumb and forefinger (Fig. 21.4), or they will release the finger and just use the non-dominant thumb on the muscle to stabilize it. Injections of 4–8 U onabotulinumtoxinA/incobotulinumtoxinA (12–24 U abobotulinumtoxinA) are often used in the belly of corrugator, 2–4 U onabotulinumtoxinA/incobotulinumtoxinA (6–12 U abobotulinumtoxinA) in the tail.

Complications can result from excessive dosage or injections placed too inferiorly, particularly in the mid-pupillary line (i.e. the region of the tail of corrugator). This can cause blepharoptosis via inferior migration of BoNT and paralysis of levator palpebrae superioris. To correct the blepharoptosis, patients can be treated with apraclonidine 0.5% eyedrops, which is an alpha-2-adrenergic agonist that causes Müller's muscle to contract (Wollina and Konrad, 2005).

Forehead

Horizontal lines in the forehead are treated by targeting the frontalis muscle. In many individuals, the central portion of the forehead above the glabellar complex is not covered by frontalis but rather by a membranous galea. In these patients, treatment of this area is not generally helpful. Frontalis is the only elevator of the upper face (brow, eyebrows, skin of the forehead). Therefore, overtreatment or incorrect targeting can lead to brow ptosis, either real or perceived.

To avoid ptosis, injections too close to the orbital rim should be avoided. Injections should be 2–3 cm above the orbital rim, and doses should be low: 2–4 U onabotulinumtoxinA/incobotulinumtoxinA (6–12 U abobotulinumtoxinA) per injection site and a total of 10–20 U onabotulinumtoxinA/incobotulinumtoxinA (30–60 U abobotulinumtoxinA) (women) or 20–30 U onabotulinumtoxinA/incobotulinumtoxinA (60–90 U

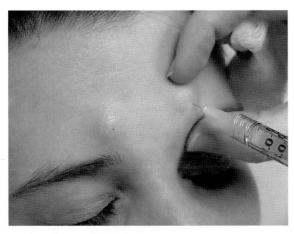

Fig. 21.4 The non-dominant thumb and forefinger are used to stabilize the target muscle. The dominant hand injects. Any erythema and distention of the skin depicted here are common following injection and are transient.

abobotulinumtoxinA) (men) total for the forehead (Fig. 21.5). Some injectors target the larger wrinkles, while others target the larger bunched muscle above or below the wrinkle. The exact amount of BoNT, as well as its placement, will be determined by the height of the forehead, the bulk of the muscle and the location of the brow at rest.

The fibers of frontalis extend laterally to the temple. If not treated adequately, a "Dr. Spock" or "comma" look can develop unilaterally or bilaterally (Fig. 21.6). Fibers of frontalis are paralyzed by 2–4 U onabotulinumtoxinA/incobotulinumtoxinA (6–12 U abobotulinumtoxinA) directed 1–2 cm above the peaked brow. If the superior fibers of frontalis are left intact, wrinkling along the hairline will mar an otherwise smooth forehead; 2 U onabotulinumtoxinA/incobotulinumtoxinA (6 U abobotulinumtoxinA) injected into the active muscle will correct the problem.

Eyes

"Crow's feet" describe the wrinkles at the lateral canthus caused by the contraction of orbicularis oculi and, to a lesser extent, the lip elevators zygomaticus major and minor and risorius. The vertically oriented fibers of orbicularis oculi are the target for BoNT in this region. Injection sites should be above the zygomatic notch to avoid affecting the zygomaticus and risorius muscles, which could cause lip ptosis. Since the fibers of orbicularis oculi are very superficial here, injection is likewise very superficial, just into the subdermal plane. Superficial, somewhat large, vessels are also common in this area; it is prudent to visualize and avoid

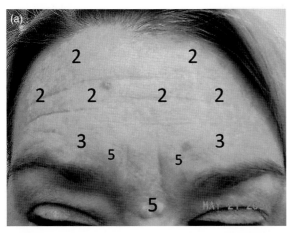
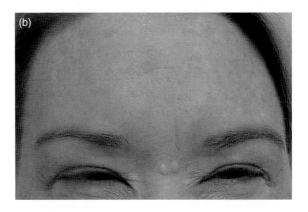

Fig. 21.5 Glabellar complex and forehead. (a) Before injection of 21 U onabotulinumtoxinA/incobotulinumtoxinA into the glabella and 12 U onabotulinumtoxinA/incobotulinumtoxinA into the frontalis. The numbers represent units of onabotulinumtoxinA/incobotulinumtoxinA and the approximate location of the injections. (b) After treatment.

the vessels in order to reduce bruising. Two to four injection points are often used, with a total of 10–15 U onabotulinumtoxinA/incobotulinumtoxinA (30–45 U abobotulinumtoxinA) injected per canthus (Fig. 21.7). We often use one injection of 8 U onabotulinumtoxinA/ incobotulinumtoxinA (24 U abobotulinumtoxinA) at the lateral eyebrow over the zygomaticofrontal suture.

Some patients have a prominent bulge with wrinkling in the infraorbital (subtarsal) area. This is secondary to the action of pretarsal fibers of orbicularis. One injection of 1–2 U onabotulinumtoxinA/incobotulinumtoxinA (3–6 U abobotulinumtoxinA) in the midpupillary line, approximately 1–2 mm below the lid margin will ameliorate the wrinkles and bulge (Figs. 21.8 and 21.9). Additionally, BoNT here tends to open the eye and produce a more almond-shaped aperture. Bruising is common in this area (Fig. 21.10), and ectropion is a risk.

Brow lift

A "furrowed" or downward brow (brow ptosis) connotes negative emotions or states: displeasure, a tired or run-down appearance. Before treating brow ptosis, it is necessary to assess brow symmetry, as an asymmetric brow is very common (Carruthers and Carruthers, 2003). After physician assessment, any brow asymmetry is demonstrated to the patient and photographed prior to injection. It is necessary to adjust the dosage of BoNT in light of the asymmetry

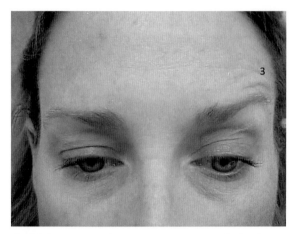

Fig. 21.6 Asymmetrically raised eyebrow following forehead injections. An additional injection of 2–3 U onabotulinumtoxinA/ incobotulinumtoxinA (6–12 U abobotulinumtoxinA) will return the brow to the desired position.

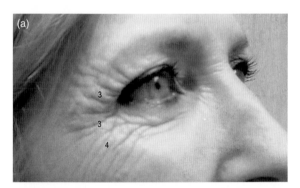

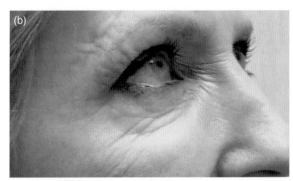

Fig. 21.7 Treatment of crow's feet. (a) Before treatment with 10 U onabotulinumtoxinA/incobotulinumtoxinA (30 U abobotulinumtoxinA). The numbers represent units of onabotulinumtoxinA/incobotulinumtoxinA used and the approximate location of the injections. (b) After treatment.

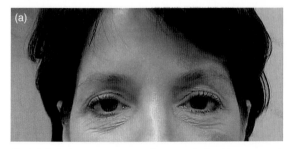

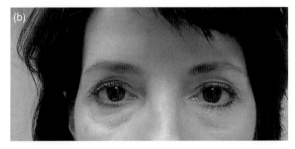

Fig. 21.8 Eyebrow asymmetry before (a) and after (b) injection of onabotulinumtoxinA to lift the brows.

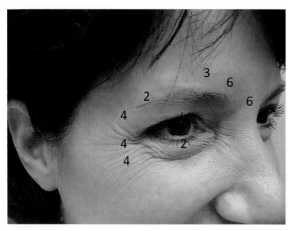

Fig. 21.9 Injection locations and units used for a brow lift and the reduction of a lower lid bulge.

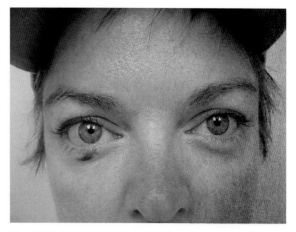

Fig. 21.10 Lower lid ecchymosis 14 days after injection of 1 U onabotulinumtoxinA/incobotulinumtoxinA (3 U abobotulinumtoxinA) in the pretarsal orbicularis oculi.

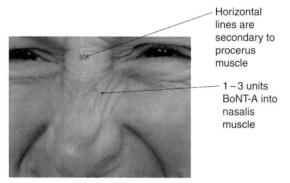

Horizontal lines are secondary to procerus muscle

1–3 units BoNT-A into nasalis muscle

Fig. 21.11 Bunny lines are produced by the nasalis muscle. Horizontal lines at the root of the nose are produced by the procerus muscle. BoNT-A, botulinum neurotoxin type A.

to avoid its perpetuation or exacerbation (Figs. 21.8 and 21.9).

Correction of brow ptosis involves treating the brow depressor muscles (glabellar complex, superolateral portions of orbicularis oculi) while maintaining the function of the elevator muscle (frontalis). As noted above, in addition to treatment of the glabella, we treat the superolateral portions of orbicularis oculi at the lateral brow over the zygomaticofrontal suture with 4–8 U onabotulinumtoxinA/incobotulinumtoxinA (12–24 U abobotulinumtoxinA). Injections of the lateral canthus (crow's feet) can also be helpful in relieving brow ptosis.

Nose

The oblique lines over the nasal dorsum ("bunny lines") are produced by the transverse action of the nasalis

muscle and are accentuated by speech, frowning and, particularly, smiling (Fig. 21.11). These lines may be present in non-treated patients or may develop after treating the glabellar complex with BoNT. Since nasalis is a very small muscle, only small doses of BoNT are needed, typically 1–3 U onabotulinumtoxinA/incobotulinumtoxinA (3–9 U abobotulinumtoxinA). The injection site is on the lateral wall of the nasal dorsum (nasal bridge) and in the subcutaneous plane. Placement is important, since levator labii superioris alaeque nasi and levator labii superioris both originate along the medial aspect of the malar prominence, and relaxation of these muscles by lateral injection of BoNT may induce upper lip ptosis.

Mouth

Small doses of BoNT can be used to rejuvenate the area around the mouth. However, optimal perioral rejuvenation usually requires more than just BoNT, for example fillers or resurfacing.

Vertical lip lines or "smoker's lines" are particularly common in women and result from repetitive contraction of the orbicularis oris muscle, from speech and particularly from pursing the lips. The permanent wrinkles that result can interfere with lipstick application, in that the lipstick runs into the lines (Fig. 21.12). Injections of 4–10 U onabotulinumtoxinA/incobotulinumtoxinA (12–30 U abobotulinumtoxinA) have been used in the upper lip and a slightly lower dose, 3–8 U onabotulinumtoxinA/incobotulinumtoxinA (9–24 U abobotulinumtoxinA), is sufficient for the lower lip. Injections should be placed 1–2 mm away

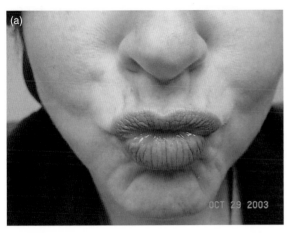
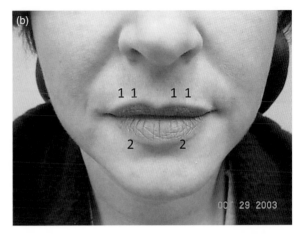

Fig. 21.12 Vertical lip lines. (a) The perioral lines can be accentuated with puckering. (b) Very small doses of botulinum neurotoxin are used to treat this area.

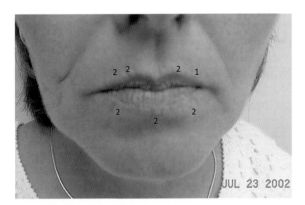
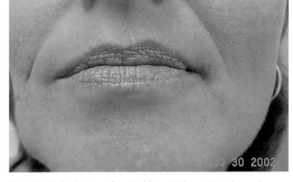

Fig. 21.13 Vertical lip lines treated with a total of 13 U onabotulinumtoxinA/incobotulinumtoxinA (39 U abobotulinumtoxinA).

Fig. 21.14 Reduction of vertical lines in the patient shown in Fig. 21.13. No fillers were used.

from the vermillion border (for patient comfort) and do not need to be placed in the lines themselves. Injecting into the lateral quarter of each lip and the cupid's bow should be avoided (Figs. 21.3, 21.13 and 21.14). Patients should be prepared for possible subtle changes in speech and word pronunciation (often not recognized by others), whih generally resolves within 2 weeks.

Frown lines or marionette lines at the corners of the mouth are another important component of the aging face, with connotations of sadness or anger. By targeting the depressor anguli oris, downturning of the corners of the mouth can be ameliorated, resulting in more neutral or upturned corners (Fig. 21.15).

Injecting into the depressor anguli oris can be moderately risky, since injection of BoNT (or its diffusion) into the more medial depressor labii inferioris can result in lower lip paralysis, which can interfere with

speech or eating. We inject into the inferiolateral aspect of the depressor anguli oris to ensure that the depressor labii inferioris is avoided. The patient is asked to frown or show his/her bottom teeth to contract the depressor anguli oris and make this triangular muscle palpable and visible. If the depressor anguli oris is not easily identifiable, injections (1–4 U onabotulinumtoxinA/incobotulinumtoxinA; 3–12 U abobotulinumtoxinA) should be made 8–10 mm lateral and 10–15 mm inferior to the lateral oral commissure (Fig. 21.13).

Chin

Chin dimpling and a prominent mental crease are caused by action of the mentalis muscle. Either 4–6 U onabotulinumtoxinA/incobotulinumtoxinA (12–18 U abobotulinumtoxinA) into the mentalis muscle at the point of chin or 2–3 U onabotulinumtoxinA/

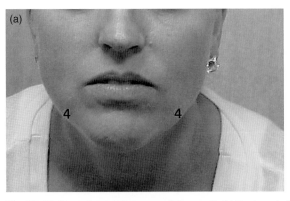

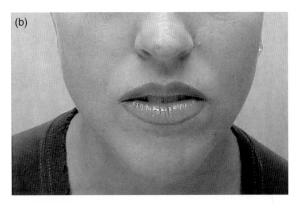

Fig. 21.15 Frown lines at the corner of the mouth. (a) Treatment of the depressor anguli oris with 1–4 U onabotulinumtoxinA/incobotulinumtoxinA (3–12 U abobotulinumtoxinA). (b) This elevates the corners of the mouth.

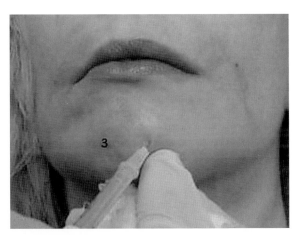

Fig. 21.16 Injection of a total of 4–6 U onabotulinumtoxinA/incobotulinumtoxinA (12–18 U abobotulinumtoxinA) into the mentalis muscle to reduce chin puckering.

incobotulinumtoxinA (6–9 U abobotulinumtoxinA) on either side of the chin can be injected. Care should be taken not to inject too much BoNT too superiorly or too laterally since the depressor labii inferioris can be affected, with consequences for speech and eating (Fig. 21.16).

Neck

Vertical neck bands (platysmal bands), sometimes inelegantly called "turkey neck," are prominent in some individuals, either at rest or with animation (Fig. 21.17). The platysma is a very superficial muscle and invests superiorly into the superficial muscular aponeurotic system. The muscle can be accentuated by having the patient show his/her bottom teeth (the same motion used to accentuate the depressor anguli

oris). Patients often have two or more prominent bands. We inject 2 U onabotulinumtoxinA/incobotulinumtoxinA (6 U abobotulinumtoxinA) every 1–2 cm along the "ridge" of the platysmal band, although other injectors will use up to 4 U onabotulinumtoxinA/incobotulinumtoxinA (12 U abobotulinumtoxinA) for each injection (Fig. 21.18). Care should be taken to inject superficially into this very superficial muscle. For patients with multiple bands, up to 40–50 U onabotulinumtoxinA/incobotulinumtoxinA (120–150 U abobotulinumtoxinA) have been used by some esthetic physicians. However, higher doses can result in neck weakness (from diffusion to the neck's strap muscles) and even in trouble swallowing.

Horizontal neck lines can be treated with BoNT, but the results are often suboptimal.

Facial sculpting and mandibular contouring

A square jaw widens the lower face and is generally considered a masculine trait. Although a square jaw can be the result of bony anatomy, it is often caused by hypertrophy of the masseter. Use of BoNT can reduce masseteric hypertrophy and return the face to a more oval (feminine) shape. Reductions of 10–38% in masseter volume or a mean decrease in thickness of up to 2.9 mm have been reported (To et al., 2001; Park et al., 2003; Choe et al., 2005; Gaofeng et al., 2010) (Fig. 21.19).

To identify the optimal injection site(s), the patient is asked to clench his/her teeth, which will accentuate the thickest part of the masseter. Doses of 10–50 U may be required. In our practice, we inject 10 U onabotulinumtoxinA/incobotulinumtoxinA (30 U

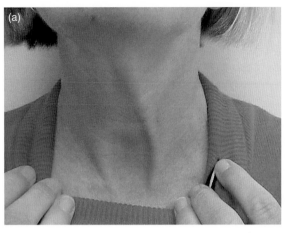
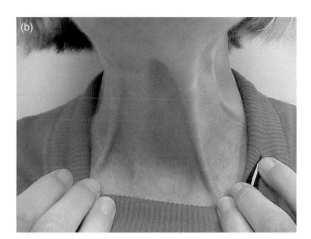

Fig. 21.17 Platysmal bands at rest (a) and with animation (b).

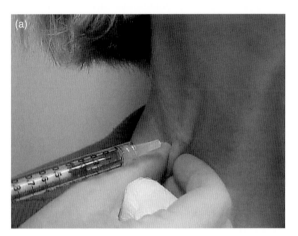
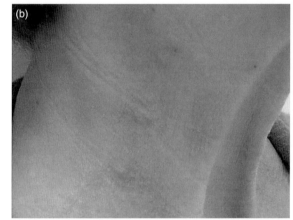

Fig. 21.18 Injection of the platysmal muscle. (a) The superficial platysma muscle is held with the non-dominant hand and 2–4 U onabotulinumtoxinA/incobotulinumtoxinA (6–12 U abobotulinumtoxinA) is injected every 1–2 cm. (b) After treatment.

abobotulinumtoxinA) into each masseter, with a total of 20 U onabotulinumtoxinA/incobotulinumtoxinA (60 U abobotulinumtoxinA) injected. We inject deep into the belly of the muscle. A few patients experience pain at the injection site 1–3 days after injection, which can be improved by the use of ice.

Over time, the jawline can obscure by the downward action of the platysma on the lower face, causing a "sagging" or "droopy" appearance. Weakening of the fibers of the platysma along the jawline releases their depressor action, allowing for unopposed elevation by the levators of the mid face. Defining the jawline in this way has been termed the "Nefertiti lift" (Levy, 2007; Gassia *et al.*, 2009) Injections of 2–3 U onabotulinumtoxinA/incobotulinumtoxinA (6–9 U abobotulinumtoxinA) should be made just under the mandible at 1–2 cm intervals, starting at the angle of the jaw and progressing anteriorly to the lateral border of depressor anguli oris (Fig. 21.20). The effects are generally longer lasting than with injections into the mid or upper face and can be particularly pronounced with injection of the platysmal bands. As with injection of the platysmal bands, care should be taken not to use excessive doses as this could result in dysphagia and neck weakness.

Side effects of botulinum neurotoxin

Adverse effects are uncommon when BoNT is injected correctly by an experienced physician. Side effects depend on the location of the injection, the patient's particular anatomy and the amount of BoNT injected. It is important to note that the injected BoNT can diffuse beyond the injection site (up to 2.7 cm in some trials; Cliff *et al.*, 2008), depending on the exact formulation of the BoNT and the volume injected.

Adverse events of short duration are:

- mild pain with injection
- headache (transient, often lasting 4–8 hours)

- bruising
- asymmetry
- focal twitching
- mild nausea (vasovagal response).

Adverse effects of longer duration, often technique dependent, are:

- blepharoptosis: injections too low in the mid-pupillary line
- brow ptosis: excessive product in the superior brow

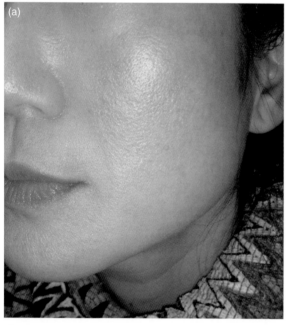
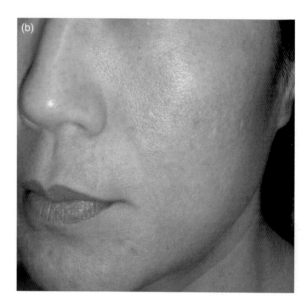

Fig. 21.19 Masseteric hypertrophy. (a) OnabotulinumtoxinA used to reduce masseter volume. (b) Four weeks after one injection of 20 U in total shows a more oval lower face.

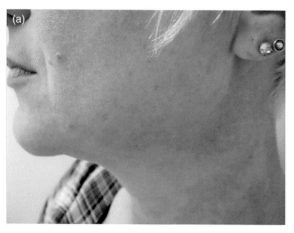
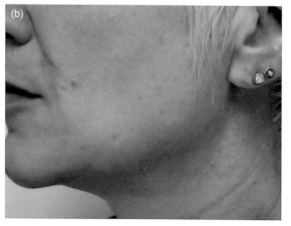

Fig. 21.20 The "Nefertiti lift." At rest, before (a) and after (b) and while contracting the platysma, before (c) and after (d). Note the more defined jawline. (Images courtesy of Dr. Phillip Levy.)

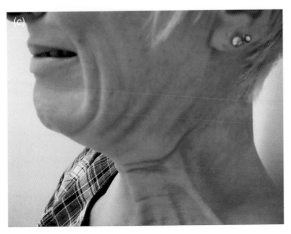
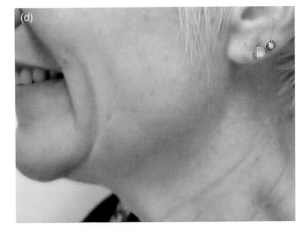

Fig. 21.20 (cont.)

- diplopia: leaking of product to the intraocular muscles
- decreased tearing and xerophthalmia: injection too medial in the lower lid
- ectropion: excessive product into the lower lid
- lagophthalmus: excessive product in the periocular area
- oral incompetence: excessive product in the perioral area
- decreased neck strength: excessive product in the platysmal area
- dysphagia: excessive product in the platysmal area.

Adverse immediate hypersensitivity reactions are extremely uncommon, but are:

- urticaria
- dyspnea
- angioedema
- anaphylaxis.

References

Alam M, Dover J, Arndl K (2002). Pain associated with injection of botulinum A exotoxin reconstituted using isotonic sodium chloride with and without preservative. *Arch Dermatol*, **138**, 510–14.

American Society for Aesthetic Plastic Surgery (2011). *Cosmetic Surgery National Data Bank. 2011*. New York: American Society for Aesthetic Plastic Surgery (http://www.surgery.org/media/statistics, accessed 17 May 2013).

Carruthers J, Carruthers A (2003). *Using Botulinum Toxins Cosmetically*. London: Martin Dunitz, pp. 17–32.

Carruthers J, Carruthers A (2007). Botulinum toxin type A treatment of multiple upper facial sites: patient-reported outcomes. *Dermatol Surg*, **33**(Suppl 1), S10–17.

Choe SW, Cho WI, Lee CK, Seo SJ (2005). Effects of botulinum toxin type A on contouring of the lower face. *Dermatol Surg*, **31**, 502–7; discussion 507–8.

Cliff SH, Judodihardjo H, Eltringham E (2008). Different formulations of botulinum toxin type A have different migration characteristics: a double-blind, randomized study. *J Cosmet Dermatol*, **7**, 50–4.

Gaofeng L, Jun T, Bo P *et al.* (2010). Evaluation and selecting indications for the treatment of improving facial morphology by masseteric injection of botulinum toxin type A. *J Plast Reconstr Aesthet Surg*, **63**, 2026–31.

Gassia V, Beylot C, Bechaux S, Michaud T (2009). Botulinum toxin injection techniques in the lower third and middle of the face, the neck and the decollete: the "Nefertiti lift". *Ann Dermatol Venereol*, **136**(Suppl 4), S111–18.

Jost WH, Kohl A, Brinkmann S, Comes G (2005). Efficacy and tolerability of a botulinum toxin type A free of complexing proteins (NT 201) compared with commercially available botulinum toxin type A (BOTOX) in healthy volunteers. *J Neural Transm*, **112**, 905–13.

Jost WH, Blümel J, Grafe S (2007). Botulinum neurotoxin type A free of complexing proteins (XEOMIN®) in focal dystonia. *Drugs.* **67**, 669–83.

Levy PM (2007). The "Nefertiti lift": a new technique for specific re-contouring of the jawline. *J Cosmet Laser Ther*, **9**, 249–52.

Oliveira de Morais O, Matos Reis-Filho E, Vilela Pereira L, Martins Gomes C, Alves G (2012). Comparison of four botulinum neurotoxin type a preparations in the treatment of hyperdynamic forehead lines in men: a pilot study. *J Drugs Dermatol*, **11**, 216–19.

Park MY, Aim KY, Jung DS (2003). Botulinum toxin type A treatment for contouring the lower face. *Dermatol Surg*, **29**, 477–83.

Rzany BD, Dill-Muller D, Grablowitz D Heckmann M, Daird D (2007). Repeated botulinum toxin A injections for the treatment of lines in the upper face: a retrospective study of 4103 treatments in 945 patients. *Dermatol Surg*, **33**(Suppl 1), S18–25.

Talarico-Filho S, Nascimento MM, De Macedo FS, De Sanctis Pecora C (2007). A double-blind, randomized, comparative study of two type A botulinum toxins in the treatment of primary axillary hyperhidrosis. *Dermatol Surg*, **33**(Suppl 1), S44–50.

To EW, Ahuja AT, Ho WS, *et al.* (2001). A prospective study of the effect of botulinum toxin A on masseteric muscle hypertrophy with ultrasonographic and electromyographic measurement. *Br J Plast Surg*, **54**, 197–200.

Wohlfarth K, Schwandt I, Wegner F *et al.* (2008). Biological activity of two botulinum toxin type A complexes (Dysport and Botox) in volunteers: a double-blind, randomized, dose-ranging study. *J Neurol*, **255**, 1932–9.

Wollina U, Konrad H (2005). Managing adverse events associated with botulinum toxin type A: a focus on cosmetic procedures. *Am J Clin Dermatol*, **6**, 141–50.

Hyperhidrosis

Henning Hamm and Markus K. Naumann

Introduction

Hyperhidrosis may generally be defined as excessive sweating or sweating beyond physiological needs. It may be divided into generalized, regional and localized/focal types and, according to whether the cause is known or not, into primary/idiopathic and secondary forms. Secondary hyperhidrosis can be induced by a number of infectious, endocrine, metabolic, cardiovascular, neurological, psychiatric and malignant conditions; it can also be caused by certain drugs and poisoning. The prevalence of hyperhidrosis in the US population has been calculated at 2.8% (Strutton *et al.*, 2004). Of those, primary axillary hyperhidrosis appears to be the most frequent type, severely affecting 0.5%.

Box 22.1 gives the diagnosis of primary focal hyperhidrosis set out by a multispecialty working group (Hornberger *et al.*, 2004). It usually starts in childhood or adolescence and mainly involves the armpits, palms, soles and craniofacial region, either alone or in various combinations. There are well-known, particularly emotional, triggers of sweating episodes, but the exact pathogenesis of the sympathetic overstimulation of eccrine sweat glands is still poorly understood apart from a clear genetic background.

As measured by standardized questionnaires, primary focal hyperhidrosis negatively affects many fields of daily life to a significant extent, including emotional status, personal hygiene, work and productivity, leisure activities and self-esteem (Hamm *et al.*, 2006). The so-called Hyperhidrosis Disease Severity Scale (HDSS) (Box 22.2), a single-item question allowing four gradations of the tolerability of sweating and its interference with daily activities, offers a simple and useful way to estimate the impairment of quality of life (Lowe *et al.*, 2007).

History taking is the most important tool in the diagnosis of primary focal hyperhidrosis and the exclusion of secondary types. Physical examination should focus on visible evidence of excessive sweating in the characteristic locations and on detection of signs that suggest a secondary cause. Laboratory tests are not needed if the presentation is characteristic and if evidence of secondary causes is lacking. In contrast, generalized forms of sweating and asymmetric patterns have to be evaluated for underlying disorders (Hornberger *et al.*, 2004). Gravimetric quantification of sweat production in predominantly involved sites is not routinely performed but may be helpful to support the diagnosis, to rate the severity and in clinical research. Minor's iodine–starch test is used to outline the sweating area prior to botulinum neurotoxin (BoNT) treatment or local surgery (see below).

Conventional treatment options

There are a large number of treatment options for primary focal hyperhidrosis, the utility of which partly depends on the site involved (Hoorens and Ongenae, 2012).

When seeking medical advice, most patients with primary axillary hyperhidrosis have already tried over-the-counter antiperspirants without success. The majority of them, particularly those with mild to moderate hyperhidrosis, can be treated effectively with topical aluminum chloride salts, which mechanically obstruct the sweat gland ducts. We prefer aluminum chloride hexahydrate 15% in aqueous solution thickened with methylcellulose (aluminum chloride hexahydrate 15 ml, methylcellulose 1.5 ml, distilled water to 100 ml) and bottled in a roll-on flask; others recommend absolute alcohol or salicylic acid gel as base for the preparation. To minimize skin irritation, the solution should be applied to dry, clean armpits at bedtime and washed off after getting up in the morning. Initially, it is used every other evening until

Manual of Botulinum Toxin Therapy, 2nd edition, ed. Daniel Truong, Mark Hallett, Christopher Zachary and Dirk Dressler. Published by Cambridge University Press. © Cambridge University Press 2013.

Box 22.1 Diagnostic criteria of primary focal hyperhidrosis

Focal, visible, excessive sweating of at least 6 months duration without apparent cause with at least two of the following characteristics:

- bilateral and relatively symmetric sweating
- impairment of daily activities
- frequency of at least one episode per week
- age of onset less than 25 years
- positive family history
- cessation of focal sweating during sleep

From Hornberger *et al.* (2004).

Box 22.2 Hyperhidrosis Disease Severity Scale

Question: How would you rate the severity of your sweating?

1. Sweating is never noticeable and never interferes with daily activities
2. Sweating is tolerable and sometimes interferes with daily activities
3. Sweating is barely tolerable and frequently interferes with daily activities
4. Sweating is intolerable and always interferes with daily activities

Note: only severity scores of 3 and 4 should be assigned to true hyperhidrosis.
From Lowe *et al.* (2007).

euhidrosis is achieved. The frequency of application can often be tapered to once every 1–3 weeks to maintain the effect. Continued treatment may even lead to atrophy of the secretory cells. If ineffective, every evening application or higher concentrations may be tried, but this will often not be tolerated by the patient. In contrast, the irritative potential of aluminum chloride salts is less severe on palms and soles and so concentrations may possibly be increased to 25–35%. Nevertheless, this treatment has proved less potent and less feasible in other than the axillary region.

Tap water iontophoresis using direct current or direct plus alternating current is regarded as the most effective non-invasive therapy for palmar and plantar hyperhidrosis. Iontophoresis is thought to work by transient disruption of ion transport in the sweat gland, but its exact mode of action is unclear. Hands or feet are placed in a shallow basin filled with tap water through which an electric current at 15–20 mA is passed for 15–30 minutes. Initially, patients undergo five to seven treatments per week, and six to ten treatments are usually required to achieve euhidrosis. Side effects include burning, tingling ("pins and needles"), irritation, erythema, skin dryness, transient paresthesia and rarely vesicles. Such reactions are best prevented by petrolatum. To maintain the effect, regular sessions about once or twice a week are necessary, which is why many patients refrain from continuation of the time-consuming procedure. The method is less practical for axillary hyperhidrosis and it is contraindicated in pregnancy and in patients with a pacemaker or metal implant.

Oral anticholinergic drugs such as methantheline bromide, propantheline bromide and bornaprine are able to suppress sweating for a short time but their effect is often accompanied by side effects, such as dry mouth, blurred vision, dizziness, urinary retention and constipation. Glycopyrrolate, oxybutynin, quetiapine, diazepam, amitriptyline, beta-blockers, diltiazem, clonidine, gabapentin and indomethacin are further oral agents that have been tried in a limited number of patients with hyperhidrosis, with variable success.

Surgery can be offered as a last choice in severe cases. Various techniques of local elimination or destruction of sweat glands have been proposed to treat axillary hyperhidrosis. En bloc excision of the entire sweating area as the simplest and most effective method has largely been abandoned since it inevitably leads to large unsightly scars. Nowadays, curettage, liposuction and combined techniques (suction curettage) performed under local or tumescent local anesthesia are favored as they have far better cosmetic results. However, bleeding, hematomas, seromas, wound infection, skin necrosis, prolonged wound healing, paresthesiae, prominent scars and wound contractures interfering with arm mobility are possible complications, and only about 70% of patients benefit from these local procedures in the long run. Microwave devices causing irreversible thermolysis of eccrine sweat glands at the interface between skin and subcutaneous tissue are an evolving treatment option that deserves further research (Glaser *et al.*, 2012).

Endoscopic thoracic sympathectomy interrupts the transmission of sympathetic nerve impulses from ganglia to nerve endings and is the most efficient but also the most invasive method to treat focal hyperhidrosis. Usually, thoracic sympathetic ganglia T_3 and T_4 are destroyed or cut through by electrocautery for

Box 22.3 Treatment algorithm for primary axillary hyperhidrosis

Treatment progresses from 1 to 4 based on success at each stage.

1. Topical over-the-counter antiperspirants
2. Topical aluminum chloride hexahydrate 10–15%
3. Intradermal injections of botulinum neurotoxin type A
4. Topical sweat gland resection by curettage or liposuction techniques

Source: adapted with permission from Hornberger *et al*. (2004).

Box 22.4 Treatment algorithm for primary palmar hyperhidrosis

Treatment progresses from 1 to 4 based on success at each stage.

1. Topical aluminum chloride 20–35% or tap water iontophoresis
2. Intradermal injections of botulinum neurotoxin type A
3. Endoscopic thoracic sympathectomy

Source: adapted with permission from Hornberger *et al*. (2004).

treatment of palmar hyperhidrosis and, in addition, T_2 in craniofacial hyperhidrosis. In about 98% of patients with palmar hyperhidrosis, immediate complete anhidrosis occurs, with only low rates of recurrence; the results in axillary hyperhidrosis are less convincing. Acute and early complications are rare but include bleeding; hemo-, pneumo- and chylothorax; pleural adhesion or effusion; neuralgia; and complete or incomplete Horner's syndrome. However, compensatory sweating mainly of the back, abdomen and legs develops regularly some weeks to months after surgery, as well as gustatory sweating, in up to half of the patients. Incapacitating compensatory sweating is claimed by about 5–10% of patients. Therefore, endoscopic thoracic sympathectomy should be reserved for patients with severe palmar hyperhidrosis who have not responded to any other treatments available.

Treatment algorithms for primary axillary and primary palmar hyperhidrosis worked out in an international consensus conference are presented in Boxes 22.3 and 22.4, respectively (Hornberger *et al*., 2004).

Botulinum neurotoxin therapy

At the turn of this century, BoNT type A (BoNT-A) evolved as a novel, minimally invasive therapeutic modality for focal hyperhidrosis. When injected intradermally, the neurotoxin blocks the release of acetylcholine from the sympathetic nerve fibers that stimulate eccrine sweat glands and causes a localized, long-lasting but reversible abolishment of sweating.

Use of BoNT-A has been evaluated most extensively in primary axillary hyperhidrosis. Three large randomized, placebo-controlled, double-blind studies and numerous open-label studies clearly document

its effectiveness and safety in this indication. In a European study enrolling 320 patients, 94% of patients treated with 50 U onabotulinumtoxinA per axilla were treatment responders at week 4 (>50% reduction in sweat production from baseline gravimetric measurement), with an average reduction in sweat production of 83.5% (Naumann and Lowe, 2001). In a 12-month follow-up study, 207 of these patients received up to three further BoNT-A injections. Response rates and satisfaction with treatment remained consistently high with no diminution of effect and no confirmed positive results for neutralizing antibodies to BoNT-A with repeated treatments (Naumann *et al*., 2003). Mean duration of benefit was about 7 months after a single treatment and 28% of patients did not require more than one injection, indicating a long-lasting benefit of at least 16 months. No major side effects occurred, with subjective increase in non-axillary sweating perceived by 4% of the patients being the most frequent complaint. Treatment with BoNT-A also markedly improved the quality of life of patients (Naumann *et al*., 2002).

In a multicenter North American trial in 322 patients comparing 50 U onabotulinumtoxinA per axilla with 75 U onabotulinumtoxinA per axilla and placebo, responders were defined as having at least a 2-grade reduction in their HDSS score. There was a 75% response rate in the treatment groups compared with a 25% response rate in the placebo-treated patients, but without significant difference between the groups treated with different onabotulinumtoxinA doses (Lowe *et al*., 2007). In the treatment groups, 80–84% had at least a 75% reduction in sweat production, compared with only 21% in the placebo group. Median duration of the BoNT-A effect was again approximately 7 months. These studies led to the licensing of Botox (onabotulinumtoxinA) for axillary hyperhidrosis in many countries worldwide.

Currently, it is the only BoNT formulation licensed for use in hyperhidrosis.

A randomized, placebo-controlled, double-blind study in 145 German patients with one axilla being treated with either 100 or 200 U abobotulinumtoxinA and the contralateral one with placebo obtained similar results with regard to efficacy and safety (Heckmann *et al.*, 2001). A significant decrease in sweat production compared with placebo was observed after 2 weeks and maintained 24 weeks after injection. The two doses proved equally effective in reducing axillary sweating.

So far, only one single-center study on the effect of the novel BoNT-A preparation incobotulinumtoxinA has been performed in hyperhidrosis. Double-blind, intraindividual side-to-side comparison of 50 U onabotulinumtoxinA and 50 U incobotulinumtoxinA in 46 patients showed no differences in onset, extent and duration of effect, as evaluated by patient and physician (Dressler, 2010). Of note, the decrease in sweat production was not assessed by gravimetrical assessment.

There are a number of smaller controlled and observational studies showing that BoNT-A (onabotulinumtoxinA, abobotulinumtoxinA) is also a valuable treatment option in palmar hyperhidrosis (Saadia *et al.*, 2001; Simonetta Moreau *et al.*, 2003). However, treatment is more complex, injections are considerably more painful, higher doses are needed, and the effect is less pronounced and less long-lasting than in axillary hyperhidrosis.

Reduction or elimination of pain during palmar injections can be achieved by median and ulnar nerve blocks performed a few centimeters proximal to the wrist. However, transient paresthesiae and the potential risk of permanent nerve damage, particularly associated with repeated treatments, are major disadvantages. In addition, patients are bothered by the sensation of disabled hands for several hours. Therefore, cryoanalgesia with ice cubes, frozen gel packs, forced cold air, liquid ethylchloride or dichlorotetrafluoroethane (Frigiderm) is preferred by most colleagues because of its convenience, low risk and minimal cost (Doft *et al.*, 2012). Precooling the hand in iced water for several minutes may have an additional benefit. Moreover, topical lidocaine cream, vibratory anesthesia, intravenous regional anesthesia (Bier block) and general sedation have been advocated to reduce or eliminate the pain.

Manufacturers generally recommend reconstitution of BoNT products in unpreserved saline. However, limited experience suggests that the use of preserved saline and solutions with local anesthetics such as lidocaine may reduce injection pain without affecting efficacy of the BoNT (Trindade de Almeida *et al.*, 2011).

The usual dose is 100 U onabotulinumtoxinA or equivalent per palm but 150 U or more may be required depending on its size. Sweating is reduced to about half the pretreatment amount, and the effect lasts about 4 months on average (Lowe *et al.*, 2002). Longer disease history seems to predict shorter duration of effect (Campanati *et al.*, 2011). Mild weakness of the intrinsic hand muscles, particularly of the thumb–index finger pinch strength, may occur in a minority of patients for up to 4–6 weeks and is usually insignificant. This most frequent side effect should be particularly pointed out to manual workers.

Injection pain and decreased hand muscle strength may be overcome by delivery of BoNT-A via iontophoresis. Two pilot studies in eight patients each showed a significant decrease of sweating in the palm treated by BoNT-A iontophoresis compared with the palm treated by normal saline iontophoresis until week 12 (Kavanagh and Shams, 2006; Davarian *et al.*, 2008). In the absence of larger studies, the relevance of this observation has to be awaited.

According to a few smaller studies injections of BoNT type B (BoNT-B) seem to be similarly effective as BoNT-A in axillary and palmar hyperhidrosis. Doses used were 2000–5000 U rimabotulinumtoxinB per axilla and 5000 U per palm. Compared with BoNT-A, side effects occur considerably more often with BoNT-B, particularly systemic adverse events, including dryness of the mouth and throat, dryness of eyes, indigestion and heartburn (Dressler *et al.*, 2002; Baumann *et al.*, 2005).

In axillary hyperhidrosis, BoNT-A treatment is now the treatment of choice if topical treatments prove ineffective. In palmar hyperhidrosis, it should be considered if topical treatments and iontophoresis have failed. Another excellent indication for BoNT-A treatment is gustatory sweating (Frey's syndrome), which is discussed in more detail in Chapter 12.

Primary hyperhidrosis of other sites has also been treated with BoNT-A, such as the scalp (Fig. 22.1) (Anders *et al.*, 2008), forehead (Kinkelin *et al.*, 2000), nose, anal fold, groins and soles (Campanati *et al.*, 2007); it has also been used in certain types of regional secondary hyperhidrosis, such as Ross syndrome (Fig. 22.2), residual limb hyperhidrosis in amputees (Charrow *et al.*, 2008), congenital eccrine nevus and compensatory sweating (Kim *et al.*, 2009). Experience in these indications is much more limited than in axillary and palmar hyperhidrosis, and no general recommendations can be given.

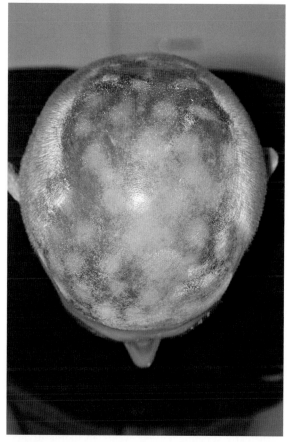

Fig. 22.1 Cranial hyperhidrosis 4 weeks after treatment with botulinum neurotoxin type A injections. Areas in which sweating is abolished are visualized by iodine–starch test.

Technique in primary axillary hyperhidrosis

Preparation for axillary BoNT-A treatment includes:

- avoidance of shaving and use of antiperspirants 48 hours prior to treatment
- exclusion of contraindications (pregnancy, lactation, severe coagulopathies, certain neuromuscular diseases, intake of aminoglycoside antibiotics and cumarins)
- provision of informed consent.

As shown in Fig. 22.3, the sequence of axillary BT-A treatment is as follows:

- clean and dry the axilla
- wipe 2% iodine solution (iodine doubly sublimated 5.0, ricinus oil 25.0, pure ethyl alcohol 80% to 250 ml) onto axillary and surrounding skin (Fig. 22.3a)
- sprinkle corn starch on to the dry iodine using a caster shaker
- wait for delineation of the sweating area by violet–black discoloration (Fig. 22.3b) and outline the sweating area with a pen
- take a picture for documentation
- clean, disinfect and wipe the axilla dry
- mark 10–15 injection points evenly distributed about 2 cm apart on the outlined area (Fig. 22.3c)
- dilute 100 U onabotulinumtoxinA (300 U abobotulinumtoxinA) with 3–5 ml of sterile normal saline
- use 1 ml tuberculin syringe with 0.05 divisions and a 30- or 32-gauge needle
- inject 3–4 U onabotulinumtoxinA (10–15 U abobotulinumtoxinA) intradermally, with the

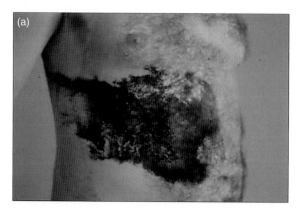

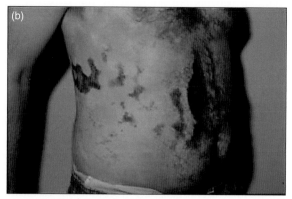

Fig. 22.2 Segmental hyperhidrosis in Ross syndrome. Sweating areas are visualized by iodine–starch test. (a) Before treatment with botulinum neurotoxin type A injections. (b) Four weeks after treatment.

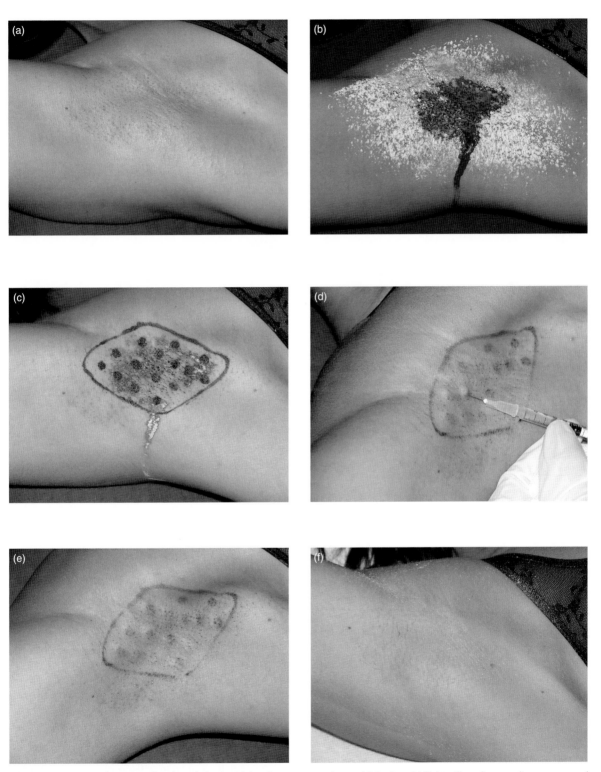

Fig. 22.3 Treatment of primary axillary hyperhidrosis with botulinum neurotoxin type A injections. (a) Right axilla and surrounding area covered with 2% iodine solution. (b) Violet–black demarcation of sweating area after application of corn starch. (c) Marking of sweating area and 15 injection points. (d) Intradermal injection of botulinum neurotoxin type A using a 1 ml syringe and 30-gauge needle. (e) Immediately after finishing the treatment procedure. (f) Iodine–starch test 4 weeks after treatment, demonstrating abolishment of sweating.

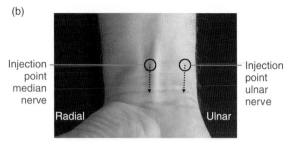

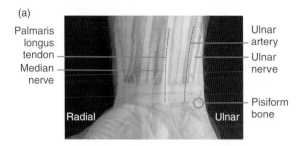

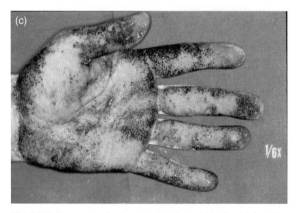

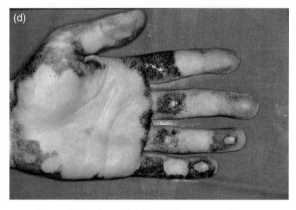

Fig. 22.4 Treatment of primary palmar hyperhidrosis with botulinum neurotoxin type A injections. (a) Anatomical stuctures of orientation for median and ulnar nerve block. (b) Points and direction of injection for median and ulnar nerve block. (c,d) Iodine–starch test before (c) and 4 weeks after (d) treatment, demonstrating virtual abolishment of sweating in treated areas.

needle bevel side up, into each injection point, giving a total of 50 U per axilla (100–150 U abobotulinumtoxinA) (Fig. 22.3d,e)

- hold the needle obliquely to reduce back flow
- clean the axilla.

Patients should be re-treated when the sweating returns at a level of concern but not within 16 weeks of the last treatment. The time interval between injections can be extended by using aluminum chloride hexahydrate.

Technique in primary palmar hyperhidrosis

Before treatment, the following should be considered:

- exclusion contraindications (see above)
- provision of informed consent (off-label use).

Nerve block for anesthesia of the palm is performed as shown in Fig. 22.4a,b:

- patient in lying position
- fill a 5 ml syringe with lidocaine or mepivacaine 1% and use a 27- or 30-gauge needle

- inject 3 ml of local anesthetic a few centimeters proximal of the wrist radial of the tendon of the palmaris longus muscle in distal direction and 2 ml of local anesthetic ulnar of the ulnar artery in direction to the pisiform bone
- exclude intravascular injection by repeated aspiration
- stop injection if the patient feels pain or sensation in the distribution of the nerve
- wait 30 minutes after anesthesia before starting treatment
- alternatively, cryoanesthesia with ice cubes or cold packs immediately before injections may be used.

The treatment procedure for palmar hyperhidrosis is as follows:

- clean and dry the palm
- iodine–starch test is usually not needed as the entire palm and volar aspects of all fingers have to be treated (Fig. 22.4c)
- mark about 20–25 injection points evenly distributed about 1.5–2 cm apart from each other

on the palm, including the ulnar side of the hand, by use of a grid or stamp

- mark five evenly distributed injection points on each finger including the finger tip
- dilute 100 U onabotulinumtoxinA (or equivalent) with 4 or 5 ml of sterile normal saline
- use 1 ml tuberculin syringe with 0.05 division and a 30- or 32-gauge needle
- inject 2–3 U onabotulinumtoxinA (or equivalent) intradermally, with the needle bevel side up, into each injection point totaling 100 U (up to 150 U) per palm
- hold the needle obliquely to reduce back flow
- clean the palm
- advise the patient not to drive a car or perform dangerous manual work on the day of treatment (in case of nerve block).

Patients should be re-evaluated about 4 weeks after treatment (Fig. 22.4d) and re-treated when the sweating returns at a level of concern but not within 16 weeks of the last treatment. The time interval between injections can be extended by using tap water iontophoresis or aluminum chloride hexahydrate.

Acknowledgment

We thank Dr. Diana Anders and Stephanie Dessoi for photodocumentation of the axillary BoNT-A-treatment.

References

Anders D, Moosbauer S, Naumann MK, Hamm H (2008). Craniofacial hyperhidrosis successfully treated with botulinum toxin type A. *Eur J Dermatol*, **18**, 87–8.

Baumann L, Slezinger A, Halem M *et al.* (2005). Double-blind, randomized, placebo-controlled pilot study of the safety and efficacy of Myobloc (botulinum toxin type B) for the treatment of palmar hyperhidrosis. *Dermatol Surg*, **31**, 263–70.

Campanati A, Bernardini ML, Gesuita R, Offidani A (2007). Plantar focal idiopathic hyperhidrosis and botulinum toxin: a pilot study. *Eur J Dermatol*, **17**, 52–4.

Campanati A, Sandroni L, Gesuita R *et al.* (2011). Treatment of focal idiopathic hyperhidrosis with botulinum toxin type A: clinical predictive factors of relapse-free survival. *J Eur Acad Dermatol Venereol*, **25**, 917–21.

Charrow A, DiFazio M, Foster L, Pasquina PF, Tsao JW (2008). Intradermal botulinum toxin type A injection effectively reduces residual limb hyperhidrosis in amputees: a case series. *Arch Phys Med Rehabil*, **89**, 1407–9.

Davarian S, Kalantari KK, Rezasoltani A, Rahimi A (2008). Effect and persistency of botulinum toxin iontophoresis in the treatment of palmar hyperhidrosis. *Australas J Dermatol*, **49**, 75–9.

Doft MA, Hardy KL, Ascherman JA (2012). Treatment of hyperhidrosis with botulinum toxin. *Aesthet Surg J*, **32**, 238–44.

Dressler D (2010). Comparing Botox and Xeomin for axillar hyperhidrosis. *J Neural Transm*, **117**, 317–19.

Dressler D, Adib Saberi F, Benecke R (2002). Botulinum toxin type B for treatment of axillar hyperhidrosis. *J Neurol*, **249**, 1729–32.

Glaser DA, Coleman WP III, Fan LK *et al.* (2012). A randomized, blinded clinical evaluation of a novel microwave device for treating axillary hyperhidrosis: the dermatologic reduction in underarm perspiration study. *Dermatol Surg*, **38**, 185–91.

Hamm H, Naumann MK, Kowalski JW *et al.* (2006). Primary focal hyperhidrosis: disease characteristics and functional impairment. *Dermatology*, **212**, 343–53.

Heckmann M, Ceballos-Baumann AO, Plewig G (2001). Botulinum toxin A for axillary hyperhidrosis (excessive sweating). *N Engl J Med*, **344**, 488–93.

Hoorens I, Ongenae K (2012). Primary focal hyperhidrosis: current treatment options and a step-by-step approach. *J Eur Acad Dermatol, Venereol* **26**, 1–8.

Hornberger J, Grimes K, Naumann M *et al.* (2004). Multi-Specialty Working Group on the Recognition, Diagnosis, and Treatment of Primary Focal Hyperhidrosis. Recognition, diagnosis, and treatment of primary focal hyperhidrosis. *J Am Acad Dermatol*, **51**, 274–86.

Kavanagh GM, Shams K (2006). Botulinum toxin type A by iontophoresis for primary palmar hyperhidrosis. *J Am Acad Dermatol*, **55**(Suppl):S115–17.

Kim WO, Kil HK, Yoon KB, Noh KU (2009). Botulinum toxin: a treatment for compensatory hyperhidrosis in the trunk. *Dermatol Surg*, **35**(5):833–8.

Kinkelin I, Hund M, Naumann M, Hamm H (2000). Effective treatment of frontal hyperhidrosis with botulinum toxin A. *Br J Dermatol*, **143**, 824–7.

Lowe NJ, Yamauchi PS, Lask GP, Patnaik R, Iyer S (2002). Efficacy and safety of botulinum toxin type A in the treatment of palmar hyperhidrosis: a double-blind, randomized, placebo-controlled study. *Dermatol Surg*, **28**, 822–7.

Lowe NJ, Glaser DA, Eadie N *et al.* (2007). North American Botox in Primary Axillary Hyperhidrosis Clinical Study Group. Botulinum toxin type A in the treatment of primary axillary hyperhidrosis: a 52-week multicenter double-blind, randomized, placebo-controlled study of efficacy and safety. *J Am Acad Dermatol*, **56**, 604–11.

Naumann MK, Lowe NJ for the Botox Hyperhidrosis Clinical Study Group (2001). Botulinum toxin type A in treatment of bilateral primary axillary hyperhidrosis: randomised, parallel group, double blind, placebo controlled trial. *BMJ*, **323**, 1–4.

Naumann MK, Hamm H, Lowe NJ for the Botox Hyperhidrosis Clinical Study Group (2002). Effect of botulinum toxin type A on quality of life measures in patients with excessive axillary sweating: a randomized controlled trial. *Br J Dermatol*, **147**, 1218–26.

Naumann MK, Lowe NJ, Kumar CR, Hamm H (2003). Botulinum toxin type A is a safe and effective treatment for axillary hyperhidrosis over 16 months: a prospective study. *Arch Dermatol*, **139**, 731–6.

Saadia D, Voustianiouk A, Wang AK, Kaufmann H (2001). Botulinum toxin type A in primary palmar hyperhidrosis: randomized, single-blind, two-dose study. *Neurology*, **57**, 2095–9.

Simonetta Moreau M, Cauhepe C, Magues JP, Senard JM (2003). A double-blind, randomized, comparative study of Dysport vs. Botox in primary palmar hyperhidrosis. *Br J Dermatol*, **149**, 1041–5.

Strutton DR, Kowalski JW, Glaser DA, Stang PE (2004). US prevalence of hyperhidrosis and impact on individuals with axillary hyperhidrosis: results from a national survey. *J Am Acad Dermatol*, **51**, 241–8.

Trindade de Almeida AR, Secco LC, Carruthers A (2011). Handling botulinum toxins: an updated literature review. *Dermatol Surg*, **37**, 1553–65.

Chapter 23

Botulinum neurotoxin A treatment for ischemic digits

Michael W. Neumeister and Kelli Webb

Raynaud's phenomenon

Raynaud's phenomenon is a vasospastic disorder that affects over 9 million people in the USA (National Institute of Arthritis and Musculoskeletal and Skin Diseases, 2006). Maurice Reynaud's description of arterial insufficiency to the fingers in 1862 led to his name being the eponym of this condition. He described the process as a "local asphyxia of the extremities" as a result of "increased irritability of the central parts of the cord presiding over vascular innervation." Raynaud's phenomenon is nine times more common in females and typically occurs between the ages of 15–40 years. These patients have an exaggerated vasoconstriction of their digital arteries in response to certain environmental triggers, which leads to pale, cold, numb and sometimes painful digits. These symptoms can last minutes to hours and may reoccur several times through the day. For the majority of patients, the symptoms are simply bothersome, but for 20% the symptoms are so severe that they seek medical attention. The digital artery vasospasm leads to diminished blood supply to the fingertips, which causes pain, ulcerations and disuse. Many patients require digit amputations for recalcitrant ulcers or exposure of the distal phalanx. The resultant digit ischemia may be also associated with considerable morbidity associated with loss of function, disability and depression.

Primary Raynaud's disease is an idiopathic condition, and secondary Raynaud's disease is associated with other connective tissue disorders. Secondary Raynaud's disease affects 90% of patients with scleroderma, 90% of patients with mixed connective tissue disease, 33% of patients with lupus and 33% of people with Sjögren's syndrome. The pathophysiology of primary versus secondary Raynaud's disease is likely different, with secondary Raynaud's disease invariably causing more severe and debilitating symptoms (Figs. 23.1 and 23.2).

Response to different treatment options varies and is difficult to predict. Initial conservative treatment methods include avoidance of exacerbating factors, particularly cold, stress and smoking. Various medications have been employed to improve blood flow and decrease pain, with variable results (Box 23.1). Pharmacologic treatments include calcium channel blockers, nitric oxide, angiotensin-converting enzyme inhibitors, selective serotonin receptor inhibitors, alpha-adrenergic blockers, anticoagulants, antithrombotics and antioxidants. Patients with severe pain and digit ulceration who have failed conservative managements are often referred to hand surgeons for further evaluation and treatment. Historically, cervical sympathectomy was a surgical treatment option but it has now fallen out of favor because of potential complications and poor long-term results (de Trafford et al., 1988). Adrian Flatt introduced digital sympathectomies for chronic ischemia, where the vessels are surgically stripped of the adventia and sympathetic innervation. The intent is to deny the digital artery of its potential to vasoconstrict. Microsurgical digital artery sympathectomy is localized surgical treatment that involves removing the adventitia from involved arteries at the level of the digital artery, palmar common digital artery, palmar arch and/or radial and ulnar arteries. Theoretically, this treatment irreversibly prevents sympathetically mediated vasoconstriction; however, it provides inconsistent relief and is often associated with surgical morbidity. Partial or full amputations may be necessary to relieve recalcitrant pain and ulcerations. The implications of amputation on quality of life are obvious. These less-than-optimal therapies leave much room for improvement for the treatment of digit ischemia associated with Raynaud's disease.

Manual of Botulinum Toxin Therapy, 2nd edition, ed. Daniel Truong, Mark Hallett, Christopher Zachary and Dirk Dressler.
Published by Cambridge University Press. © Cambridge University Press 2013.

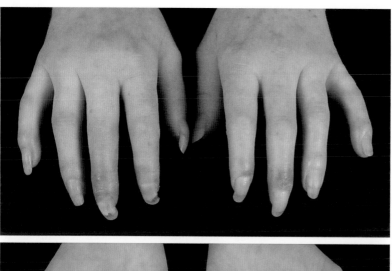

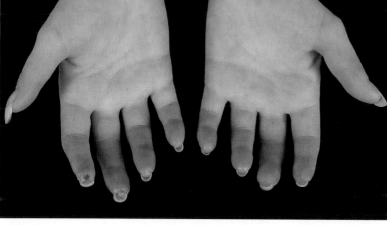

Fig. 23.1 Clinical appearance of a patient with Raynaud's disease. Discoloration and ulcerations are common physical findings.

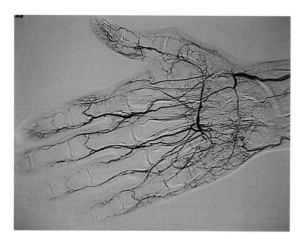

Fig. 23.2 A typical angiogram of a patient with Raynaud's disease showing diffuse vasospasm of digital arteries.

Botulinum neurotoxin for Raynaud's disease

There have been five studies since 2004 that have evaluated the use of botulinum neurotoxin type A (BoNT-A) for the treatment of Raynaud's disease (Sycha *et al.*, 2004; Van Beek *et al.*, 2007; Fregene *et al.*, 2009; Neumeister *et al.*, 2009; Neumeister, 2010) (Table 23.1). Although these studies have many limitations, such as lack of controls, varying severity of disease and variability of dosing, all reported favorable clinical results, with overall improvement in patient pain and reduction in soft tissue ulceration. There is no information in the literature about BoNT-B.

In 2004, Sycha *et al.* reported encouraging results in a pilot study of BoNT-A injections into the hands

Box 23.1 Medications used in Raynaud's phenomenon

Sympatholytics
- clonidine
- phentolamine
- prazosin
- phenoxybenzamine
- propanolol
- Calcium channel blockers

Anticoagulants
- aspirin
- dipyridamole

Nitrates

Angiotensin-converting enzyme inhibitors

Anticonvulsants
- gabapentin
- phenytoin
- carbamazepine
- clonazepam
- valproic acid

Antidepressants

Selective serotonin receptor inhibitors

Calcitonin

of two patients with Raynaud's phenomenon. Van Beek *et al.* (2007) published an article describing BoNT-A injections in the hands of 11 patients with Raynaud's phenomenon. They found that injecting BoNT-A reduced patients' rest pain, promoted healing of digit ulcerations and reduced overall frequency of attacks. In 2009, Fregene *et al.* described BoNT-A injections in the hands of 26 patients with Raynaud's phenomenon. They found that 75% of patients experienced a significant reduction in pain; 56% experienced improvement in transcutaneous oxygen saturation; 48% of ulcers healed within 9.5 weeks; and 89% of patients experienced improvements after one treatment. In July 2009, Neumeister and colleagues described the effects of BoNT-A in 19 patients, 16 of whom reported resolution of pain. All chronic ulcers healed within 60 days of injection, and 84% of patients noticed an immediate increase in finger perfusion. Neumaister in 2010 reported 28 of 33 patients treated with BoNT-A experienced improved blood flow and pain relief.

Although the US Food and Drug Administration has approved eight different uses for BoNT-A, numerous off-label uses have been documented in the literature. The neurotoxin inhibits muscle contraction through its initial uptake into the nerve terminal and the eventual blockade of acetylcholine release. This process typically has a delay of 1 to 4 days and has an effect that lasts 2–4 months. Unlike the paralytic effect of BoNT in muscle, the treatment of patients with chronic ischemia and pain has almost immediate and prolonged effects. In Raynaud's disease, BoNT-A may work with a different mechanism. It has been postulated that BoNT-A may affect several pain-related neurotransmitters, including norepinephrine, substance P, glutamate and calcitonin gene-related protein. The effects of BoNT-A injections may be related to the local or central blockade of neurotransmitters that are upregulated in states of chronic nerve irritation and pain. Additionally, the effects of BoNT-A in improving vascularity of the ischemic digits may be sympathetically mediated. If BoNT-A blocks substance P, it may decrease or abolish the self-perpetuating cycle of pain and sympathetic stimulation. Finally, there may also be direct or indirect crosstalk between the A and C fibers in the dorsal root ganglion, a method of communication known as "ephapses." In fact, numerous chemical and anatomical changes have been observed within the dorsal root ganglion in chronic pain models. It is conceivable that BoNT-A has more than one mode of pain inhibition and may be acting at a number of sites. Whether by the blockade of neurotransmitters, by blockade of ectopic sodium channels on chronically irritated nerves or through its effect on microvascularity, BoNT-A has a distinct role in pain reduction in patients with Raynaud's disease.

Interestingly, the pain associated with the Raynaud's disease resolves almost immediately for the majority of patients, even those patients who had ulcerations. The mechanism of improved blood flow, therefore, may be different than the mechanism responsible for resolution of pain.

Technique for injecting botulinum neurotoxin in Raynaud's phenomenon

The following are recommended:

- use the same room with an ambient temperature for each patient
- reconstitute vial with 10 ml of preservative-free saline (100 U in 10 ml)

Table 23.1 Summary of findings from all retrospective studies using injected botulinum neurotoxin A to treat Raynaud's disease with ischemic digits

Study	No. patients (M/F)	No. with Raynaud's phenomenon (1°/2°)	Average age (years [range])	Symptomatic relief (% [No.])	Follow-up (average months [maximum])	Duration pain relief (average months [range])	Complications (No.[%])
Sycha et al. (2004)	2 (0/2)	1/1	50.5 (19–63)	100 (2/2)	1.75 (2)	1.75 (1.5–2)	None
Van Beek et al. (2007)	11 (2/9)	1/10	50.8 (23–70)	100 (11/11)	9.6 (30)	NR	Temporary intrinsic muscle weakness, 3 (27%)
Fregene et al. (2009)	26 (12/14)	15/11	55 (37–72)	75 (19/6)	18 (45)	NR	Temporary intrinsic muscle weakness, 6 (23%) Transient dysthesia, in distribution of injection, 1 (4%)
Neumeister et al. (2009)	19 (7/12)	13/6	44.1 (15–72)	84 (16/19)	NR (59)	23.4 (0.5–59)	Temporary intrinsic muscle weakness, 3 (16%)
Neumeister (2010)	33 (14/19)	23/10	43.0 (15–72)	84 (28/33)	(103)	(0.5–103)	Temporary intrinsic muscle weakness, 7 (21%)

1°, primary; 2°, secondary; NR, not reported.

- inject 50–100 U BoNT-A into the hand (1–2 ml around each neurovascular bundle)
- target the neurovascular bundles (Fig. 23.3)
- use a wrist block with local anesthetic to decrease the pain of injections

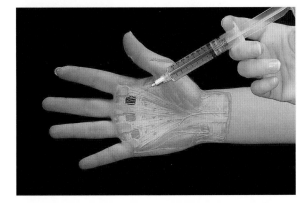

Fig. 23.3 Botulinum neurotoxin is reconstituted in 100 ml of normal saline and 1–2 ml of the solution is injected around the neurovascular bundles at the level of the metacarpophalangeal joint.

- laser Doppler scan before and 20 minutes after injection to quantify increased perfusion
- assess using pain scales on a 1–10 range
- assess using magnetic resonance angiography.

Figures 23.4 to 23.8 show pre- and post-injection status with onabotulinumtoxinA for Raynaud's disease.

Indications for BoNT-A in patients with ischemic digits are:

- Raynaud's phenomenon
- vascular insufficiency not amenable to bypass surgery.

Contraindications for BoNT-A in patients with ischemic digits:

- known allergies
- pregnancy
- breast-feeding mothers
- active infection
- myasthenia gravis

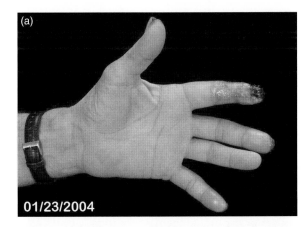

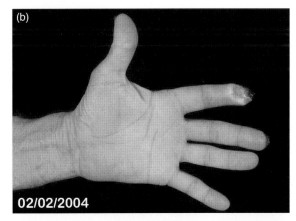

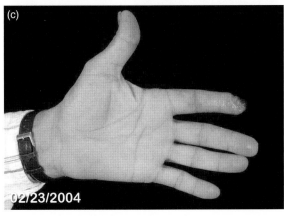

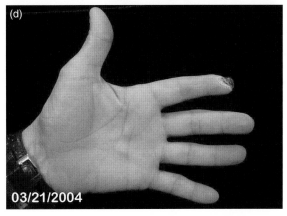

Fig. 23.4 OnabotulinumtoxinA for ischemic digits. (a) Pre-injection; (b–d) post-injection over the next 2 months. Perfusion is enhanced, with a corresponding symptomatic relief of pain.

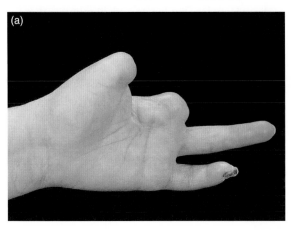
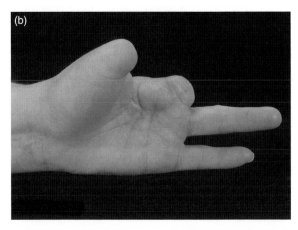

Fig. 23.5 OnabotulinumtoxinA in a 37-year-old woman with Raynaud's disease. She had previous amputations for ulcerations and exposed bone and presented with severe pain and ischemia to the remaining digits. She feared further amputations. (a) Pre-injection; (b) post-injection. The onabotulinumtoxinA injections increased perfusion, ameliorated the pain and prevented further amputations.

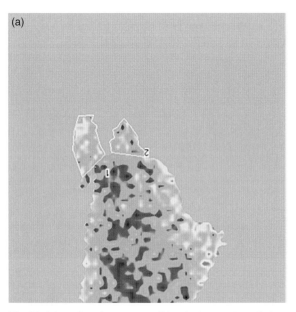
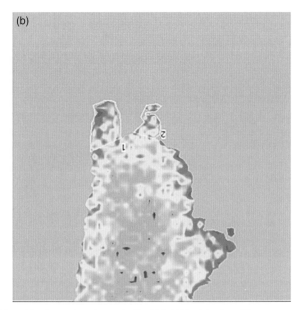

Fig. 23.6 Laser Doppler scan quantifying the increase in perfusion achieved for the patient shown in Fig. 23.5. (a) Pre-injection; (b) post-injection The lighter shades denote greater perfusion after the injections.

- patients on medications that decrease neuromuscular transmission
  - calcium channel blockers
  - penicilamine
  - aminoglycosides
  - licoamides
  - polymixins
  - magnesium sulfate
  - anticholinesterases
  - succinylcholine
  - quinidine.

References

de Trafford JC, Lafferty K, Potter CE, Roberts VC, Cotton LT (1988). An epidemiological survey of Raynaud's phenomenon. *Eur J Vasc Surg*, **2**, 167–70.

Fregene A, Ditmars D, Siddiqui A (2009). Botulinum toxin type A: a treatment option for digital ischemia in patients

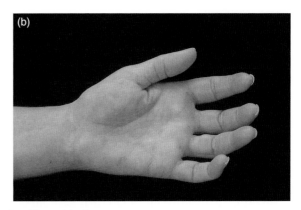

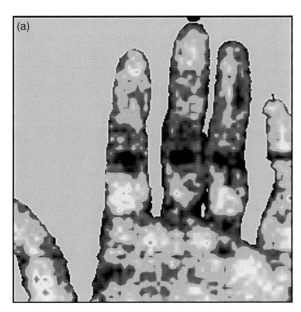

Fig. 23.7 Injection of 50 U onabotulinumtoxinA per hand. (a) Pre-injection; (b) post-injection.

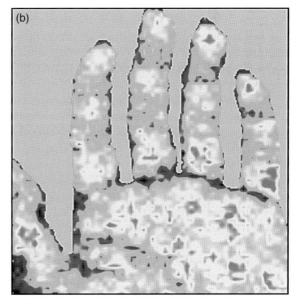

Fig. 23.8 Laser Doppler scan quantifying the increase in perfusion achieved for the patient shown in the patient in Fig. 23.7. (a) Pre-injection; (b) post-injection. The dark shades demonstrate poor perfusion while lighter shades demonstrate a much greater perfusion.

with Raynaud's phenomenon. *J Hand Surg Am*, **34**, 446–52.

National Institute of Arthritis and Musculoskeletal and Skin Diseases (2006). *Questions and Answers about Raynaud's Phenomenon* (NIH Publication No. 06–4911). Bethesda, MD: National Institutes of Health.

Neumeister MW (2010). Botulinum toxin type A in the treatment of Raynaud's phenomenon. *J Hand Surg*, **35**, 2085–92.

Neumeister MW, Chambers CB, Herron MS *et al.* (2009). Botox therapy for ischemic digits. *Plast Reconstr Surg*, **124**, 191–201.

Sycha T, Graninger M, Auff E, Schnider P (2004). Botulinum toxin in the treatment of Raynaud's phenomenon: a pilot study. *Eur J Clin Invest*, **34**, 312–13.

Van Beek AL, Lim PK, Gear AJL, Pritzker MR (2007). Management of vasospastic disorders with botulinum toxin A. *Plast Reconstr Surg*, **119**, 217.

Chapter 24

Botulinum neurotoxin in wound healing

Holger G. Gassner

Introduction

Visible scars, particularly on the face, may have important social and psychological implications and are a significant concern for patients before undergoing surgery. Many new developments in science and medicine have been driven by the desire to minimize or eliminate scars, including endoscopic, minimally invasive and robotic surgeries. Despite these innovations, many procedures still require open incisions, resulting in visible scars, and research into scarless healing continues.

To optimize healing and minimize scarring, an understanding of the wound-healing process is of critical importance. The first phase of wound healing, the inflammatory phase, generally lasts a few days and is characterized by vasodilation and cellular response. The wound must be thoroughly irrigated and meticulously cleaned to maintain asepsis and discourage the persistence of macrophages and other inflammatory cells that prolong inflammation.

The second phase of wound healing, the proliferative phase, is characterized by epithelial regeneration and collagen synthesis. This phase lasts several weeks and may overlap the inflammatory phase. Epithelial regeneration is greatly improved if wounds are closed by primary intention; wounds that heal by secondary intention take much longer for this process.

Preserving secretions in the wound has been shown to enhance epithelial regeneration during the proliferative phase in two ways. First, desiccation is avoided. Second, the presence of important cytokines that orchestrate the wound-healing process is ensured. Therefore, occlusive and semi-occlusive dressings have become an established clinical practice in the care of healing wounds until epithelialization is complete.

The final stage of wound healing is characterized by the maturation of the scar. With time, it becomes finer and less erythematous because its collagen content is more organized. This process is susceptible to external stimuli such as sun exposure and mechanical irritation. Hence, these external factors should be eliminated or minimized to improve healing and to minimize the risk of scar hypertrophy and pigment changes.

Clinical wound care

Many measures have become routine in the care of healing wounds and have been shown or proven to positively affect the final appearance of the resulting scar. These measures include cleaning and irrigation of the wound, disinfection, aseptic technique, application of the right suture material, performing exact anatomical closure, application of semi-occlusive dressings and the instruction of the patient to avoid sun exposure.

Tension

Tension is the overriding factor adversely affecting all phases of wound healing. Repetitive tension leads to inflammation, which in turn causes increased collagen synthesis and deposition of glycosaminoglycans, resulting in prolonged erythema and scar hypertrophy. Even under ideal circumstances, a wound will invariably produce scarring if the wound edges are under tension. Continuous and static tensions are caused by static tissue qualities. An immobile wound that is closed after resection of a lesion may be under static tension if the resulting defect has not been adequately closed.

Much research has been performed to better understand the static tension of healing wounds, such as work by Larrabee and colleagues (Larrabee,

Manual of Botulinum Toxin Therapy, 2nd edition, ed. Daniel Truong, Mark Hallett, Christopher Zachary and Dirk Dressler. Published by Cambridge University Press. © Cambridge University Press 2013.

1986; Larrabee and Sutton, 1986) investigating the biomechanical characteristics of skin. Important implications for the design of operative techniques and local flaps have emanated from these studies. These data have provided us with a better understanding about undermining, multilayered closure, the design of local flaps, the application of external dressings and stenting devices.

Anatomical location

The underlying musculature generates dynamic tension on a healing wound and may vary greatly depending on the anatomical location of the wound. Particularly for the face, muscles exert tension on the overlying skin through mass movement and, more importantly, through direct internal insertions into the skin. The effect of repetitive tension on a healing wound is particularly pronounced in areas overlying the frontalis and smaller forehead muscles. Similarly, the perioral musculature is strong, active and directly exerts tension onto the overlying skin. The same principles apply to a lesser degree to the chin and cheeks.

In the neck, the anatomical situation is somewhat different. The platysma is a broad, plain muscle without dermal attachments into the skin. Instead, there are important gliding planes in the neck. Hence the effects of contraction of the platysma on the overlying skin are less direct than those observed in certain areas of the face. The importance of these varying influences on the underlying musculature of the overlying skin is evidenced by the varying degrees and intensity of wrinkle lines and relaxed skin tension lines.

Implications of relaxed skin tension lines

Dupuytren was the first to observe that the skin has inherent elastic properties that cause round wounds to deform and become elliptical. Further research led to the conclusion that in most cases the effect of the underlying musculature results in texture changes of the overlying skin, which are not permanent.

An important clinical example supports this point. The skin of the forehead shows horizontal rhitids. A round wound of the forehead also deforms and becomes a horizontally aligned ellipse. These effects are greatly reduced in patients with long-standing facial paralysis.

It is broadly accepted that wounds that are aligned parallel with the relaxed skin tension lines heal with favorable scars. By the same token, wounds that cross the relaxed skin tension lines at unfavorable angles

tend to heal with scar hypertrophy. The likely cause is repetitive tension on the wound edges by the underlying musculature. In the case of the favorably aligned wounds, the underlying musculature pulls perpendicular to the wound edges and assists the wound in reapproximation. The unfavorably aligned wound is subject to oblique tension of the underlying muscle. This causes shearing forces and distortion of the wound edges and likely maintains a subclinical inflammatory response, which eventually leads to erythema and scar hypertrophy.

Chemo-immobilization of cutaneous wounds

The principle of chemo-immobilization of cutaneous wounds was introduced by our group at the Mayo Clinic. Initially, a primate model was utilized to study the effects of chemo-immobilizing unfavorably aligned wounds. The forehead was used as a model as the frontalis muscle directly affects the overlying skin (Gassner et al., 2000).

In this animal model, one side of the forehead was determined as experimental. A blinded surgeon performed standardized excisions on both sides of the forehead. Subsequently, saline and botulinum neurotoxin (BoNT) were injected in the experimental and control sides of the forehead, respectively (Fig. 24.1).

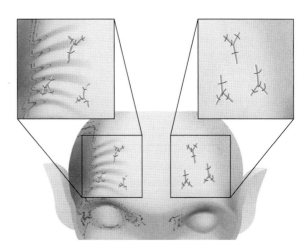

Fig. 24.1 The forehead of the animal was divided into two symmetric halves. The left side was injected with botulinum neurotoxin , the other with saline. Subsequently, standardized excisions were performed and closed in a standardized fashion by a blinded facial plastic surgeon. Immobilization of the experimental wounds was observed 1 week after the treatment, while the wounds on the experimental side continued to be distorted by the activity of the underlying frontalis muscle (top frames).

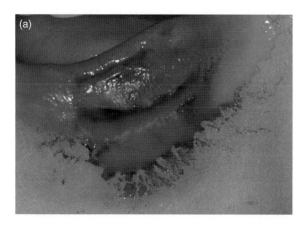

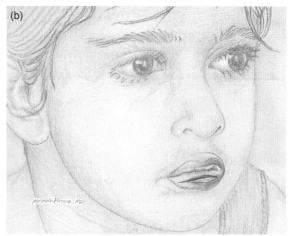

Fig. 24.2 Through-and-through defect of the lower lip in a 1-year old infant.

Three months after surgery, a blinded panel of three facial plastic surgeons evaluated the appearance of the scar using a standardized visual analog scale. The pharmacologically immobilized wounds were rated as more favorable in appearance than the ones in the control site. The resulting data form the basis for clinical trials in humans.

Human use of chemo-immobilization

Initial case reports of human use included traumatic wounds of the forehead and subsequently of the peri-oral region. They were followed by use for surgical wounds of the rest of the face and of the neck. No adverse effects or complications were reported. Of note, many patients opted for aggressive immobiliza-tion even of functionally important areas such as the lip, in the hopes of maximizing the therapeutic effect. For example, temporary paralysis of the lip was discussed as an example of the treatment effect and not of being an untoward effect or a complication. With further positive experiences, the indications were broadened and included pediatric applications.

Figure 24.2 shows a lower lip wound in a 1-year-old infant. The lower wound is a complete through-and-through defect; the upper wound is about a 50% depth defect. Figure 24.3 shows anatomical closure of the wound in a layered fashion. After appropriate informed consent of the off-label use of the therapy and also of the somewhat limited experience in infants, the wound was aggressively immobilized by intramus-cular injection of BoNT. The infant was observed to have decreased mobility of the lower lip for about 8 to

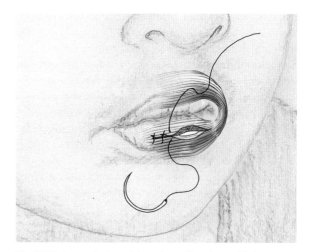

Fig. 24.3 Anatomical repair is performed in a layered fashion utilizing resorbable suture material.

10 weeks after the treatment. Food intake and articu-lation was not compromised. Figure 24.4 shows the intramuscular treatment of the wound with BoNT during surgery. The wound healed uneventfully and the cosmetic result seemed very favorable. Figure 24.5 shows the wound with 5 years of follow-up.

Clinical trial

The first clinical trial of chemo-immobilization was performed at the Mayo Clinic (Gassner and Sherris, 2000). Surgical and traumatic wounds of the forehead were included in the study. According to a randomized protocol, patients were injected with normal saline or with BoNT. Dosages of 15 U/2 cm wound length were applied. This dosage is large compared with the

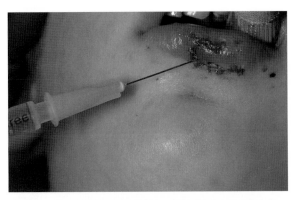

Fig. 24.4 The underlying orbicularis oris muscle is injected with botulinum neurotoxin A.

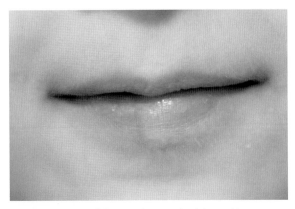

Fig. 24.5 Five-year follow-up photograph of the resulting scar.

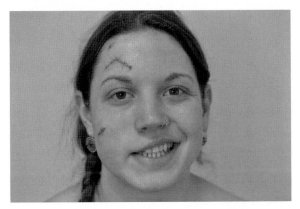

Fig. 24.6 Immobilized soft tissue wounds of the forehead and cheek in a 21-year-old female. The frontalis, zygomaticus and buccinator muscles were injected with a total dosage of 60 U botulinum neurotoxin A.

cosmetic use of BoNT; it has been the author's long-term observation that chemo-immobilization for healing wounds requires a higher dosage and more aggressive treatment than the immobilization used for forehead wrinkles. This may be because a relatively broad area around the scar requires treatment for adequate immobilization of the wound edges. After completion of the study, close-up photographs taken at the 6-month follow-up were presented to a blinded panel of evaluators, who then graded the cosmetic appearance of the resulting wound taking into account the original wound and trauma. The experimentally immobilized wounds were rated as cosmetically more favorable compared with the control wounds, which led to the conclusion that aggressive immobilization of wounds located on the forehead has a favorable effect on the eventual scarring.

Gassner and Sherris (2000) noted that the effect of BoNT on immobilization varied greatly depending on the anatomical area. Figures 24.6 to 24.9 illustrate this observation. This 21-year-old woman sustained soft tissue cuts to the forehead and the cheek. Both wounds were deep; the forehead wound reached the periosteum and was more complex than the somewhat shallower cut on the cheek. Both wounds were meticulously closed in a layered fashion and subsequently aggressively immobilized with a total dose of 60 U BoNT serotype A (Fig. 24.6). At 6 months, both scars were in the maturation phase. The cheek scar showed more pronounced erythema and widening compared with the forehead scar (Figs. 24.7–24.9). The forehead and the perioral area seem to be particularly well suited for BoNT-induced immobilization, the suitability of the cheek and neck appearing more limited. Consequently, caution should be employed in extrapolating from these results to other parts of the body.

Current studies and data

The initial studies were followed by additional research on the use of BoNT in wound healing and scarring.

Mason et al. (1996) described the use of BoNT to improve the healing of anal fissures. This application is likely based on a different principle. Here the likely mechanism is not repetitive mechanical tension on wound edges. More likely, contracture and static tension likely cause secondary metabolic changes that then eventuate in chronic anal fissure. Similarly, Patti and Almasio (2005) reported a double-blind randomized study showing that BoNT improved wound healing after hemorrhoidectomy.

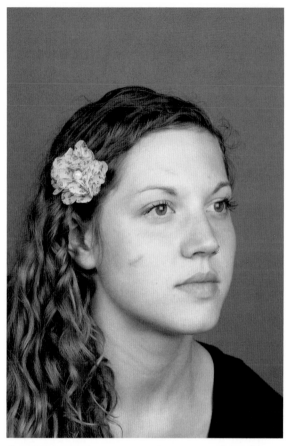

Fig. 24.7 Despite the greater irregularity and complexity of the forehead laceration, the cheek wound responded less well to the chemo-immobilization treatment and was healing with more pronounced widening and erythema at 6 months.

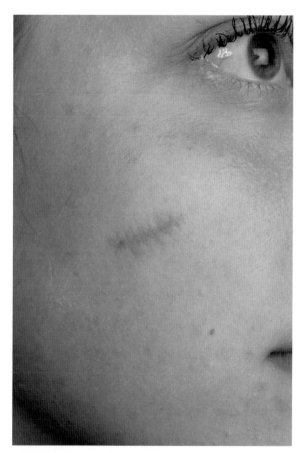

Fig. 24.8 Close-up photograph of the cheek wound.

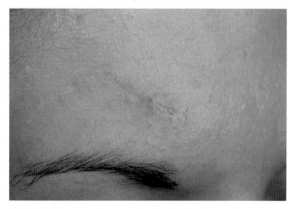

Fig. 24.9 Close-up photograph of the forehead wound.

The role of BoNT in urethral wound healing was studied in an animal model (Sahinkanat *et al.*, 2009). Blinded trials showed that pretreatment with BoNT positively affected the results of skin laser resurfacing in the face. Principle and mechanism of action are likely identical to the effects of BoNT observed in facial wound healing (Zimbler *et al.*, 2001).

The use of BoNT to affect the healing of bony fractures or tendon injuries showed inconsistent results. It could not be conclusively shown that BoNT-induced immobilization favorably modulated the healing of bones and tendons in various studies (Kubat and Rekant, 2008; Hettrich *et al.*, 2011; Hao *et al.*, 2012).

Xiao *et al.* (2009) have shown possible beneficial effects of BoNT injections into mature, hypertrophic cutaneous scars. The mechanical action of this effect is not well understood. This report was followed by additional research, including experimental studies on rabbits, since a positive effect of BoNT on hypertrophic scarring cannot be explained by mechanical immobilization (Wang *et al.*, 2009).

After performing extensive cytokine analyses of a cell culture model of cutaneous scarring in the laboratory, no effects of BoNT on any of the investigated cytokines were found (Haubner *et al.*, 2012). There is incomplete evidence to suggest that BoNT plays a role in enhancing wound healing beyond the initial phases that are susceptible to mechanical influences; therefore, the recommendation for BoNT treatment of wounds would be within the first 3 to 4 weeks after wounding, at the very latest.

Conclusions

Immobilization of healing cutaneous wounds with BoNT has been shown in multiple studies to have a positive effect on healing in certain anatomical regions. The best available evidence exists for the forehead and the periorbital region, where the anatomical interactions of the underlying mimetic musculature and the overlying skin is most direct, secondary to tendinous insertions of the musculature into the skin. Further studies are indicated to evaluate the suitability of wounds in other anatomical regions, such as the neck. The application of BoNT to enhance the healing of skeletal structures, such as bone and tendon, shows promise but requires further research.

References

Gassner HG, Sherris DA (2000). Addition of an anesthetic agent to enhance the predictability of the effects of botulinum toxin type A injections: a randomized controlled study. *Mayo Clin Proc*, **75**, 701–4.

Gassner HG, Sherris DA, Otley CC (2000). Treatment of facial wounds with botulinum toxin A improves cosmetic outcome in primates. *Plast Reconstr Surg*, **105**, 1948–53.

Hao Y, Ma Y, Wang X, Jin F, Ge S (2012). Short-term muscle atrophy caused by botulinum toxin-A local injection impairs fracture healing in the rat femur. *J Orthop Res*, **30**, 574–80.

Haubner F, Ohmann E, Müller-Vogt U *et al.* (2012). Effects of botulinum toxin A on cytokine synthesis in a cell culture model of cutaneous scarring. *Arch Facial Plast Surg*, **14**, 122–6.

Hettrich CM, Rodeo SA. Hannafin JA *et al.* (2011). The effect of muscle paralysis using Botox on the healing of tendon to bone in a rat model. *J Shoulder Elbow Surg*, **20**, 688–97.

Kubat WD, Rekant M (2008). Botulinum toxin use as an adjunctive modality in a patient with multiple flexor tendon ruptures. *Hand (N Y)*, **3**, 237–9.

Larrabee WF Jr.(1986). A finite element model of skin deformation. I. Biomechanics of skin and soft tissue: a review. *Laryngoscope*, **96**, 399–405.

Larrabee WF Jr., Sutton D (1986). A finite element model of skin deformation. II. An experimental model of skin deformation *Laryngoscope*, **96**, 406–12.

Mason PF, Watkins MJ, Hall HS, Hall AW (1996). The management of chronic fissure in-ano with botulinum toxin. *J R Coll Surg*, **41**, 235–8.

Patti R, Almasio PL (2005). Improvement of wound healing after hemorrhoidectomy: a double-blind, randomized study of botulinum toxin injection. *Dis Colon Rectum*, **48**, 2173–9.

Sahinkanat T, Ozkan KU, Ciralik H, Ozturk S, Resim S (2009). Botulinum toxin-A to improve urethral wound healing: an experimental study in a rat model. *Urology*, **73**, 405–9.

Wang L, Tai NZ, Fan ZH (2009). Effect of botulinum toxin type A injection on hypertrophic scar in rabbit ear model. *J Plastic Surg*, **25**, 284–7.

Xiao Z, Zhang F, Cui Z (2009). Treatment of hypertrophic scars with intralesional botulinum toxin type A injections: a preliminary report. *Aesthetic Plast Surg*, **33**, 409–12.

Zimbler MS, Holds JB, Kokoska MS *et al.* (2001). Effect of botulinum toxin pretreatment on laser resurfacing results: a prospective, randomized, blinded trial. *Arch Facial Plast Surg*, **3**, 165–9.

Chapter 25

Use of botulinum neurotoxin in neuropathic pain

Szu-Kuan Yang and Chaur-Jong Hu

Introduction

Botulinum neurotoxin (BoNT) has been used effectively to alleviate pain in many pain disorders and has been proven to be a good choice for treatment of neuropathic pain. There have been no major side effects, only minor local infection. Randomized controlled studies and open-label studies indicate BoNT is beneficial in diabetic neuropathic pain, trigeminal neuralgia and postherpetic neuralgia (Piovesan *et al.*, 2005; Ranoux *et al.*, 2008; Yuan *et al.*, 2009; Xiao *et al.*, 2010). This chapter discusses the putative mechanisms of BoNT action and injection methodology for these three conditions.

Peripheral and central sensitization processes are involved in the pathophysiology of neuropathic pain (Baron, 2006; Pace *et al.*, 2006). Abnormal muscle contraction, released substance P and calcitonin gene-related peptide also play significant roles in hyperalgesia of neuropathic pain. An ideal therapy for neuropathic pain should block these pain-inducing pathways as completely as possible. Muscle paralytic mechanisms, vasodilatation, pain-related neurotransmitter blockage, peripheral inflammatory pain inhibition and the inhibition of central pain perception contribute to the effectiveness of BoNT for neuropathic pain (Ranoux *et al.*, 2008; Yuan *et al.*, 2009; Neumeister *et al.*, 2009).

Pathophysiology of neuropathic pain

Neuropathic pain refers to pain associated with peripheral nervous system injury. It is a common form of chronic pain, which usually also includes nociceptive pain, visceral pain and the mixed etiology. Diabetic neuropathy, postherpetic neuralgia, radiculopathy pain, trigeminal neuralgia and complex regional pain syndrome are all neuropathic pain syndromes. Other pain syndromes, such as migraine headache and myofascial pain, share some clinical and pathophysiologic features with neuropathic pain. In addition to pain, patients with chronic neuropathic pain usually suffer from numbness, tingling, stinging, itching and burning sensations.

Both peripheral and central sensitization processes are involved in the pathophysiology of neuropathic pain (Baron, 2006; Pace *et al.*, 2006) (Fig. 25.1). After tissue damage, mast cells and macrophages are activated and some blood-borne immune cells are recruited. Many kinds of inflammation mediators are released, including tumor necrosis factor-alpha, interleukin-1β, interleukin-6, nitric oxide, prostaglandins, nerve growth factor and cyclooxygenase 2. These inflammatory mediators are related to pain either directly through action on nociceptors or indirectly by enhancing the release of other pain-related mediators. The resultant damage of afferent C and Aδ nerve fibers also causes ectopic discharges, with a subsequent reduction in nociceptor thresholds as a result of the accumulation of sodium channels through neuroplasticity and alteration of the modulatory systems. Ectopic discharges further induce a central sensitization that enhances neuropathic pain. The NMDA (*N*-methyl-D-aspartate) receptor for the excitatory neurotransmitter glutamate appears to play a significant role in the development of central sensitization. In addition, abnormal muscle contraction and released substance P and calcitonin gene-related peptide also mediate hyperalgesia.

Botulinum neurotoxin for pain relief

Botulinum neurotoxin has been used effectively to alleviate pain in certain pain disorders, including migraine,

---

Manual of Botulinum Toxin Therapy, 2nd edition, ed. Daniel Truong, Mark Hallett, Christopher Zachary and Dirk Dressler.
Published by Cambridge University Press. © Cambridge University Press 2013.

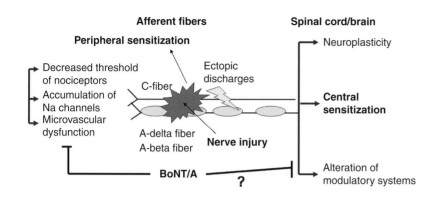

Fig. 25.1 Botulinum neurotoxin A (BoNT/A) may have various ways in relieving neuropathic pain. However, the central effect is still debated.

myofascial pain syndrome, plantar fasciitis, arthritis and carpal tunnel syndrome (Jabbari and Machado, 2011). This has extended the field of traditional pain therapy, particularly for the unsatisfactory treatment of neuropathic pain. In fact, BoNT can suppress both nociceptor sensitization and neuropathic pain and has been shown to have a pain-relieving effect in peripheral neuropathic pain of various conditions (Ranoux et al., 2008; Yuan et al., 2009).

Botulinum neurotoxin also has a role in the treatment of ischemic pain in vasospastic disorders (Neumeister et al., 2009).

How botulinum neurotoxin works with neuropathic pain

Abnormal muscle contractions contribute to chronic pain (Gunn, 2001). Botulinum neurotoxin serotypeA (BoNT-A) is well known to have an effect on inhibition of muscle contraction and this may partially explain its effect on chronic pain. It has also been hypothesized that BoNT-A blocks the neurovascular smooth muscle cells, thereby causing vasodilatation (Van Beek et al., 2007).

In preclinical models, BoNT-A was found to effectively block the release of several pain-related neurotransmitters, including norepinephrine, substance P, glutamate and calcitonin gene-related peptide, from afferent nerve terminals (Cui et al., 2004; Aoki, 2005). These pain-related neurotransmitters can stimulate depolarization of C fibers, which are responsible for propagation of chronic pain. The experimental studies showed that interruption of the release of pain-related neurotransmitters could block the peripheral sensitization of pain.

Extracellular ATP is implicated in a considerable number of sensory processes, including pain. Evidence shows that activation of P2X3 purine receptor by ATP leads to a much stronger nociceptive effect in inflamed tissue; BoNT-A has been reported to block these receptors, which are almost exclusively expressed in the sensory neurons (Paukert et al., 2001; Ford et al., 2006).

BoNT-A also blocks the translocation of the capsaicin receptor (vanilloid receptor; a member of the transient receptor potential cation channel subfamily V), a protein that is responsible for perception of peripheral inflammatory pain in peripheral nociceptor terminals (Morenilla-Palao et al., 2004). In a formalin-induced pain study, BoNT-A was found to have an antinociceptive effect, which was associated with the inhibition of glutamate release from the primary afferent terminals (Cui et al., 2004). The excitatory amino acid glutamate is also involved in the induction and maintenance of central sensitization of pain by exerting its postsynaptic effect via NMDA receptors (Petrenko et al., 2003). These findings raise the possibility of potential indirect central effects of BoNT.

In summary, BoNT may act to relieve neuropathic pain via multiple mechanisms (Fig. 25.1). Easing muscle contraction, improving microvascularity, blockade of neurotransmitter release and inhibiting central perception all contribute to the effectiveness of BoNT for neuropathic pain.

Diabetic neuropathic pain

Chronic pain is one of the most common complications of diabetic neuropathy. The prevalence of painful peripheral neuropathy in type 2 diabetes is more than 25% (Davies et al., 2006). There is still no comprehensive understanding of the underlying biologic process responsible for diabetic neuropathic pain. However, it is believed that both neuropathic pain and microangiopathy-related ischemic pain play significant roles.

A randomized double-blind crossover trial demonstrated the pain-relieving effect of BoNT for diabetic foot pain (Yuan *et al.*, 2009). This pilot study included 20 patients with type 2 diabetes who suffered from neuropathic pain in both feet and had been diagnosed with diabetes for at least 3 years. The recruited patients were assessed to confirm the diagnosis of polyneuropathy by (1) physical examination, (2) the neuropathic pain diagnostic questionnaire DN4, and (3) nerve conduction velocity examinations. Participants were randomly assigned to receive either BoNT-A or saline injections as their first treatment and were crossed over to the alternate treatment in the second half of the study. The injections were given at 12 evenly spaced sites across the dorsum of each foot. Each injection comprised either approximately 4 U BoNT-A or 0.9% saline, 0.10 ml, using a 8 mm (5/16-inch) 30-gauge needle. Since the dorsal area of each foot is over 100 cm^2 for most people, the average dosage adopted for this trial was below 0.5 U/cm^2 (Fig. 25.2). This dosage is much lower than the therapeutic dosage in the study of BoNT-A for trigeminal neuralgia (Piovesan *et al.*, 2005). The visual analog scale (VAS), the Chinese version of the Pittsburgh Sleep Quality Index (CPSQI), and the Short Form-36 (SF-36) quality-of-life questionnaire were given at intervals of 1, 4, 8 and 12 weeks after the initial injection. The second (i.e. crossover) injection was given in the 12th week.

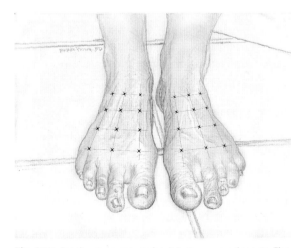

Fig. 25.2 Botulinum neurotoxin for diabetic neuropathic pain: The injections were given at 12 evenly spaced sites across the dorsum of each foot. Each injection comprised approximately 4 U onabotulinumtoxinA/incobotulinumtoxinA. The average dosage adopted for this trial was below 0.5 U/cm^2.

At 4, 8 and 12 weeks, significant reductions in VAS occurred in the BoNT-A group compared with the placebo group. Within the BoNT-A treatment group, 44.4% experienced good responses (a reduction in VAS by ≥3) within 3 months after the initial injection, whereas no good responses were found in the placebo group. The BoNT-A treatment began to show a trend toward significantly improving after the 4th week, with the effect ultimately lasting for 12 weeks. The improvement in sleep quality scored by CPSQI in the BoNT-A treatment group only appeared transiently at 4 weeks after initial injection. There were no significant differences in the changes in scores for the physical and mental components of the SF-36 between the two groups at the same time points. There was one patient with a mild local skin infection at the injection site at 1 day after injection. In this trial, BoNT-A therapy was found to be effective and safe for relieving diabetic neuropathic pain in the feet. The improvement lasted for at least 3 months. However, the improvement of neuropathic pain induced by BoNT-A injections might be insignificant for changing quality of life and sleep quality.

Trigeminal neuralgia

Several studies have provided evidence that BoNT has beneficial effects on the treatment of trigeminal neuralgia (Piovesan *et al.*, 2005; Turk *et al.*, 2005). Piovesan *et al.* (2005) used transcutaneous BoNT-A injection to treat 13 patients with trigeminal neuralgia in an open-label pilot study. The injection sites were chosen according to the patients' descriptions and anatomically outlined pain sites. The mean therapeutic dose for all branches and patients was approximately 3.22 U/cm^2. After BoNT-A, there was a significant reduction of the pain area and VAS assessment (Fig. 25.3). All patients reduced their use of preventive medication and some were medication free.

Postherpetic neuralgia

Herpes zoster is induced by reactivation of dormant varicella zoster virus (Sampathkumar *et al.*, 2009). Herpetic neuralgia usually lasts 2 to 4 weeks and occasionally precedes the onset of rash by 7 to 10 days (Argoff *et al.*, 2004). For most patients, herpetic neuralgia disappears in a few weeks, but about

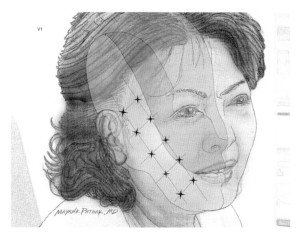

Fig. 25.3 Botulinum neurotoxin for trigeminal neuralgia. The injection sites are chosen according to the patient's description and the anatomically outlined pain sites. The injections are subcutaneous and in a grid manner. The mean therapeutic dosage for all branches of nerves and patients is approximately 3.22 U/cm^2 (onabotulinumtoxinA). The number of units and the sites to be injected varies for each patient. Stars indicate injection sites.

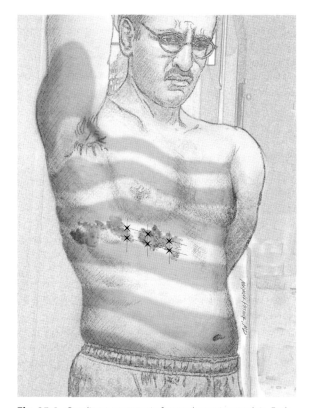

Fig. 25.4 xBotulinum neurotoxin for postherpetic neuralgia. Each vial containing 100 U botulinum neurotoxin A (onabotulinumtoxinA) is diluted with 4 ml saline, resulting in a concentration of 25 U/ml. About 5 U is injected subcutaneously over 1–2 cm^2 in a chessboard fashion over the affected area. A total of 20 sites (100 U) are injected for every individual. Black points indicate injection sites.

10% develop postherpetic neuralgia, which is defined as pain persisting for longer than 4 months after the onset of the skin rash. The mechanisms for conversion to postherpetic neuralgia from acute herpes neuralgia are still unclear (Opstelten *et al.*, 2002).

The pathophysiology of postherpetic neuralgia involves processes within the peripheral and central nervous systems. During the acute stage, reactivated dormant virus replicates and propagates along the nerve. It induces an inflammation and immune responses, which results in damage in peripheral and central neurons (Argoff *et al.*, 2004). As a result, both peripheral and central sensitizations are triggered.

Administration of BoNT-A has been found to significantly decrease VAS pain scores in postherpetic neuralgia compared with lidocaine and placebo at day 7 and 3 months post-treatment (Xiao *et al.*, 2010). In that trial, BoNT-A 100 U/20 ml saline was given subcutaneously with single-use tuberculin syringes (1 ml), 1 ml for every injection site within 1.0–2.0 cm radius of skin.

In our clinic, we dilute each vial of 100 U onabotulinumtoxinA with 4 ml of saline, resulting in a concentration of 25 U/ml. For postherpetic neuralgia, approximately 5 U is injected subcutaneously for each 1–2 cm^2 in a chessboard fashion over the affected area. A total of 20 sites (100 U) are injected for each individual (Fig. 25.4).

Technique for botulinum neurotoxin treatment of neuropathic pain

For neuropathic pain, the BoNT-containing solution is injected subcutaneously or intradermally, in a chessboard manner, over the affected area.

For intradermal injection, the needle is inserted at an angle of 10 to 15 degrees with the bevel of the needle pointing up. The injection should be shallow enough that the bevel is just covered by skin and the needle should be easily visible under the skin. The solution is slowly injected and a small bubble of skin will rise if intradermal injection is done correctly (Fig. 25.5).

The recommended dilution method and dose for neuropathic pain is given in Table 25.1

There have been no major side effects. A minor side effect is local infection.

219

Table 25.1 Recommended dilution and dose for onabotulinumtoxinA (Botox)

	Dilution	Dose
Diabetic neuropathic pain	100 U/2 ml saline (50 U/ml)	0.2 ml/injection site, 0.5 U every cm^2
Trigeminal neuralgia	100 U/2 ml saline	0.2 ml/injection site, 3 U every cm^2
Postherpetic neuralgia	100 U/4–20 ml saline (5–25 U/ml)	0.2 ml/injection site, 0.5–3 U every cm^2

Source: Allergan, Irvine, CA, USA.

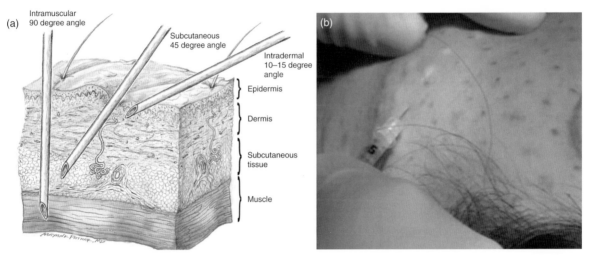

Fig. 25.5 Botulinum neurotoxin for neuropathic pain. It is suggested that the botulinum neurotoxin -containing solution is injected subcutaneously or intradermally. (a) For intradermal injection, the needle is inserted at an angle of 10–15 degrees with the bevel (angled hole) of the needle pointing up. The injection should be shallow enough that the bevel is just covered by the skin and the needle should be easily visible under the skin. (b) The solution is injected slowly and a small bubble of skin will rise if an intradermal injection is properly achieved.

References

Aoki KR (2005). Review of a proposed mechanism for the antinociceptive action of botulinum toxin type A. *Neurotoxicology*, **26**, 785–93.

Argoff CE, Katz N, Backonja M (2004). Treatment of postherpetic neuralgia: a review of therapeutic options. *J Pain Symptom Manage*, **28**, 396–411.

Baron R (2006). Mechanisms of disease: neuropathic pain a clinical perspective. *Nat Clin Pract Neurol*, **2**, 95–106.

Cui M, Khanijou S, Rubino J, Aoki KR (2004). Subcutaneous administration of botulinum toxin A reduces formalin-induced pain. *Pain*, **107**, 125–33.

Davies M, Brophy S, Williams R, Taylor A (2006). The prevalence, severity and impact of painful diabetic peripheral neuropathy in type 2 diabetes. *Diabetes Care*, **29**, 1518–22.

Ford AP, Gever JR, Nunn PA *et al.* (2006). Purinoceptors as therapeutic targets for lower urinary tract dysfunction. *Br J Pharmacol*, **147**, S132–43.

Gunn CC (2001). Neuropathic myofascial pain syndromes. In Loeser, JD (ed.) *Bonica's Management of Pain*. Philadelphia, PA: Lippincott, Williams & Wilkins, pp. 522–9.

Jabbari B, Machado D (2011). Treatment of refractory pain with botulinum toxins: an evidence-based review. *Pain Med*, **12**, 1594–606.

Morenilla-Palao C, Planells-Cases R, García-Sanz N, Ferrer-Montiel A (2004). Regulated exocytosis contributes to protein kinase C potentiation of vanilloid receptor activity. *J Biol Chem*, **279**, 25665–72.

Neumeister MW, Chambers CB, Herron MS *et al.* (2009). Botox therapy for ischemic digits. *Plast Reconstr Surg*, **124**, 191–201.

Opstelten W, Mauritz JW, de Wit NJ *et al.* (2002). Herpes zoster and postherpetic neuralgia: incidence and risk indicators using a general practice research database. *Fam Pract*, **19**, 471–5.

Pace MC, Mazzariello L, Passavanti MB *et al.* (2006). Neurobiology of pain. *J Cell Physiol*, **209**, 8–12.

Paukert M, Osteroth R, Geisler HS *et al.* (2001). Inflammatory mediators potentiate ATP-gated channels through the P2X(3) subunit. *J Biol Chem*, **276**, 21077–82.

Petrenko AB, Yamakura T, Baba H, Shimoji K (2003). The role of *N*-methyl-D-aspartate (NMDA) receptors in pain a review. *Anesth Analg*, **97**, 1108–16.

Piovesan EJ, Teive HG, Kowacs PA *et al.* (2005). An open study of botulinum A toxin treatment of trigeminal neuralgia. *Neurology*, **65**, 1306–8.

Ranoux D, Attal N, Morain F, Bouhassira D (2008). Botulinumtoxin typeA induces direct analgesic effects in chronic neuropathic pain. *Ann Neurol*, **64**, 274–83.

Sampathkumar P, Drage LA, Martin DP (2009). Herpes zoster (shingles) and postherpetic neuralgia. *Mayo Clin Proc*, **84**, 274–80.

Turk U, Ilhan S, Alp R, Sur H (2005). Botulinum toxin and intractable trigeminal neuralgia. *Clin Neuropharmacol*, **28**, 161–2.

Van Beek AL, Lim PK, Gear AJL, Pritzker MR (2007). Management of vasospastic disorders with botulinum toxin A. *Plast Reconstr Surg*, **119**, 217–26.

Xiao L, Mackey S, Hui H *et al.* (2010). Subcutaneous injection of botulinum toxin A is beneficial in postherpetic neuralgia. *Pain Med*, **11**, 1827–33.

Yuan RY, Sheu JJ, Yu JM *et al.* (2009). Botulinum toxin for diabetic neuropathic pain a randomized double-blind crossover trial. *Neurology*, **72**, 1473–8.

Chapter 26

The use of botulinum neurotoxin in the management of headache disorders

Stephen D. Silberstein

Clinical aspects of headache disorders

Headache affects more than 45 million individuals in the USA, which makes it one of the most common nervous system disorders (National Institute of Neurological Disorders and Stroke, 2002). The International Headache Society's diagnostic criteria for headache disorders (ICHD-II, Headache Classification Committee, 2004) classifies primary headache disorders as those in which headache itself is the illness, with no other etiology diagnosed. Examples include migraine and tension-type headache (TTH). Headache disorders can be further classified as episodic (<15 headache days per month) or chronic (≥15 headache days per month for more than 3 months).

Migraine is a primary headache disorder characterized by enhanced sensitivity of the nervous system (Silberstein, 2000) associated with a combination of neurological, gastrointestinal and autonomic disturbances (Silberstein, 2004). The ICHD-II has provided criteria for a total of seven subtypes of migraine (including migraine with and migraine without aura). The ICHD-II diagnostic criteria for migraine without aura (Headache Classification Committee, 2004) include

- headache associated with at least two of the following: unilateral location, pulsating quality, moderate or severe pain intensity and aggravation by or causing avoidance of routine physical activities
- at least one of the following during headache: nausea and/or vomiting, photophobia and phonophobia
- headache not attributable to another disorder.

It is estimated that 28 million Americans, including 18% of women and 7% of men, are afflicted with severe, disabling migraines (Lipton et al., 2001). The World Health Organization (2012) ranked migraine as one of the world's most disabling illnesses, profoundly impacting quality of life and causing functional impairment and disruption of household or social activities. The economic burden of the disease to society is also considerable. In the USA, the yearly medical costs exceed 1 billion dollars, and costs to employers due to migraine-related absenteeism and reduced productivity is 13 billion dollars (Hu et al., 1999).

Chronic daily headache is a heterogeneous group of headache disorders that can include chronic migraine and chronic TTH, as well as other headache types that occur 15 days or more per month in the absence of structural or systemic disease (Silberstein et al., 2005). It affects 4–5% of the general population worldwide (Castillo et al., 1998; Scher et al., 1998; Wang et al., 2000). Patients with chronic daily headache often overuse acute headache medications (Silberstein et al., 2005) and have greater disability and lower quality of life than patients with episodic headache (Meletiche et al., 2001; Bigal et al., 2003; Lipton et al., 2011).

Tension-type headache is the most common of the primary headache disorders, with an annual prevalence as high as 38% (Schwartz et al., 1998). Tension-type headache is associated with bilateral pain that is pressing or tightening in quality and mild to moderate in intensity. It is not associated with nausea and vomiting or routine physical activity, but it may be associated with photophobia or phonophobia (Headache Classification Committee, 2004). Frequent episodic TTH (at least 10 episodes occurring on ≥1 but <15 days per month) or chronic TTH (≥15 days per month) is associated with greatly decreased quality of life and high disability (Schwartz et al., 1998; Headache Classification Committee, 2004).

Manual of Botulinum Toxin Therapy, 2nd edition, ed. Daniel Truong, Mark Hallett, Christopher Zachary and Dirk Dressler.
Published by Cambridge University Press. © Cambridge University Press 2013.

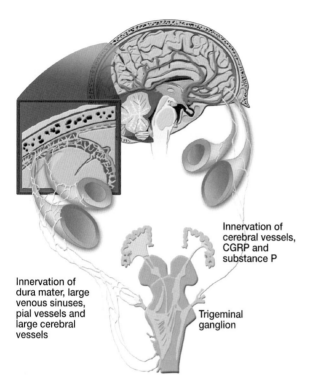

Fig. 26.1 Craniovascular innervation. CGRP, calcitonin gene-related peptide. (Reproduced with permission from Goadsby PJ (2001). Pathophysiology of headache. In Silberstein SD, Lipton RB, Dalessio DJ (eds.) *Wolff's Headache and Other Head Pain*, 7th edn. New York: Oxford University Press; 2001, p. 59.)

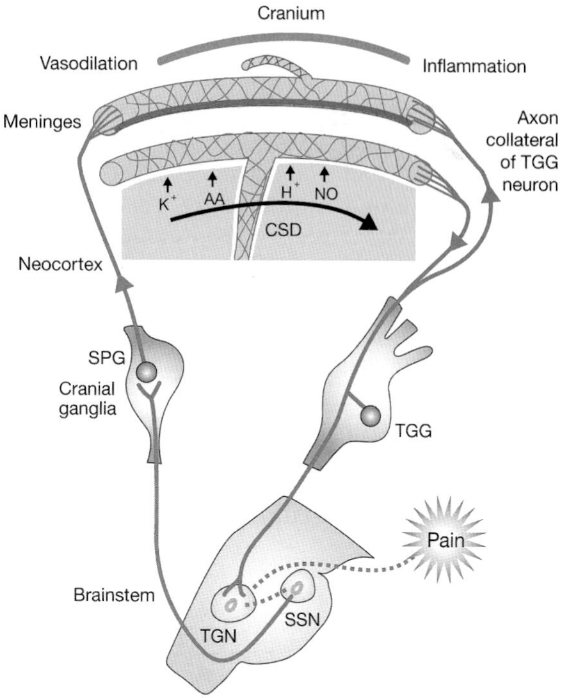

Labels in figure: Innervation of cerebral vessels, CGRP and substance P; Innervation of dura mater, large venous sinuses, pial vessels and large cerebral vessels; Trigeminal ganglion

Labels in Fig. 26.2: Cranium; Vasodilation; Inflammation; Meninges; Axon collateral of TGG neuron; K⁺; AA; H⁺; NO; CSD; Neocortex; SPG; Cranial ganglia; TGG; Pain; Brainstem; TGN; SSN

Fig. 26.2 Cortical spreading depression. AA, arachidonic acid; NO, nitric oxide; CSD, cortical spreading depression; TGG, trigeminal ganglion; SPG, sphenopalatine ganglion; TGN, trigeminal nucleus; SSN, superior sagittal sinus. (Reproduced with permission from Silberstein SD. Migraine. *Lancet*, 2004;363:381–91.)

Pathophysiology of headache disorders

Migraine is believed to arise from activation of meningeal and blood vessel nociceptors, along with a change in central pain modulation mediated by the trigeminal system (Silberstein, 2004). In response to stimulation of the trigeminal sensory neurons, perivascular nerve fibers that innervate blood vessels release peptide mediators, neurokinin A, substance P and calcitonin gene-related peptide, which transmit nociceptive activity to the brainstem autonomic nuclei via glutamate-mediated transduction (Fig. 26.1). The trigeminovascular system can be activated by cortical spreading depression, a process characterized by shifts in cortical steady-state potential; transient increases in potassium, nitric oxide and glutamate; and transient increases followed by sustained decreases in cortical blood flow (Fig. 26.2) (Silberstein, 2004). Trigeminal activation results in release of vasoactive peptide-producing neurogenic inflammation, vasodilation, sensitization of nerve fibers and, ultimately, pain and associated symptoms (Silberstein, 2004). Migraine

pain is likely a result of the combination of activation of pain-producing intracranial structures and reduction in endogenous pain control pathways (Silberstein, 2004; Silberstein *et al.*, 2008).

The pathophysiology underlying TTH is not well understood. The relative contributions of peripheral and central pain mechanisms to TTH remain unclear (Silberstein *et al.*, 2006).

Treatment of headache

Acute (abortive) migraine treatments, which patients take in an attempt to relieve pain and disability and prevent progression, include migraine-specific medications, such as ergots or triptans, and non-specific agents, such as analgesics or opioids (Silberstein, 2004). Patients with acute TTH typically self-medicate with over-the-counter analgesics, such as aspirin, acetaminophen, or non-steroidal anti-inflammatory drugs (NSAIDs), which could lead to drug overuse. They may also use prescription NSAIDs or combination analgesics.

Preventive treatments are designed to reduce the frequency, severity or duration of migraine attacks. These are indicated when acute medications are ineffective or overused or headaches are very frequent or disabling. Preventive agents include beta-adrenergic blockers, antidepressants, calcium channel and serotonin antagonists, anticonvulsants and NSAIDs (Silberstein, 2004). While daily oral-prophylactic treatments have proven effective, issues such as lack of compliance with daily dosing regimens and adverse effects have limited their usefulness (Blumenfeld *et al.*, 2003; Silberstein, 2004) and this resulted in a search for other modalities and agents, including botulinum neurotoxin (BoNT), as potential preventive treatments.

Botulinum neurotoxin in headache disorders

Formulations

The seven BoNT serotypes (A1, A2, A3, B, C1, D, E, F and G) produced by *Clostridium botulinum* are synthesized as single-chain polypeptides. All serotypes inhibit acetylcholine release, although their intracellular target proteins, physiochemical characteristics and potencies are different (Aoki and Guyer, 2001; Mauskop, 2004). Serotype A (BoNT-A) has been the most widely studied serotype for therapeutic purposes (Aoki and Guyer, 2001). A major clinical advantage of BoNT-A arises from its extraordinarily prolonged duration of action due to the longevity of its protease (90 days in rats and probably much longer in human neurons). A di-leucine in the light chain of BoNT-A underlies its long duration of action by inhibiting its degradation (Wang *et al.*, 2011).

Currently, BoNT-A is available for clinical use in the USA as onabotulinumtoxinA (Botox, Allergan, Irvine, CA, USA), abobotulinumtoxinA (Dysport, Ipsen, Slough, UK) and incobotulinumtoxinA (Xeomin, Merz Pharmaceuticals, Greensboro, NC, USA). Serotype B is available as rimabotulinumtoxinB (NeuroBloc/Myobloc, Solstice Neurosciences, South San Francisco, CA, USA). Lyophilized Botox is available in vials containing 100 or 200 U and is diluted with 2 or 4 ml of preservative-free 0.9% saline to yield a concentration of 5.0/0.1 ml or 2.5 U/0.1 ml, respectively (Allergan, 2004a). Reconstituted solutions of Botox can be refrigerated but must be used within 4 hours (Allergan, 2004a). Lyophilized incobotulinumtoxinA is available in vials containing 50 or 100 U and is diluted

with preservative-free 0.9% saline. Dysport is reconstituted with 1.0 ml of 0.9% saline to yield a solution of 500 U/ml and the reconstituted product may be stored in a refrigerator for up to 8 hours before use (Allergan, 2004b). NeuroBloc/Myobloc is available in 0.5, 1 and 2 ml vials containing 5000 U/ml (Mauskop, 2004).

There is no formula for establishing dosage equivalence for onabotulinumtoxinA and abobotulinumtoxinA, which have different dosing, safety and efficacy properties. It has been difficult to establish dose conversion factors for BoNT-A preparations. In general, these formulations lack bioequivalence and interchangeability (Aoki and Guyer, 2001). In fact, the Botox package insert states that units of activity cannot be compared with nor converted into units of other BoNT preparations (Allergan, 2004a).

Mechanism of action of botulinum neurotoxin in headache

Botulinum neurotoxin binds to motor and sympathetic nerve terminals. It enters the nerve terminals and inhibits the release of acetylcholine. This inhibition occurs as the BoNT cleaves one of several proteins integral to the successful docking and release of acetylcholine from vesicles situated within nerve endings. This results in blocking of neuromuscular transmission at the neuromuscular junction. Following intramuscular injection, BoNT produces partial chemical denervation of the muscle, resulting in a localized reduction in muscle activity (Aoki and Guyer, 2001; Mauskop, 2004).

The association between BoNT use and the alleviation of migraine headache symptoms was discovered during initial clinical trials of BoNT-A treatment for hyperfunctional facial lines (Binder *et al.*, 2000). Treatment with BoNT has been used for a variety of disorders associated with painful muscle spasms. Because migraine attacks are frequently associated with muscle tenderness (Jensen *et al.*, 1998), it was generally believed that intramuscular BoNT might prevent abnormal sensory signals in the affected muscle from reaching the central nervous system. If abnormal muscle physiology can trigger migraine, one would predict that BoNT treatment would work prophylactically only in patients whose migraine attacks develop on the heels of episodic or chronic muscle tenderness.

Jakubowski *et al.* (2006) explored neurological markers that might distinguish patients with migraine who would benefit from BoNT treatment from those who would not. The prevalence of neck tenderness, aura, photophobia, phonophobia, osmophobia, nausea and throbbing was similar between responders and non-responders. However, the two groups offered different accounts of their pain. Among non-responders, 92% described a build up of pressure inside their head (exploding headache). Among responders, 74% perceived their head to be crushed, clamped or stubbed by external forces (imploding headache), and 13% attested to an eye-popping pain (ocular headache). The finding that exploding headache is not as responsive to extracranial BoNT injections is consistent with the view that migraine pain is mediated by intracranial innervation. The amenability of imploding and ocular headaches to BoNT treatment suggests that these types of migraine pain also involve extracranial innervation (Jakubowski *et al.*, 2006). The precise mechanisms by which BoNT alleviates headache pain are unclear. Its inhibition of the release of glutamate and the neuropeptides substance P and calcitonin gene-related peptide from nociceptive neurons suggests that its antinociceptive properties are distinct from its neuromuscular activity (Dodick *et al.*, 2005).

Botulinum neurotoxin may inhibit central sensitization of trigeminovascular neurons, which is believed to be key to migraine's development and maintenance (Aoki, 2003; Cui *et al.*, 2004; Oshinsky *et al.*, 2004; Dodick *et al.*, 2005). Oshinsky *et al.* (2004) used a preclinical model of sensitizing dorsal horn neurons in the trigeminal nucleus caudalis following chemical stimulation of the dura as a model for testing the effects of BoNT on central sensitization. They used single neuron electrophysiology of second sensory neurons in the trigeminal nucleus caudalis with cutaneous receptive fields and microdialysis of the trigeminal nucleus caudalis to evaluate the effects of pretreatment of the periorbital region of the rat with BoNT-A. In saline-treated animals, extracellular glutamate increased steadily after 100 minutes following the application of inflammatory soup to the dura. The increase in glutamate reached approximately three times the basal level at 3 hours after the inflammatory soup. Electrophysiologic recordings of neurons in the trigeminal nucleus caudalis before and after sensitization confirmed these data. Following the inflammatory soup, there was an increase in the magnitude of the response to sensory stimuli and an increase in the cutaneous receptive field of the second sensory neurons in the trigeminal nucleus caudalis.

Afferent–efferent communication happens in the nerve through axon–axon glutamate secretion, and at the level of the ganglion through non-synaptic release of glutamate and peptides (substance P and calcitonin gene-related peptide). Following a 5-minute chemical stimulation of the dura in a rat, the extracellular level of glutamate increases two- to three-fold. This increase was blocked by pretreating the face of the rat with BoNT-A. Producing the large changes in extracellular glutamate in the central nervous system requires a massive sensory activation. The afferents of the dura may recruit the afferents of the face and head, which leads to the sensitization of these areas seen in human and animal studies. Use of BoNT may block the axon–axon and interganglionic communication of the afferents and thus prevent central and peripheral sensitization outside of the dura. Electrophysiological studies confirmed that there is no change in the magnitude of the sensory response in the trigeminal nucleus caudalis neurons or their receptive field in the BoNT-A-treated rats following the inflammatory soup. These data show that peripheral application of BoNT-A prevents central sensitization elicited by stimulation of the dura with inflammatory mediators (Oshinsky *et al.*, 2004).

Oshinsky *et al.* (2004) have proposed the following hypothesis: Following chemical stimulation of the dura (during a migraine attack and in this rat model), the dural afferents communicate with other trigeminal afferents on the ophthalmic division of the trigeminal nerve and recruit them to secrete glutamate and neuropeptides. This would recruit more afferents, spreading activation and sensitization. The number of afferents activated on the dura is small compared with the total number of afferents in the whole trigeminal system, so activation of the dural afferents alone may not be sufficient to produce the large changes in the central nervous system that lead to central sensitization.

Treatment guidelines

Therapy with BoNT-A is now indicated for patients with chronic migraine. It may also be effective for patients with a high frequency of episodic migraine. Its use is contraindicated for patients with sensitivity to BoNT. It must be used with caution in patients with neuromuscular disorders, such as myasthenia gravis (Blumenfeld *et al.*, 2003).

Treatment techniques

Sterile technique should be observed for the entire BoNT injection procedure. Injections do not have to be intramuscular, but the muscles are used as reference sites for injections, which are most commonly administered in the glabellar and frontal regions, the temporalis muscle, the occipitalis muscle and the cervical paraspinal region.

The injection protocols commonly used are: (1) the fixed-site approach, which uses fixed, symmetrical injection sites and a range of predetermined doses; (2) the follow-the-pain approach, which often employs asymmetrical injections and adjusts the sites and doses depending on where the patient feels pain and where the examiner can elicit pain and tenderness on palpation of the muscle; and (3) a combination approach, which uses injections at fixed frontal sites supplemented with follow-the-pain injections (this approach typically uses higher doses of BoNT-A) (Blumenfeld et al., 2003).

Based on exploratory phase secondary chronic migraine studies (Castillo et al., 1998; Evers et al., 2004), the PREEMPT clinical program established a successful modified follow-the-pain protocol treatment paradigm (Elkind et al., 2006). OnabotulinumtoxinA (155 U) is administered as 31 fixed-site, fixed-dose injections across seven specific head and neck muscle areas. A sterile 1 ml Luer Lock syringe with a 30-gauge 0.5 inch (1.25 cm) needle is used. Each injection is 0.1 ml, which contains 5 U BoNT-A. Up to 40 U additional onabotulinumtoxinA can be administered, using a follow-the-pain strategy, into the temporalis, occipitalis and/or trapezius muscles, with a maximum dose of 195 U administered to 39 sites (Table 26.1). When deciding on dose and location of additional onabotulinumtoxinA, the location of the patient's predominant pain and the severity of palpable muscle tenderness should be considered (Table 26.1 lists and Figs. 26.3–26.8 illustrate the recommended anatomical sites of injection for headache and the onabotulinumtoxinA (Botox) dose per site used in the PREEMPT trials).

Clinical comparison of efficacy of botulinum neurotoxin formats in headache disorders

Most studies on the efficacy and safety of BoNT in headache treatment have used onabotulinumtoxinA (Botox). No large, well-controlled studies using other preparations have been published. The following discussion will focus on relevant studies with onabotulinumtoxinA. Clinical trial results discussed

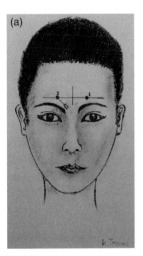
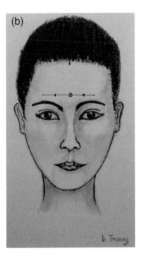

Fig. 26.3 The corrugator and procerus injection sites. (a) The corrugator injection sites (bilateral) are above the medial superior edge of the orbital ridge (bony landmark). (b) The procerus site is above and midline to the medial superior aspect of the orbital ridge (bony landmark) of each eye.

Table 26.1 OnabotulinumtoxinA dosing for chronic migraine by muscle

Head/neck area	Total dose (U [No. intramuscular injection sites[a]])	
	Minimum dose	Maximum dose
Frontalis	20 (4)	20 (4)
Corrugator	10 (2)	10 (2)
Procerus	5 (1)	5 (1)
Occipitalis	30 (6)	≤40 (5 U/site) (≤8)
Temporalis	40 (8)	≤50 (5 U/site) (≤10)
Trapezius	30 (6)	≤50 (5 U/site) (≤10)
Cervical paraspinal muscle group	20 (4)	20 (4)
Total dose	155 (31)	195 (≤39)

[a] Each intramuscular injection site received 0.1 ml (5 U) onabotulinumtoxinA.

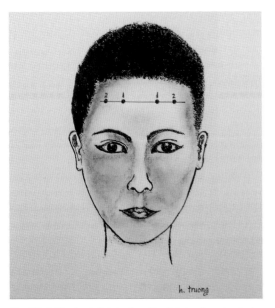

Fig. 26.4 The frontalis injection sites (bilateral) are located just beneath the skin surface of the central and forehead regions.

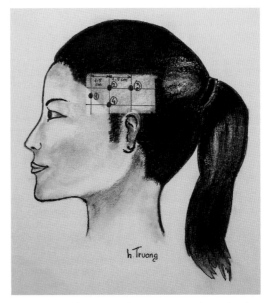

Fig. 26.5 The first temporalis injection site is located in the anterior aspect of the temporalis muscle. The second and fourth sites are within the medial aspect and the third site is located in the posterior aspect of this muscle. These injections should be repeated on the left side for a total of eight injections into the temporalis muscle. Additional injections can be distributed between the right and left temporalis muscles in areas of maximal tenderness and/or pain.

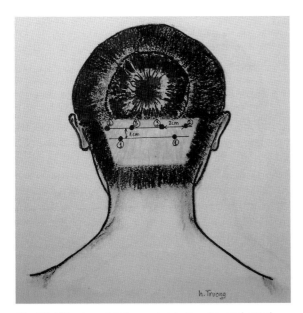

Fig. 26.6 The six occipitalis muscle injection sites are located superior to the supranuchal ridge on either side of the occipital protuberance. In the areas of maximal tenderness and/or pain, up to two additional injections can be distributed across the right and left occipitalis muscles.

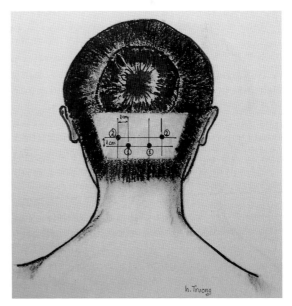

Fig. 26.7 The first cervical paraspinal injection site is lateral to the midline and inferior to the occipital protuberance. The second site is lateral and superior to the first injection. These injections should be repeated symmetrically on the contralateral side for a total of four injections.

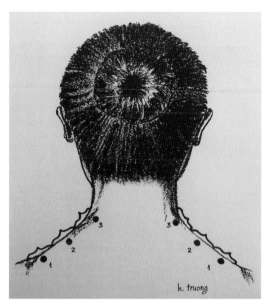

Fig. 26.8 The first of the three trapezius muscle injection sites is located in the lateral aspect of the muscle. The second site is within the mid-portion of the muscle and the third site is within the superior aspect of the muscle. Symmetrical injections should be repeated on the contralateral side for a total of six injections. Up to four additional injections can be distributed between the right and left trapezius muscles in areas identified as having maximal tenderness.

below are summarized in Table 26.2 (Schulte-Mattler and Leinisch, 2008).

Some studies support the efficacy of BoNT-A in migraine treatment. A double-blind, vehicle-controlled trial of 123 patients with moderate to severe migraine found that subjects treated with a single injection of 25 U BoNT-A (but not those treated with 75 U) showed significantly fewer migraine attacks per month, as well as reductions in migraine severity, number of days requiring acute medication, and incidence of migraine-induced vomiting. The lack of significant effect in the higher-dose group may be related to baseline group differences, such as fewer migraines or a longer time since migraine onset (Silberstein *et al.*, 2000). Another double-blind, placebo-controlled, region-specific study found a significant reduction in migraine pain among patients who received simultaneous injections of BoNT-A in the frontal and temporal regions, as well as an overall trend toward BoNT-A superiority to placebo in reducing migraine frequency and duration (Brin *et al.*, 2000). A randomized, double-blind, placebo-controlled study compared the efficacy of placebo, 16 U BoNT-A and 100 U BoNT-A as

migraine prophylaxis when injected into the frontal and neck muscles (Evers *et al.*, 2004). While there were no statistically significant differences in reduction of migraine frequency among the groups, the accompanying symptoms of migraine were reduced in the group receiving 16 U BoNT-A (Evers *et al.*, 2004).

New studies, however, have failed to demonstrate significant improvements over placebo. A study of 232 patients with moderate to severe episodic migraine (four to eight episodes/month) compared placebo with regional (frontal, temporal, or glabellar) or combined (frontal/temporal/glabellar) treatment with BoNT-A (Saper *et al.*, 2007). Reductions from baseline in migraine frequency, maximum severity and duration occurred with BoNT-A and placebo, but there were no significant between-group differences. Elkind *et al.* (2006) conducted a series of three sequential studies of 418 patients with a history of four to eight moderate to severe migraines per month, with further randomization at each stage, and BoNT-A doses ranging from 7.5 to 50 U. Placebo and BoNT-A produced comparable decreases from baseline in migraine frequency at each time point examined, with no consistent, statistically significant between-group differences observed.

Several randomized, double-blind, placebo-controlled studies support the efficacy of BoNT for the treatment of chronic daily headache. In a large, placebo-controlled study of 355 patients, Mathew *et al.* (2005) found that BoNT-A did not differ from placebo in the primary efficacy measure (change from baseline in headache-free days at day 180); however, there were significant differences in several secondary endpoints, including a greater percentage of patients with a 50% or more decrease in headache frequency and a greater mean change from baseline in headache frequency at day 180. A subgroup analysis of 228 patients not taking concomitant preventive agents found that the BoNT-A group had a greater decrease in headache frequency compared with placebo after two and three injections and at most time points from day 180 to 270 (Dodick *et al.*, 2005). In a similar study of 702 patients by Silberstein *et al.* (2005), which utilized several doses of BoNT-A (75, 150, 225 U), the primary efficacy endpoint (mean improvement from baseline in headache frequency at day 180) was also not met. However, all groups responded to treatment, and patients taking 150 and 225 U BoNT-A had a greater decrease in

Table 26.2 Summary of randomized, double-blind, controlled studies of the efficacy of botulinum neurotoxin A in the treatment of headache

Headache type	Outcome
Migraine	
Silberstein *et al.* (2000)	Decreased migraine frequency and severity and acute medication use with BoNT-A 25 U but not with BoNT-A 75 U
Brin *et al.* (2000)	Decreased migraine pain compared with PBO with simultaneous frontal and temporal BoNT-A injections
Evers *et al.* (2004)	No difference from PBO in decreased frequency of migraine; greater decrease in migraine-associated symptoms with BoNT-A 16 U
Saper *et al.* (2007)	Decreased frequency and severity of migraine in BoNT-A and PBO groups with no between-group differences
Elkind *et al.* (2006)	Comparable decreases in migraine frequency in both BoNT-A and PBO groups with no between-group differences
Chronic migraine	
Mathew *et al.* (2005)	No difference from PBO on primary efficacy endpoint: change in headache-free days from baseline at day 180; a significantly higher percentage of BoNT-A group had a ≥50% decrease in headache days/month at day 180 compared with PBO
Dodick *et al.* (2005)	Greater decrease in headache frequency after 2 and 3 injections compared with PBO
Silberstein *et al.* (2005)	No difference from PBO on primary efficacy endpoint (change in headache frequency from baseline at day 180); greater decrease in headache frequency for BoNT-A 225 U and 150 U than PBO
Aurora *et al.* (2010); Diener *et al.* (2010); Dodick *et al.* (2010)	Two large double-blind placebo-controlled trials (PREEMPT) using follow-the-pain approach; BoNT-A both safe and effective
Chronic tension-type headache	
Silberstein *et al.* (2006)	No difference from PBO on primary efficacy endpoint (mean change from baseline in chronic tension-type headache days); greater percentage of BoNT-A group than PBO group with ≥50% reduction in headache frequency at 90 and 120 days for several doses of BoNT-A

BoNT-A, botulinum neurotoxin A; PBO, placebo.

headache frequency at day 240 than did those taking placebo.

The PREEMPT clinical program confirmed onabotulinumtoxinA as an effective, safe and well-tolerated headache prophylaxis treatment for adults with chronic migraine. Two phase III, multicenter studies (PREEMPT 1 and 2; Aurora *et al.*, 2010; Diener *et al.*, 2010), which each had a 24-week, double-blind, parallel-group, placebo-controlled phase followed by a 32-week open-label phase, enrolled 1384 patients with chronic migraine. All patients received the minimum intramuscular dose of 155 U onabotulinumtoxinA administered to 31 injection sites across seven head and neck muscles using a fixed-site, fixed-dose injection paradigm. In addition, up to 40 U onabotulinumtoxinA, administered intramuscularly to eight injection sites across three head and neck muscles, was allowed using a modified follow-the-pain approach. Therefore, the minimum dose was 155 U and the maximum dose was 195 U (Table 26.2). Statistically significant reductions from baseline for frequency of headache days after BoNT-A treatment compared with placebo treatment in both PREEMPT 1 ($p = 0.006$) and PREEMPT 2 ($p > 0.001$) were observed. Statistically significant improvement from baseline after onabotulinumtoxinA treatment compared with placebo treatment was seen for headache episodes in PREEMPT 2 ($p = 0.003$). Pooled analysis demonstrated that onabotulinumtoxinA treatment significantly reduced mean frequency of headache days (-8.4 onabotulinumtoxinA, -6.6 placebo; $p < 0.001$) and episodes (-5.2 onabotulinumtoxinA, -4.9 placebo; $p = 0.009$). Additionally, significant between-group differences favoring onabotulinumtoxinA existed for several other efficacy variables (migraine episodes, migraine days, moderate or severe headache days, cumulative hours of headache on headache days, and proportion of patients with severe disability). The PREEMPT results showed highly significant improvements in multiple headache symptom measures and demonstrated improvement in patients' functioning, vitality, psychological distress and overall quality of life. Multiple treatments of 155 U up to 195 U per treatment cycle administered every 12 weeks were shown to be safe and well tolerated (Aurora *et al.*, 2010; Diener *et al.*, 2010; Dodick *et al.*, 2010).

Studies evaluating the efficacy of BoNT-A in chronic TTH have been inconsistent. A double-blind, randomized, placebo-controlled study (Silberstein *et al.*, 2006) of 300 patients found that while all treatment groups, including placebo, improved at day 60 in mean change from baseline in chronic TTH-free days per month (primary endpoint), BoNT-A did not demonstrate improvement compared with placebo at any dose or regimen (50 to 150 U). However, a significantly greater percentage of patients in the three BoNT-A groups at day 90 and two BoNT-A groups at day 120 had a 50% or greater decrease in chronic TTH days than the placebo group. Furthermore, a review evaluating clinical studies of TTH supports the benefit of BoNT-A in reducing headache frequency and severity, improving quality of life and disability scale assessment and reducing the need for acute medication (Mathew *et al.*, 2005). Another review, which also included studies with both onabotulinumtoxinA and abobotulinumtoxinA, concluded that randomized, double-blind, placebo-controlled trials present contradictory results that could be attributable to variable doses, injection sites and treatment frequency (Rozen and Sharma, 2006).

Adverse events associated with botulinum neurotoxin use

More than two decades of clinical use have established BoNT-A as a safe drug, with no systemic reactions in clinical trials for headache. Rash and flu-like symptoms can rarely occur as a result of an allergic reaction (Mauskop, 2004). However, serious allergic reactions have never been reported. Injection of anterior neck muscles can cause dysphagia (swallowing difficulties) in some patients (Mauskop, 2004). Dysphagia and dry mouth appear to be more common with injections of BoNT-B (rimabotulinumtoxinB) because of its wider

migration pattern (Mauskop, 2004). The most common side effects when treating facial muscles are cosmetic and include ptosis or asymmetry of the position of the eyebrows. Another possible, but rare, side effect is difficulty in holding the head erect because of neck muscle weakness (Mauskop, 2004). Patients with headache disorders occasionally develop a headache following the injection procedure, although some have immediate relief of an acute attack. The latter is most likely caused by a trigger point injection effect (Mauskop, 2004). Worsening of headaches and neck pain can occur and last for several days or, rarely, weeks after the injections because of the irritating effect of the needling and delay in the muscle-relaxing effect of BoNT (Mauskop, 2004).

Summary

Headache disorders, including migraine, chronic migraine and chronic TTH, are common debilitating conditions that profoundly impact quality of life. Existing preventive and acute pharmacotherapies, which may provide some relief to headache sufferers, vary in efficacy and may be associated with adverse events. Clinical studies suggest that BoNT is a safe treatment and is efficacious for the prevention of some forms of migraine (i.e. chronic migraine and perhaps high-frequency episodic migraine). Further research is needed to understand the mechanism of action of BoNT in headache, further establish its safety and efficacy for these indications and fully develop its therapeutic potential.

References

Allergan (2004a). *Botox package insert*. Irvine, CA: Allergan.

Allergan (2004b). *Dysport package insert*. Irvine, CA: Allergan.

Aoki KR (2003). Evidence for antinociceptive activity of botulinum toxin type A in pain management. *Headache*, **43**, S109–15.

Aoki KR, Guyer B (2001). Botulinum toxin type A and other botulinum toxin serotypes; a comparative review of biochemical and pharmacological actions. *Eur J Neurol*, **8**(Suppl 5), 21–9.

Aurora SK, Dodick DW, Turkel CC *et al.* (2010). OnabotulinumtoxinA for treatment of chronic migraine: results from the double-blind, randomized, placebo-controlled phase of the PREEMPT 1 trial. *Cephalalgia*, **30**, 793–803.

Bigal ME, Rapoport AM, Lipton RB, Tepper SJ, Sheftell FD (2003). Assessment of migraine disability using the

Migraine Disabiilty Assessment (MIDAS). Questionnaire: a comparison of chronic migraine with episodic migraine. *Headache* **43**, 336–42.

Binder WJ, Brin MF, Blitzer A, Shoenrock LD, Pogoda JM (2000). Botulinum toxin type A (Botox) for treatment of migraine headaches: an open-label study. *Otolaryngol Head Neck Surg*, **123**, 669–76.

Blumenfeld AM, Binder W, Silbrestein SD, Blizter A (2003). Procedures for administering botulinum toxin type A for migraine and tension-type headache. *Headache*, **43**, 884–91.

Brin MF, Swope DM, O'Brien C, Abbasi S, Pogoda JM (2000). Botox for migraine: double-blind, placebo-controlled, region-specific evaluation. *Cephalalgia* **20**, 421–2.

Castillo J, Munoz P, Guitera V, Pascual J (1998). Epidemiology of chronic daily headache in the general population. *Headache*, **38**, 378.

Cui M, Khanijou S, Rubino J, Aoki KR (2004). Subcutaneous administration of botulinum toxin A reduces formalin-induced pain. *Pain*, **107**, 125–33.

Diener HC, Dodick DW, Aurora SK et al. (2010). OnabotulinumtoxinA for treatment of chronic migraine: results from the double-blind, randomized, placebo-controlled phase of the PREEMPT 2 trial. *Cephalalgia*, **30**, 804–14.

Dodick DW, Mauskop A, Elkind AH et al. (2005). Botulinum toxin type A for the prophylaxis of chronic daily headache: subgroup analysis of patients not receiving other prophylactic medications (a randomized, double-blind, placebo-controlled study). *Headache*, **45**, 315–24.

Dodick DW, Turkel CC, DeGryse RE et al. (2010). OnabotulinumtoxinA for treatment of chronic migraine: pooled results from the double-blind, randomized, placebo-controlled phases of the PREEMPT clinical program. *Headache*, **50**, 921–36.

Elkind AH, O'Carroll P, Blumenfeld A, deGryse R, Dimitrova R (2006). A series of three sequential, randomized, controlled studies of repeated treatments with botulinum toxin type A for migraine prophylaxis. *J Pain*, **7**, 688–96.

Evers S, Vollmer-Haase J, Schwaag S et al. (2004). Botulinum toxin A in the prophylactic treatment of migraine: a randomized, double-blind, placebo-controlled study. *Cephalalgia*, **24**, 838–43.

Goadsby PJ (2001). Pathophysiology of headache. In Silberstein SD, Lipton RB, Dalessio DJ (eds.) *Wolff's Headache and Other Head Pain*, 7th edn. New York: Oxford University Press, pp. 57–72.

Headache Classification Committee (2004). The International Classification of Headache Disorders, 2nd edition. *Cephalalgia*, **24**, 1–160.

Hu XH, Markson LE, Lipton RB, Stewart WF, Berger ML (1999). Burden of migraine in the United States: disability and economic costs. *Arch Intern Med*, **159**, 813–18.

Jakubowski M, McAllister PJ, Bajwa ZH et al. (2006). Exploding vs. imploding headache in migraine prophylaxis with botulinum toxin A. *Pain*, **125**, 286–95.

Jensen R, Bendtsen L, Olesen J (1998). Muscular factors are of importance in tension-type headache. *Headache*, **38**, 10–17.

Lipton RB, Stewart WF, Diamond S, Diamond ML, Reed M (2001). Prevalence and burden of migraine in the United States: data from the American Migraine Study II. *Headache*, **41**, 646–57.

Lipton RB, Varon SF, Grosberg B et al. (2011). OnabotulinumtoxinA improves quality of life and reduces impact of chronic migraine. *Neurology*, **77**, 1465–72.

Mathew NT, Frishberg BM, Gawel M et al. (2005). Botulinum toxin type A (BOTOX) for the prophylactic treatment of chronic daily headache: a randomized, double-blind, placebo-controlled trial. *Headache*, **45**, 293–307.

Mauskop A (2004). The use of botulinum toxin in the treatment of headaches. *Pain Physician*, **7**, 377–87.

Meletiche DM, Lofland JH, Young WB (2001). Quality of life differences between patients with episodic and transformed migraine. *Headache*, **41**, 573–8.

National Institute of Neurological Disorders and Stroke (2002). *Headache: Hope Through Research* (NIH publication 02-158). Bethesda, MD: National Institutes of Health.

Oshinsky M, Poso-Rosich P, Luo J, Hyman S, Silberstein SD (2004). Botulinum toxin A blocks sensitization of neurons in the trigeminal nucleus caudalis. *Cephalalgia*, **24**, 781.

Rozen D, Sharma J (2006). Treatment of tension-type headache with botox: a review of the literature. *Mt Sinai J Med*, **73**, 493–8.

Saper JR, Mathew NT, Loder EW, deGryse R, VanDenburgh AM (2007). A double-blind, randomized, placebo-controlled comparison of botulinum toxin type A injection sites and doses in the prevention of episodic migraine. *Pain Med*, **8**, 478–85.

Scher AI, Stewart WF, Liberman J, Lipton RB (1998). Prevalence of frequent headache in a population sample. *Headache*, **38**, 497–506.

Schulte-Mattler WJ, Leinisch E (2008). Evidence based medicine on the use of botulinum toxin for headache disorders. *J Neural Transm*, **115**, 647–51.

Schwartz BS, Stewart WF, Simon D, Lipton RB (1998). Epidemiology of tension-type headache. *JAMA*, **279**, 381–3.

Silberstein SD (2000). Practice Parameter. Evidence-based guidelines for migraine headache (an evidence-based review): Report of the Quality Standards Subcommittee of the American Academy of Neurology for the United States Headache Consortium. *Neurology*, **55**, 754–62.

Silberstein SD (2004). Migraine. *Lancet*, **363**, 381–91.

Silberstein SD, Mathew N, Saper J, Jenkin S (2000). Botulinum toxin type A as a migraine preventive treatment: for the Botox Migraine Clinical Research Group. *Headache*, **40**, 445–50.

Silberstein SD, Stark SR, Lucas SM *et al.* (2005). Botulinum toxin type A for the prophylactic treatment of chronic daily headache: a randomized, double-blind, placebo-controlled trial. *Mayo Clin Proc*, **80**, 1126–37.

Silberstein SD, Gobel H, Jensen R *et al.* (2006). Botulinum toxin type A in the prophylactic treatment of chronic tension-type headache: a multicentre, double-blind, randomized, placebo-controlled, parallel-group study. *Cephalalgia*, **26**, 790–800.

Silberstein SD, Lipton RB, Dodick DW (eds) (2008). *Wolff's Headache and Other Head Pain*, 8th edn. Oxford: Oxford University Press.

Wang J, Zurawski TH, Meng J *et al.* (2011). A dileucine in the protease of botulinum toxin A underlies its long-lived neuroparalysis: transfer of longevity to a novel potential therapeutic. *J Biol Chem*, **286**, 6375–85.

Wang SJ, Fuh JL, Lu SR *et al.* (2000). Chronic daily headache in Chinese elderly: prevalence, risk factors and biannual follow-up. *Neurology*, **54**, 314–19.

World Health Organization (2012). *Headache Disorders* (Fact sheet No. 277). Geneva: World Health Organization (http://www.who.int/mediacentre/factsheets/fs277/en/, accessed 26 May 2013).

The use of botulinum neurotoxin in musculoskeletal pain and arthritis

Jasvinder A. Singh

Prevalence and impact of arthritis

Arthritis affects nearly 50 million adults in the USA and is projected to increase in prevalence to 67 million adults, or 25% of those aged 18 years and older, by the year 2030 (Centers for Disease Control and Prevention, 2010a).

Arthritis is associated with significant healthcare and cost burden on society. In the USA alone, arthritis results in about 1 million annual hospitalizations (Helmick *et al.*, 2008) and 44 million annual outpatient visits (American Academy of Orthopedic Surgeons, 2008). In 2003, the total cost of arthritis was $128 billion in the USA, including $81 billion in direct medical costs and $47 billion in indirect costs (lost earnings) (Centers for Disease Control and Prevention, 2007). Osteoarthritis alone is responsible for between $3.4 and $13.2 billion job-related costs each year (Buckwalter *et al.*, 2004; Centers for Disease Control and Prevention, 2010b). Consequently, arthritis constitutes a public health problem associated with significant socioeconomic burden.

Osteoarthritis is the most common type of non-inflammatory arthritis that affects the aging population, but it can also present at a younger age in those with trauma or obesity. It primarily affects hands, knees and hips but can be generalized and affect other joint areas. It is characterized by cartilage lesions leading to symmetric narrowing of joint space, over-production of bone leading to osteophytes and bony deformities. Inflammatory arthritis is characterized by swelling of the joint lining, which leads to joint destruction and bony erosions when not optimally treated. Two common types of inflammatory arthritis are rheumatoid arthritis and gout, which have predilection for different joints and have a different pathophysiology. Both are also associated with significant joint swelling, warmth and tenderness.

Available treatments for arthritis and challenges

Significant therapeutic advances have been made in the last few decades in patients with inflammatory arthritis such as rheumatoid arthritis (Siddiqui, 2007); these have targeted inflammatory cytokines such as tumor necrosis factor and others, as well as various cell types (T- and B-cells and macrophages). Treatment includes disease-modifying antirheumatic drugs (DMARDs) and, since 1998, several biologic agents that can be used in combination with DMARDs or alone for the treatment of rheumatoid arthritis. However, fewer advances have occurred in the treatment of osteoarthritis. The treatment of refractory musculoskeletal pain, including refractory joint pain (regardless of any underlying cause), remains a big challenge. Few therapies are available and commonly used approaches include oral therapies, intra-articular therapies, topical treatments and physical therapy.

Use of common oral therapies such as non-steroidal anti-inflammatory drugs (NSAIDs), opioid medications and analgesics (e.g. acetaminophen) is associated with significant adverse events (Ge *et al.*, 2006), particularly in the elderly. The common adverse events include gastrointestinal side effects, including peptic ulcer disease with its complications (bleeding, perforation), renal failure and liver toxicity in patients using NSAIDs; sedation, confusion, constipation and falls in those taking narcotics; and liver toxicity in patients taking acetaminophen. Intra-articular corticosteroids, intra-articular hyaluronic acid and topical preparations have limited efficacy in patients with osteoarthritis. Physical therapy is effective; however compliance with therapy has not been assessed and feasibility remains a challenge. Many patients are unable to do physical

Manual of Botulinum Toxin Therapy, 2nd edition, ed. Daniel Truong, Mark Hallett, Christopher Zachary and Dirk Dressler. Published by Cambridge University Press. © Cambridge University Press 2013.

therapy because of personal preference, comorbidities and/or distance from the therapy site. Therefore, effective and safe therapeutic options are limited for the treatment of refractory musculoskeletal pain and arthritis-related joint pain, and new therapeutic options for these conditions are needed.

Neurobiology of joints and current understanding of chronic joint pain

Recent reviews have summarized the current understanding of joint pain and the various mechanisms involved. Joints are innervated with articular nerves that contain Aδ, Aβ and C fibers. All joint structures except articular cartilage have these nerve endings. In normal healthy individuals, these nociceptors have high threshold for excitation in response to mechanical and thermal stimuli, such that normal activities of walking, stair climbing, sports (and palpation of the joint) are not associated with pain/unpleasant sensation. However, in the presence of joint injury or inflammation, many of these nerve fibers lower their excitation threshold. This leads to enhanced responses to both innocuous and noxious mechanical, chemical and thermal stimuli. This phenomenon is called peripheral sensitization (Schaible et al., 2009). Chronic joint inflammation is also associated with hyperexcitability of spinal nociceptive neurons, referred to as central sensitization (Neugebauer et al., 1993). A variety of mediators can sensitize joint nerves and nociceptors to mechanical stimuli, including bradykinin, prostaglandin E_2, prostaglandin I_2, serotonin, substance P and neuropeptide Y (Schaible et al., 2006). Another contributor to joint pain and inflammation is neurogenic inflammation – a process where articular nerves, stimulated by inflammation, release neuropeptides from nerve terminals following axon reflexes, postganglionic sympathetic nerves release neuropeptides following sympathetic reflexes, and local inflammatory cells release neuropeptides as the result of cytokine or neuropeptide stimulation (Schaible et al., 2005). It is likely that these processes underlie the clinical observed signs and symptoms of pain and mechanical hyperalgesia in inflamed joints.

Activation of glial cells, other immune cells, cytokines and neuropeptides contributes to the generation of pain. The role of pain pathways, pain receptors and various other contributors to both inflammatory and neuropathic pain have been described in Woolf and Costigan (1999).

Antinociceptive effects of botulinum neurotoxin

The following text summarizes the studies that provide the initial evidence for the antinociceptive effect of botulinum neurotoxin (BoNT), followed by existing evidence related to use of BoNT in various musculoskeletal pain conditions including refractory arthritis.

Clinical observations

Various clinical studies of cutaneous pain support the antinociceptive action of BoNT (Kramer et al., 2003; Ranoux et al., 2008; Yuan et al., 2009), while some studies found no such evidence (Blersch et al., 2002; Voller et al., 2003; Sycha et al., 2006). The evidence is summarized in Table 27.1. In summary, the evidence for antinociceptive effect of intradermal BoNT for cutaneous pain is mixed and contradictory, with some positive and some negative studies. However, a majority of these studies had small sample size, suggesting that they may be unpowered and may have had false negative results. More studies with adequate sample sizes need to be performed to assess if BoNT has antinociceptive action after an intradermal injection.

Refractory osteoarticular joint pain

Table 27.2 summarizes the efficacy data from two non-randomized studies (Mahowald et al., 2006; Singh et al., 2009a) followed by data from randomized controlled trials (RCTs) in refractory shoulder joint pain (one study) and refractory knee joint pain (two randomized studies) caused by osteoarthritis or inflammatory arthritis (Singh et al., 2009b; Mahowald et al., 2009; Boon et al., 2010). These studies have all used onabotulinumtoxinA (Botox). In one RCT comparing a single intra-articular injection of 100 U onabotulinumtoxinA with placebo for shoulder pain in osteoarthritis onabotulinumtoxinA was superior to placebo in pain reduction and quality of life improvement (Singh et al., 2009b). In a RCT comparing a single intra-articular injection of two doses (100 or 200 U) of onabotulinumtoxinA with intra-articular methylprednisolone acetate for knee osteoarthritis pain, onabotulinumtoxinA was as effective as the corticosteroid in improving pain, function and quality of life (Boon et al., 2010). In a RCT comparing a single intra-articular injection of 100 U onabotulinumtoxinA with intra-articular placebo, significantly greater

Table 27.1 Clinical and translational studies suggesting antinociceptive action of botulinum neurotoxin

Reference	Trial type and duration	Intervention and comparison	Participants, mean age, gender	Main result, efficacy
Kramer et al. (2003)	RCT, double-blind, 14 days	Intradermal Botox 5–20 U or saline (contralateral side) on volar forearm	15 healthy volunteers, 25 years (SD, 4), 8M/7F	Botox caused an anhidrotic skin area in all patients, and had a significantly smaller axon reflex flare and lower pain rating, but similar amount of hyperalgesia to pinprick and allodynia after electrical stimulation, compared with placebo
Yuan et al. (2009)	RCT, double-blind crossover trial, 12 weeks	Intradermal Botox 50 U or saline; 12 injections into feet	18 patients with diabetic neuropathic pain, 65.6 years (SD, 9.2), 6M/12F	Significant reduction in pain assesssed by VAS by 0.83 at 1 week, 2.22 at 4 weeks, 2.33 at 8 weeks and 2.53 at 12 weeks after injection in the Botox group, compared with changes of 0.39, −0.11, 0.42 and 0.53 for the placebo group at the same time points ($p < 0.05$).
Ranoux et al. (2008)	RCT, double-blind, 24 weeks	Intradermal injection 20–190 U Botox versus placebo into the painful area	29 patients with focal painful neuropathies, 54 years (SD, 13.9), 10M/19F	Botox was associated with persistent sustained effects on spontaneous pain intensity, neuropathic symptoms and general activity from 2 weeks after the injection to 14 weeks, compared with placebo
Sycha et al. (2006)	RCT, double-blind, 1 month	Intradermal Dysport 100 U or saline placebo (contralateral side) on upper ventral leg	6 healthy volunteers, 30–40 years, 5M/1F	No significant differences between groups in heat or cold pain perception threshold, skin blood flow, mechanical pain threshold or mechanical allodynia. Dysport, but not saline, produced changes in sudomotor function by leading to substantial anhidrotic area
Blersch et al. (2002)	RCT, double-blind, 2-month	Subcutaneous Dysport 100 U or saline placebo in the two forearms	50 healthy volunteers, 26 years (range, 17–48), 25M/25F	No differences were found between the groups with regards to pain thresholds for heat or cold at 4 and 8 weeks; no differences in electric stimulation pain thresholds between the groups
Voller et al. (2003)	RCT, double-blind, 28 days	Intradermal Botox 30 U or saline placebo in the two forearms	16 healthy volunteers, 29 years (SD, 5), 8M/8F	No significant difference between groups at day 28 in heat pain perception and tolerance thresholds, electric pain perception and tolerance thresholds, area of secondary hyperalgesia after capsaicin application and capsaicin-induced flare

Botox, onabotulinumtoxinA; Dysport, abobotulinumtoxinA; SD, standard deviation; RCT, randomized controlled trial; M, male; F, female; VAS, visual analog scale.

reduction in pain was seen in the group with severe pain (≥7 on 0–10 scale) with onabotulinumtoxinA compared with placebo. No deaths, anaphylactic reaction or septic arthritis were reported in any group in any studies and strength testing did not reveal any significant changes at any time point in treatment groups. None of the common adverse events were significantly different between groups, in the three RCTs (Mahowald et al., 2009; Singh et al., 2009b; Boon et al., 2010). These three small trials were powered for efficacy but not safety outcomes.

In summary, three RCTs and three non-randomized studies support the efficacy of a single intra-articular injection of BoNT in patients with refractory joint pain. However, larger dose-ranging studies with safety assessments are needed.

Knee injection can be performed by diluting 100 U onabotulinumtoxinA into 1 or 2 ml of normal saline and injecting it into the knee joint using a 21- or 22-gauge needle and any of the approaches (medial, lateral, superior or inferior) according to personal preference. Other formulations of BoNT can presumably be used, but

Table 27.2 Studies of botulinum neurotoxin in osteoarticular pain, showing efficacy and outcomes

Reference	Trial type and duration	Intervention and comparison	Participants, mean age, gender	Main result, efficacy
Non-randomized studies				
Mahowald et al. (2006)	Open-label	25–100 U IA Botox	15 refractory painful shoulder, 11 lower extremity joint pain (pain duration, 3–40 years); 42–82 years; 9M/2F	Botox: lower extremity and shoulder pain decreased from 7 to 2.7 and 8.2 to 2.4, respectively; shoulder flexion improved from 68 to 113 degrees; shoulder abduction improved from 50 to 74 degrees. Timed stands test (time to stand up 10 times from a sitting position) improved from 36 to 23 seconds. Pain relief began by 2 weeks in most patients; duration of pain relief 3–10 months
Singh et al. (2009a)	Open-label	30–150 U IA Botox	Long-term follow-up of 11 patients from Mahowald et al. (2006) study (pain duration, 3–40 years); 42–82 years; 9M/2F	Re-injections associated with pain reduction in 9/10, as seen with the first injection. Pain severity decreased from 6.6 (SD, 1.2) to 3.3 (SD, 2.7) on 0–10 NRS, which was statistically significant (p = 0.003); pain relief lasted 3–17 months
RCTs				
Singh et al. (2009b)	RCT, double-blind, 1 month	100 U IA Botox + 1 ml 2% lidocaine (in 21) or IA saline + 1 ml 2% lidocaine (in 22)	36 patients with 43 painful shoulders (pain duration, 8–11 years); Botox 72 years (SEM, 2), placebo 70 years (SEM, 3), 35M/1F	Significantly greater reduction in VAS pain in Botox (2.4) than placebo (0.8) (p = 0.02). Higher proportion dropped out at 1 month from placebo (45%) than Botox (19%) (p = 0.13). SF-36 scores improved significantly more in Botox than placebo in 5/8 subscales (p = 0.04–0.001). McGill affective dimension scores were significantly greater in Botox than placebo group (p = 0.047). Trend towards significance in SPADI disability scores (p = 0.083). No significant differences in active flexion, active abduction, SPADI pain and total and McGill sensory and total scores
Boon et al. (2010)	RCT, double-blind, 8 weeks	IA Botox at 100 U (in 20) or 200 U (in 20), IA methylprednisolone acetate 40 mg (in 20)	60 patients with 60 knees (pain duration, 6–10 years); Botox 100 U, 64 years (SD, 13); Botox 200 U, 61 years (SD, 9); corticosteroid: 61 years (SD, 10); 25M/35F	Significant reduction in VAS pain with injection in each of the 3 groups, but no significant difference between groups: Botox (2.4) and, placebo (0.8). 2-point reduction in VAS pain in 60% Botox 100 U, 26% in Botox 200 U and 42% in corticosteroid group (p = 0.10). Significant reduction in WOMAC pain, function and stiffness scales and 40-m walk with injection in each of the 3 groups, but no significant difference between groups

| Mahowald et al. (2009) | RCT, double-blind, 1 month | 100 U IA Botox + lidocaine (in 21) or IA saline + lidocaine (in 21) | 42 with refractory chronic painful knees | Short-form McGill pain scores changes similar in Botox (−4.7; $p = 0.048$) and placebo (−5.6; $p = 002$) groups at 1 month; at 3 months, change in total McGill pain was significant only in the Botox (−4.2; $p = 0.002$) but not placebo (−4.6; $p = 0.09$) groups Baseline severe pain group (NRS ≥ 7: $n = 23$): 48% decrease in the total pain score from 23.8 (SD, 2.6) to 14.9 (SD, 2.9) at 1 month ($p = 0.011$) and 15.8 at 3 months ($p = 0.002$) in Botox group; no significant change in IA-placebo group Baseline moderate pain group (NRS, 4.5–6.9; $n = 19$): little change with either treatment and no between group differences |

Botox, onabotulinumtoxinA; RCT, randomized controlled trial; M. male' F. female; VAS, visual analog scale; SPADI, Shoulder Pain and Disability Index; WOMAC, Western Ontario McMaster Osteoarthritis Index; NRS, numeric rating scale; SD, standard deviation; SEM, standard error of mean; IA, intra-articular.

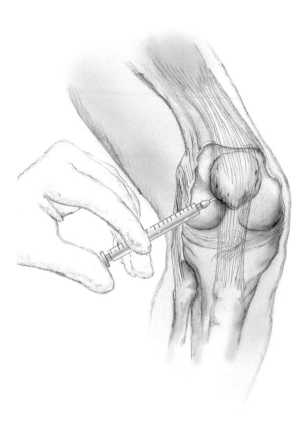

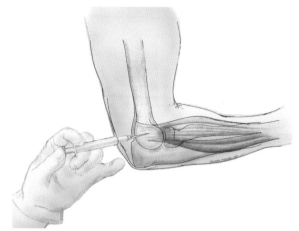

Fig. 27.2 Technique for injection for tennis elbow (lateral epicondylitis of the elbow).

Fig. 27.1 Technique for intra-articular injection of the knee joint using the medial approach.

there is less experience with them. The shoulder can be similarly injected with a 21- or 22-gauge needle using posterior, anterior or lateral approach to the glenohumeral joint, according to personal preference. Although not recommended by the manufacturer, some clinicians prefer using 1% lidocaine to dilute the BoNT instead of normal saline to confirm the correct delivery of the medication by improvement in pain 5 minutes after the injection (Fig. 27.1).

Tennis elbow

The efficacy of local injection of BoNT into the extensor tendons inserting on the external epicondyle for improving pain was examined in an open-label case series of 14 patients with "treatment-resistant" tennis elbow with follow-up at 6–8 months (Morre *et al.*, 1997). This was confirmed in a 12-week RCT of 60 patients comparing BoNT with placebo (Wong *et al.*, 2005) (Table 27.3). Four patients in the abobotulinumtoxinA (Dysport)

group had paresis of the fingers at 4 weeks (in one patient persisting to week 12) compared with none in the placebo group, but grip strength was similar in both groups at the two time points (Wong *et al.*, 2005). Another RCT in 40 patients with tennis elbow found that a single injection of 40 U onabotulinumtoxinA seemed to be as effective as surgical release for improvement of pain, but led to a better range of motion at 3 and 6 months (Keizer *et al.*, 2002) (Table 27.3). A third RCT compared a single injection of 50 U onabotulinumtoxinA into the extensor tendons with placebo (Hayton *et al.*, 2005). There were no statistically significant differences by treatment in pain (difference of 1.1 between groups; $p = 0.54$), grip strength (difference of 0.57 kg between groups; $p = 0.90$), or quality of life; 12 of the 18 patients in the onabotulinumtoxinA group had a transient extensor lag of the long finger at 1 week that disappeared 3 months after the injection (Hayton *et al.*, 28).

Injection for tennis elbow is performed by inserting a 21- or 22-gauge needle 5 cm distal to the area of maximal tenderness at the lateral epicondyle, deep to the forearm fascia and injecting 50 U onabotulinumtoxinA constituted in 2 ml of normal saline (or corresponding doses of other formulations) (Fig. 27.2).

Temporomandibular joint pain

In three non-randomized studies, intramuscular injections of 150–200 U abobotulinumtoxinA into masseter and/or temporalis muscles were associated with significant improvement in pain, functional disability and tenderness (von Lindern, 2001) (Table 27.4). The

Table 27.3 Studies of botulinum neurotoxin in tennis elbow

Reference	Trial type and duration	Intervention and comparison	Participants, mean age, gender	Main result, efficacy
Non-randomized studies				
Morre et al. (1997)	Open label	20–40 U BoNT[a] injected into extensor digitorum communis muscle	14 patients (mean pain duration: 2.4 years, range 0.6–6), 43 years (range 34–60), 5 M/9 F	>50% pain relief in 9/14, complete pain relief in 4/14 during the 6–8 months of follow-up Pain relief began by 2 weeks in 10 patients, 3 weeks in 1 and after 4 weeks in 3
RCTs				
Wong et al. (2005)	RCT, double-blind, 3 month	1 injection of 60 U Dysport versus placebo in muscle and subcutaneous tissue	60 patients (mean pain duration: Dysport 12 years [SD,9]; placebo 19 years [SD,21]); Dysport 46 years (SD, 9), placebo 44 years (SD, 6); 11M/49F	Dysport: VAS pain 25.3 mm at 4 weeks; 23.5 mm at 12 weeks Placebo: VAS pain 50.5 mm at 4 weeks; 43.5 mm at 12 weeks Differences significant at both 4 ($p < 0.0001$) and 12 ($p = 0.0006$) weeks
Keizer et al. (2002)	RCT, not blinded, 24 months	Surgical release versus 1 or 2 injections of 30–40 U Botox into extensor carpi radius brevis	40 patients (mean pain duration: 11 months; range, 6–48), 43 years (range, 25–72), 19M/21F	No difference in pain between groups Range of motion significantly better in Botox than in surgery group at 3 and 6 months; no difference at 12 or 24 months Sick leave lower in surgery group than in BoNT group at 3 months ($p = 0.01$), but no difference at 6, 12 and 24 months Overall score was similar in the two groups at 3, 6, 12 and 24 months
Hayton et al. (2005)	RCT, double-blind, 3 months	1 intramuscular injection of 50 U Botox versus saline placebo	40 patients (>6 months' pain as inclusion criteria), 48 years (range, 37–71), 21M/19F	No significant differences in pain scores, grip strength and SF-12 between Botox and placebo at 3 months

[a] BoNT; the type of neurotoxin and the preparation was not specified.
Botox, onabotulinumtoxinA; Dysport, abobotulinumtoxinA; SF-12, Short Form 12; RCT, randomized controlled trial; VAS, visual analog scale; SD, standard deviation; M, male; F, female.

effect lasted 2–12 months, and few side effects were reported. In a subsequent single-blinded randomized study with 90 patients with temporomandibular joint pain, 60 received intramuscular injections of 35 U onabotulinumtoxinA and 30 received placebo (von Lindern et al., 2003). A greater proportion of patients in onabotulinumtoxinA compared with the placebo group had a 2 point or greater improvement on a

visual analog pain scale during the follow-up. No speech impairment or systemic botulism was reported.

Injections for temporomandibular joint pain are administered intramuscularly, usually within the mouth into the masseter and temporalis muscles (see Fig. 9.1). A total of 150–200 U onabotulinumtoxinA is diluted in 1–2 ml of normal saline and injections of 50 U each are made into multiple painful and tender

Table 27.4 Studies of botulinum neurotoxin in temporomandibular joint disorder, anterior knee pain and hip pain

Reference	Trial type and duration	Intervention and comparison	Participants, mean age, gender	Main result, efficacy
Facial pain and temporomandibular joint disorder				
von Lindern (2001)	Open-label, 12 months	200 U Botox injected intramuscularly	41 patients (failed conservative treatment for 3–12 months), no age/gender data	80% patients had improvement in pain; mean pain severity decreased from 6.4 to 3.5 on a VAS; 13 patients had a "major improvement" as evident by disappearance of pain; relief lasted 3–12 months for most
Freund et al. (2000)	Open-label, 8-weeks	150 U Botox in each masseter and 25 U in each temporalis muscle	46 patients (median pain duration, 8 years), 41 years, 7M/39F	Comparing pre-injection to post-injection at 8 weeks: significant improvement in pain VAS from a median of 8 to 5, functional disability index from 5.3 to 3.9, tenderness to palpation from 15.5 to 6, jaw opening from 29.5 to 34.5 mm ($p < 0.05$ for all)
Freund et al. (1999)	Open label, 8 weeks	150 U Botox in each masseter and 50 U in each temporalis muscle	15 patients (mean pain duration 10 years), 39 years, 2M/13F	Compared pre-injection to post-injection at 8 weeks: significant improvement in pain VAS from a mean of 7.3 to 4, functional disability index from 5.5 to 3.1, tenderness to palpation from 17 to 7.6, jaw opening from 27 to 34 mm ($p < 0.05$ for all).
von Lindern et al. (2003)	RCT, double-blind, 1–3 months	35 U Botox versus placebo in masticatory muscles	90 patients (failed conservative treatment for 3–34 months), no age/gender data	Reduction in VAS pain at 1–3 months post-injection was significantly more in Botox than placebo group ($p < 0.01$) Greater proportion with ≥2-point reduction in VAS pain in Botox (76%) than placebo group (10%; no statistical comparison)
Anterior knee pain				
Singer et al. (2006) 8 women	Open-label, 1-year	300 to 500 U Dysport into vastus lateralis muscle	8 patients (mean pain duration 5 years, range, 1–19), 29 years, 8F	Patients reported decrease in knee pain (individual changes shown, not means), increase in function with improvement in force production in affected limb from 22.7 to 24.3 kg and an improvement in the time taken to ascend and descend a flight of 11 stairs from 12 to 10 seconds; improvements were maintained at 24 weeks
Hip pain				
Marchini et al. (2010)	Open-label, 12 weeks	400 U Dysport into adductor longus and adductor magnus muscles	39 patients (mean pain duration 6.7 years, SD, 7), 68 years (SD, 9; range 41–82), 20M/19F	Significant improvement in Harris Hip Score at 2, 4 and 12 weeks after the Dysport injection ($p < 0.0001$) Decrease in pain 2, 4 and 12 weeks after the Dysport injection ($p < 0.001$) Significant improvement in SF-36 score 4 and 12 weeks after treatment

Botox, onabotulinumtoxinA; Dysport, abobotulinumtoxinA; RCT, randomized controlled trial; VAS, visual analog scale; SF-36, Short Form 36; SD, standard deviation; M, male; F, female.

areas of masseter muscles bilaterally and 25 U each into temporalis muscle bilaterally.

Summary and conclusions

This chapter has reviewed studies using BoNT for osteoarticular pain. Most studies used either intra-articular or intramuscular administration in patients with refractory pain who had failed multiple other treatment interventions. Preclinical laboratory evidence supports an independent antinociceptive mechanism of action for BoNT. While there are several osteoarticular conditions for which BoNT has been studied in an RCT compared with placebo, for several conditions, such as low-back pain, plantar fasciitis, temporomandibular disorder and carpal tunnel syndrome, the evidence is based on limited data at this time. For other conditions, such as osteoarthritis of knee/shoulder and tennis elbow, data from several RCTs and non-randomized studies are available. Most RCTs reviewed in this chapter had several limitations. Most studies were single center, had a small sample size, short follow-up and, in some cases, non-standardized injection techniques. In addition, observation of larger effect size in non-randomized studies compared with RCTs indicates bias and placebo effect, as reported previously for other conditions. Few side effects, mostly transient and mild, were reported from these studies of small sample size. Evidence from larger multicenter studies of longer duration that test various dosages, regimens and routes of administration of BoNT are needed to better define its role in management of osteoarticular pain.

References

American Academy of Orthopedic Surgeons (2008).*United States Bone and Joint Decade: The Burden of Musculoskeletal Diseases in the United States*. Rosemont, IL: American Academy of Orthopedic Surgeons.

Blersch W, Schulte-Mattler WJ, Przywara S *et al.* (2002). Botulinum toxin A and the cutaneous nociception in humans: a prospective, double-blind, placebo-controlled, randomized study. *J Neurol Sci*, **205**, 59–63.

Boon AJ, Smith J, Dahm DL *et al.* (2010). Efficacy of intra-articular botulinum toxin type A in painful knee osteoarthritis: a pilot study. *PM R*, **2**, 268–76.

Buckwalter JA, Saltzman C, Brown T (2004). The impact of osteoarthritis: implications for research. *Clin Orthop Relat Res*, **427**(Suppl), S6–15.

Centers for Disease Control and Prevention (2007). National and state medical expenditures and lost earnings attributable to arthritis and other rheumatic conditions: United States, 2003. *MMWR*, **56**, 4–7.

Centers for Disease Control and Prevention (2010a). Prevalence of doctor-diagnosed arthritis and arthritis-attributable activity limitation: United States, 2007–2009. *MMWR*, **59**, 1261–5.

Centers for Disease Control and Prevention (2010b). *Arthritis Foundation. A National Public Health Agenda for Osteoarthritis*. Atlanta, GA: Centers for Disease Control and Prevention (http://www.cdc.gov/arthritis/docs/OAagenda.pdf, accessed 24 May 2013).

Freund B, Schwartz M, Symington JM (1999). The use of botulinum toxin for the treatment of temporomandibular disorders: preliminary findings. *J Oral Maxillofac Surg*, **57**, 916–20; discussion 920–1.

Freund B, Schwartz M, Symington JM (2000). Botulinum toxin: new treatment for temporomandibular disorders. *Br J Oral Maxillofac Surg*, **38**, 466–71.

Ge Z, Hu Y, Heng BC *et al.* (2006). Osteoarthritis and therapy. *Arthritis Rheum*. **55**, 493–500.

Hayton MJ, Santini AJ, Hughes PJ *et al.* (2005). Botulinum toxin injection in the treatment of tennis elbow. A double-blind, randomized, controlled, pilot study. *J Bone Joint Surg Am*, **87**, 503–7.

Helmick CG, Felson DT, Lawrence RC *et al.* (2008). Estimates of the prevalence of arthritis and other rheumatic conditions in the United States. Part I. *Arthritis Rheum*. **58**, 15–25.

Keizer SB, Rutten HP, Pilot P *et al.* (2002). Botulinum toxin injection versus surgical treatment for tennis elbow: a randomized pilot study. *Clin Orthop Relat Res*. 125–31.

Kramer HH, Angerer C, Erbguth F, Schmelz M, Birklein F. (2003). Botulinum toxin A reduces neurogenic flare but has almost no effect on pain and hyperalgesia in human skin. *J Neurol*, **250**, 188–93.

Mahowald ML, Singh JA, Dykstra D (2006). Long term effects of intra-articular botulinum toxin A for refractory joint pain. *Neurotox Res*. **9**, 179–88.

Mahowald ML, Krug HE, Singh JA, Dykstra D (2009). Intra-articular Botulinum toxin type A: a new approach to treat arthritis joint pain. *Toxicon*. **54**, 658–67.

Marchini C, Acler M, Bolognari MA *et al.* (2010). Efficacy of botulinum toxin type A treatment of functional impairment of degenerative hip joint: Preliminary results. *J Rehabil Med*, **42**, 691–3.

Morre HH, Keizer SB, van Os JJ (1997). Treatment of chronic tennis elbow with botulinum toxin. *Lancet*, **349**, 1746.

Neugebauer V, Lucke T, Schaible HG (1993). N-Methyl-D-aspartate (NMDA) and non-NMDA receptor antagonists block the hyperexcitability of dorsal horn neurons during development of acute arthritis in rat's knee joint. *J Neurophysiol*, **70**, 1365–77.

Ranoux D, Attal N, Morain F, Bouhassira D (2008). Botulinum toxin type A induces direct analgesic effects in chronic neuropathic pain. *Ann Neurol*, **64**, 274–83.

Schaible HG, Del Rosso A, Matucci-Cerinic M (2005). Neurogenic aspects of inflammation. *Rheum Dis Clin North Am*, **31**, 77–101.

Schaible HG, Schmelz M, Tegeder I (2006). Pathophysiology and treatment of pain in joint disease. *Adv Drug Deliv Rev*, **58**, 323–42.

Schaible HG, Richter F, Ebersberger A *et al.* (2009). Joint pain. *Exp Brain Res*, **196**, 153–62.

Siddiqui MA (2007). The efficacy and tolerability of newer biologics in rheumatoid arthritis: best current evidence. *Curr Opin Rheumatol*, **19**, 308–13.

Singer BJ, Silbert PL, Dunne JW, Song S, Singer KP. (2006). An open label pilot investigation of the efficacy of Botulinum toxin type A [Dysport] injection in the rehabilitation of chronic anterior knee pain. *Disabil Rehabil*, **28**, 707–13.

Singh JA, Mahowald ML, Kushnaryov A, Goelz E, Dykstra D (2009a). Repeat injections of intra-articular botulinum toxin A for the treatment of chronic arthritis joint pain. *J Clin Rheumatol*, **15**, 35–8.

Singh JA, Mahowald ML, Noorbaloochi S (2009b). Intra-articular botulinum toxin A for refractory shoulder pain: a randomized, double-blinded, placebo-controlled trial. *Transl Res*, **153**, 205–16.

Sycha T, Samal D, Chizh B *et al.* (2006). A lack of antinociceptive or antiinflammatory effect of botulinum toxin A in an inflammatory human pain model. *Anesth Analg*. **102**, 509–16.

Voller B, Sycha T, Gustorff B *et al.* (2003). A randomized, double-blind, placebo controlled study on analgesic effects of botulinum toxin A. *Neurology*, **61**, 940–4.

von Lindern JJ (2001). Type A botulinum toxin in the treatment of chronic facial pain associated with temporo-mandibular dysfunction. *Acta Neurol Belg*, **101**, 39–41.

von Lindern JJ, Niederhagen B, Berge S, Appel T (2003). Type A botulinum toxin in the treatment of chronic facial pain associated with masticatory hyperactivity. *J Oral Maxillofac Surg*, **61**, 774–8.

Wong SM, Hui AC, Tong PY *et al.* (2005). Treatment of lateral epicondylitis with botulinum toxin: a randomized, double-blind, placebo-controlled trial. *Ann Intern Med*, **143**, 793–7.

Woolf CJ, Costigan M (1999). Transcriptional and posttranslational plasticity and the generation of inflammatory pain. *Proc Natl Acad Sci USA*, **96**, 7723–30.

Yuan RY, Sheu JJ, Yu JM *et al.* (2009). Botulinum toxin for diabetic neuropathic pain a randomized double-blind crossover trial. *Neurology*, **72**, 1473–8.

Chapter 28

Treatment of plantar fasciitis with botulinum neurotoxins

Bahman Jabbari and Shivam Om Mittal

Introduction

Plantar fasciitis (PF) is the most common cause of chronic heel pain and is a major health issue in runners and long-distance walkers. It affects 2 million people in the USA and results in approximately 1 million visits to the physician office, 62% of which are to primary care physicians. The annual cost of treatments is estimated to be between $192 and $376 million (Tu and Bytomski, 2011). Overuse injury may lead to repetitive microtears of the plantar fascia near the calcaneus, irritating pain fibers and producing secondary inflammation. Other risk factors include obesity, flat or overarched feet and improper shoes. The pain usually involves the inferior and medial aspect of the heel (calcaneus), at the medial aspect of the calcaneal tubercle. However, the entire course of the plantar fascia may be involved. Patients typically have intense heel pain, described as aching, jabbing or burning pain, with the first couple of steps in the morning. Pain is reproduced by palpation of the median tubercle of the calcaneum and with dorsiflexion of the toes (Windlass test) (Young, 2012). In many patients, the application of ice and/or the use of heel cup orthosis activity modification and a stretching/strengthening exercise program reduce the pain satisfactorily. Further measures include deep-tissue massage therapy, night splints and periods of immobilization. Persistent problems may respond to treatment with posterior night splints, ultrasound, iontophoresis, phonophoresis, extracorporal shock wave therapy or even local corticosteroid injections (Goff and Crawford, 2011). Where medical approaches fail, surgery is advocated but has modest results. Approximately 10–12% of patients fail to achieve pain relief from medical and/or surgical treatment.

Anatomy of the plantar fascia

The plantar fascia comprises dense collagen fibers that extend longitudinally from the calcaneus to the base of each proximal phalanx (Fig. 28.1a). The fascia has medial, central and lateral parts, underneath which the flexor digitorum brevis and the abductor hallucis muscles reside (Fig. 28.1b). The plantar fascia serves to anchor muscles and tendons on the concave surface of the sole and digits, facilitates excursion of the tendons, prevents excessive compression of digital vessels and nerves and may even aid in venous return (Williams et al., 1995). The central band of the plantar fascia, abductor hallucis and flexor digitorum brevis attach to the medial calcaneal tubercle, the site of most pain in PF. Anatomical changes described in PF include marked thickening of the plantar fascia (Mahowald et al., 2011), microtears related to repeated trauma and secondary inflammation. The pain may be caused by one or more of the following: mechanical irritation of pain fibers by plantar fascia thickened from repeated trauma, ischemic pain from chronic pressure of a thickened fascia against digital vessels, and an enhanced reaction to a local pain neurotransmitter/chemical found in the inflammatory response (such as substance P or glutamate). Furthermore, like any other chronic pain condition, peripheral and central sensitization as well as sympathetic overactivity may play a role in pain persistence.

Rationale for using botulinum neurotoxin for treatment of plantar fasciitis

The data from animal studies and early observations of pain relief with onabotulinumtoxinA (Botox in cervical dystonia) prompted investigations on the analgesic

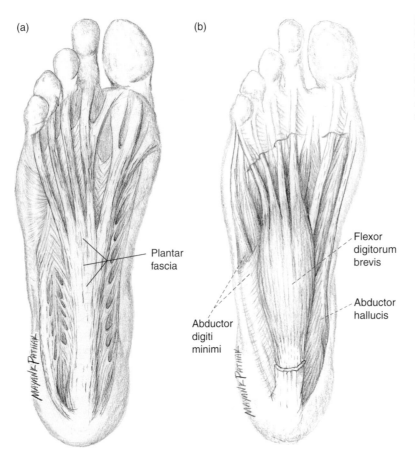

(a)

(b)

Fig. 28.1 Anatomy of the plantar fascia. (a) The plantar fascia extends from the heal to the base of all toes. (b) Superficial muscles of the foot after the plantar fascia is removed. Flexor digitorum brevis lies directly beneath the fascia at the middle of the foot. Abductor hallucis and abductor digiti minimi are seen close to the heal on either side of flexor digitorum brevis.

Plantar fascia

Flexor digitorum brevis

Abductor hallucis

Abductor digiti minimi

effect of botulinum neurotoxin (BoNT) in human pain disorders. In the rat formalin model, injection of onabotulinumtoxinA into the paw a week before formalin injection significantly reduced the inflammatory peak of pain and accumulation of glutamate locally (Cui *et al.*, 2004). A number of other mechanisms also are described based on animal investigations (Aoki and Francis, 2011). In humans, BoNT treatment of chronic pain of cervical dystonia and migraine are approved by US Food and Drug Administration and double-blind, placebo-controlled studies indicate probable efficacy (class B evidence) in postherpetic and post-traumatic neuralgia, piriformis syndrome and total knee arthroplasty (Jabbari and Machado, 2011).

Randomized, prospective studies of botulinum neurotoxin treatment

At the present time, based on two class II, placebo-controlled, double-blind studies, onabotulinumtoxinA

is considered "probably effective" in treatment of PF, meeting level B evidence according to the criteria of the American Academy of Neurology (French and Gronseth, 2008). In the first study (Babcock *et al.*, 2005), 27 patients were randomized into group A (toxin) and group B (placebo). The onabotulinumtoxinA solution was prepared by mixing 100 U with 1 ml of preservative-free normal saline. Patients in group A received 70 U (0.7 ml) in two divided doses: 40 U (0.4 ml) in the tender region of the heel medial to the base of the plantar fascia insertion and 30 U (0.3 ml) in the most tender point of the arch of the foot (between the heel and middle of the foot) (Fig. 28.2). A 27-gauge, 20 mm (0.75 inch) needle was used for injections. Group B received normal saline at the same locations and of similar volume. Pain relief was measured by visual analog scale (VAS), pressure algometry and the Maryland foot score at baseline (before treatment) and at 3 and 8 weeks after injection. Twenty seven patients participated in the study (11 with unilateral and 16 with

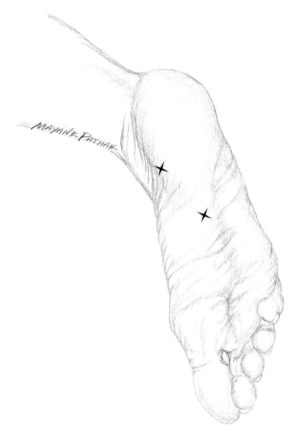

Fig. 28.2 Injection sites in plantar fasciitis.

bilateral PF). In patients with bilateral PF, one foot received onabotulinumtoxinA and the other placebo. The pain response to BoNT compared with placebo was statistically significant at both 3 and 8 weeks ($p < 0.005$, <0.001, <0.0003 for VAS, pressure algometry and Maryland foot score, respectively). None of the patients reported any side effects.

In the second study (Huang et al., 2010), the effect of onabotulinumtoxinA was compared with placebo in 50 patients (25 in each treatment group). Under ultrasonographic guidance, 50 U onabotulinumtoxinA was injected into the fascia via a posterior approach below the calcaneus. Follow-up evaluation at 3 weeks and 3 months demonstrated significant improvement in VAS pain score and plantar fascia thickness ($p < 0.001$), with significant improvement in pressure velocity (gait assessment) at 3 months ($p < 0.05$). Thus, both studies showed significant improvement of heel and foot pain at designated time points.

In another randomized controlled study (Diaz-Llopis et al., 2012), the efficacy of onabotulinumtoxinA

(70 U, injected using the technique of Babcock et al. [2005]) was compared with corticosteroids in 56 patients (28 in each treatment group). After 6 months, there was significant pain relief ($p = 0.001$), improvement in foot function ($p < 0.001$), wearing shoes ($p = 0.004$) and self-perceived foot health ($p < 0.001$) in the onabotulinumtoxinA-treated group compared with the corticosteroid group.

Technique for botulinum neurotoxin treatment: the Yale/Walter Reed protocol

We use the technique reported in our 2005 study (Babcock et al., 2005). As noted above, this method includes two injection sites (Fig. 26.2) covering both the area of most common pain (medical aspect of the heel) and the central band of plantar fascia with its major underlying muscle (flexor digitorum brevis). We encourage physical therapy along with BoNT treatment and no changes in patient's medications during the first month of treatment.

References

Aoki KR, Francis J (2011). Updates on the antinociceptive mechanism hypothesis of botulinum toxin A. *Parkinson Relat Disord*, **17**, S28–33.

Babcock MS, Foster L, Pasquina P, Jabbari B (2005). Treatment of pain attributed to plantar fasciitis with botulinum toxin A: a short-term, randomized, placebo-controlled, double-blind study. *Am J Phys Med Rehabil*, **84**, 649–54.

Cui M, Khanijou S, Rubino J, Aoki KR (2004). Subcutaneous administration of botulinum toxin A reduces formalin-induced pain. *Pain*, **107**, 125–33.

Diaz-Llopis IV, Rodrguez-Ruiz CM, Mulet-Perry S (2012). Randomized controlled study of the efficacy of the injection of botulinum toxin type A versus corticosteroids in chronic plantar fasciitis: results at one and six months. *Clin Rehabil*, **26**, 594–606.

French J, Gronseth G (2008). Lost in a jungle of evidence: we need a compass. *Neurology*, **71**, 1634–8.

Goff JD, Crawford R (2011). Diagnosis and treatment of plantar fasciitis. *Am Fam Physician*, **84**, 676–82.

Huang YC, Wei SH, Wang HK, Lieu FK (2010). Ultrasonographic guided botulinum toxin type A treatment for plantar fasciitis: An outcome-based investigation for treating pain and gait changes. *J Rehabil Med*, **42**, 136–40.

Jabbari B, Machado D (2011). Treatment of refractory pain with botulinum toxins: an evidence-based review. *Pain Med*, **12**, 1594–606.

Mahowald S, Legge BS, Grady JF (2011). The correlation between plantar fascia thickness and symptoms of plantar fasciitis. *J Am Podiatr Med Assoc*, **101**, 385–9.

Tu P, Bytomski JR (2011). Diagnosis of heel pain. *Am Fam Physician*, **84**, 909–16.

Williams PL, Banister LH, Berry MM (1995). Plantar fasciitis and plantar muscles of the foot. *Gray's Anatomy*, 38th edn. Edinburgh: Churchill Livingstone, pp. 1284–6.

Young C (2012). In the clinic. Plantar fasciitis. *Ann Intern Med*, **156**, 1–16.

Chapter 29

Use of botulinum neurotoxin in the treatment of low-back pain

José De Andrés and Gustavo Fabregat

Introduction

Chronic low-back pain is one of the leading causes of physician office visits and work absenteeism in developed countries. It is estimated that from 49% to 70% of the adult population will suffer at least one episode of low-back pain over their lifetime (Koes *et al.*, 2006).

Although the etiopathogenesis of non-specific low-back pain is unknown, multiple factors may be involved in pain occurrence. Involvement of the muscles directly or indirectly stabilizing the lumbar spine may play a significant role in the occurrence and maintenance of low-back pain syndromes (Porterfield and DeRosa, 1998).

This chapter reviews the pathophysiology, diagnosis and treatment with botulinum neurotoxin (BoNT) of myofascial pain of muscles involved in lumbosciatic conditions (quadratus lumborum, iliopsoas and paravertebral) (Table 29.1). The piriformis muscle is reviewed in the next chapter.

Quadratus lumborum muscle

Dysfunction of the quadratus lumborum muscle is considered the most common cause of low-back pain by many authors (Travell and Simmons, 1983). Its impairment may be severely disabling as it plays an important stabilizing role in the spine, and makes the load of standing body weight intolerable.

Review of anatomy

The quadratus lumborum muscle is found on the posterolateral aspect of the lumbar spine and has a flat, quadrilateral morphology. It inserts below the outer border of the iliac crest, above the lower border of the 12th rib and in its medial portion on the tips of the transverse processes of L1–L5 (Fig. 29.1).

It is formed by fibers that cross one another in three directions:

- costotransverse fibers stretch from the transverse processes of L1 to rib 12
- iliotransverse fibers run from the iliac crest to the transverse processes of the last four lumbar vertebrae
- iliocostal fibers extend from the iliac crest to the lower border of rib 12.

When the subject is erect, the muscle acts to stabilize the lumbar spine on the pelvis. Unilateral contraction flexes the lumbar spine to the same side. With the spine fixed, the muscles' function is to elevate the hip on the same side. Bilateral contraction allows extension of the lumbar spine and trunk. It is also an accessory respiratory muscle.

The nerve supply for the quadratus lumborum muscle is provided by thoracic nerve T_{12} and the lumbar plexus (L_1 to L_3 spinal nerves).

Symptoms

Pain is reported by patients as deep and worsens with standing or unsupported sitting. The typical pain distribution caused by quadratus lumborum muscle dysfunction is depicted in Fig. 29.2.

Typically, pain may extend to the groin and genital areas and sometimes simulate a distribution compatible with sciatic nerve dysfunction, with referred pain over the area of the sacroiliac joints and lower buttocks.

The upper trigger points show a typical pattern of pain toward the sacroiliac joints and trochanteric region. The lower trigger points radiate toward the buttocks. It is important in these cases to consider differential diagnosis with pain originating in the lumbar zygapophyseal joints and pain from nerve

Manual of Botulinum Toxin Therapy, 2nd edition, ed. Daniel Truong, Mark Hallett, Christopher Zachary and Dirk Dressler. Published by Cambridge University Press. © Cambridge University Press 2013.

Table 29.1 Summary of key points in the anatomy of the different muscles commonly involved in low-back pain

	Quadratus lumborum	Iliopsoas	Paravertebral muscle
Origin	Iliac crest	*Iliacus*: iliac fossa *Psoas major*: vertebral body and transverse processes of L1–L5	*Deep*: transverse processes *Superficial*: sacral thoracolumbar aponeurosis
Insertion	12th rib and transverse processes of L1 to L4	Lesser trochanter of the femur	*Deep*: spinous processes *Superficial*: ribs and dorsolumbar transverse processes
Function	*Bilaterally*, extensor of lumbar spine *Unilaterally*: lateral rotator of spine Also accessory respiratory muscle	Hip flexion and abduction	Extensors and rotators of vertebral column
Nerve supply	T_{12} costal nerve and lumbar plexus (L_1 to L_3)	Lumbar plexus (L_2 to L_4)	Posterior branch of spinal nerve (lateral division to superficial muscles and medial division to deep muscles)

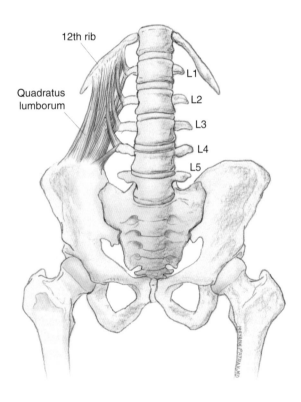

12th rib

L1

L2

L3

L4

L5

Quadratus lumborum

Fig. 29.1 Anterior view showing the insertion sites of the quadratus lumborum muscle.

root involvement (particularly S_1), which may show similar patterns of pain radiation. The severity of pain may become completely disabling for the patient.

Patients have difficulty in flexing the trunk, rotating it to the contralateral side of the affected side or leaning toward any position when lying in a supine position. They may also report difficulty in rising from a sitting position without using the arms. In acute cases, coughing or sneezing may be painful.

Examination

An examination should be performed for rotation and lateral flexion mobility of the lumbar spine; both will be painful, but lateral flexion will be the most affected. Contracture of the quadratus lumborum may cause a functional lumbar scoliosis of convexity contralateral to the affected side as well as declination of the contralateral hemipelvis (Travell and Simmons, 1983).

For examination of the trigger points, the patient is placed in lateral decubitus position on the contralateral side. With patient in this position, a rolled sheet is placed in the lower part of the lumbar spine, leaving the upper leg behind the other until the knee touches the table; the upper arm is extended above the head to grip the edge of the table, so that the space between the last rib and the iliac crest is opened to the maximum, permitting optimal access to the muscle (Fig. 29.3). In this position, trigger points are examined by pressing down on the areas next to the iliac crest and the 12th rib (superficial trigger points), which causes pain that radiates to the trochanter, and external side of the thigh and in the area next to the lumbar spine, which causes pain that radiates to the sacroiliac joints and buttocks.

(a) (b)

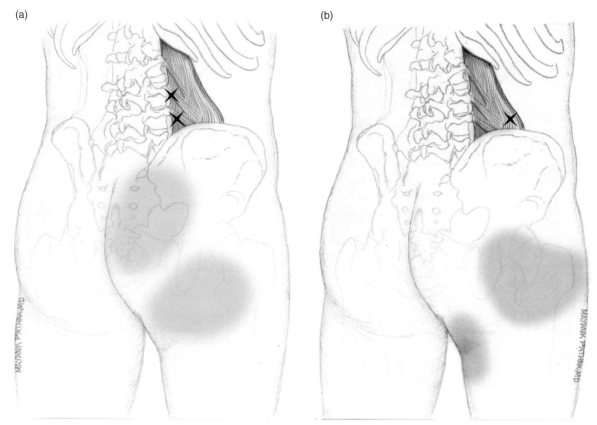

Fig. 29.2 Patterns of referred pain of the trigger points of the quadratus lumborum muscle. (a,b) Pain pattern of superficial trigger points, palpable below and next to the 12th rib (a) and above the iliac crest (b). (c) Pain pattern of deep trigger points next to the lumbar transverse processes.

Treatment

The doses of the different types of BoNT used for treatment of quadratus lumborum muscle dysfunction are summarized in Table 29.2.

The technique to infiltrate the quadratus lumborum muscle is classically performed under X-ray guidance. With the patient in a prone position, the X-ray unit is placed in anteroposterior projection and the highest point of the iliac crest is located. The space between the spinal processes of L4 and L5 is located and a mark is made on the skin above the highest point of the crest at the height of the L4–L5 space (Fig. 29.4a).

The skin is infiltrated with a small amount of local anesthetic using a Quincke-type, 22-gauge, 90 mm spinal needle inserted perpendicular to the skin.

Once the needle is firmly secured and tunnel vision is obtained, the X-ray unit is placed in lateral view, and the needle is advanced in this projection until it reaches the midpoint of the lamina of the corresponding vertebra (Fig. 29.4b).

The X-ray is placed again in anteroposterior projection and 0.2 ml of water-soluble contrast medium is injected, and an image of intramuscular distribution should be obtained in anteroposterior (Fig. 29.4c) and lateral (Fig. 29.4d) view. Once the image is obtained, injection of BoNT is performed.

This procedure has also been described using ultrasound guidance (Curatolo and Eichenberger, 2007).

The main risk when performing infiltration of the quadratus lumborum muscle is penetrating into the abdominal cavity with the needle or causing damage to structures such as the kidneys since this muscle is one of the muscles making up the posterior abdominal wall (Fig. 29.5).

Iliopsoas muscle

Review of anatomy

The psoas major muscle is inserted proximally on the sides of the vertebral bodies of the last thoracic

Table 29.2 Doses of the different types of botulinum neurotoxin used in the treatment of low-back pain

	Quadratus lumborum (IU)	Iliopsoas (IU)	Paravertebral (IU)
Type A			
OnabotulinumtoxinA (Botox)	50–150	50–200	40–50 per level (max. 400–500)
AbobotulinumtoxinA (Dysport)	150–400	150–600	120–150 per level (max. 1200–1500)
Type B			
RimabotulinumtoxinB (NeuroBloc)	2500–5000	3000–7500	800–1000 per level (max. 8000–10000)

(c)

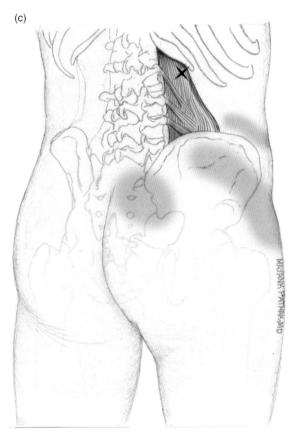

Fig. 29.2 (cont.)

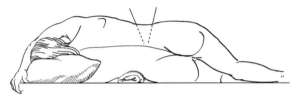

Fig. 29.3 Patient position to examine the quadratus lumborum muscle. Complete opening of the iliocostal space is achieved by placing a pillow below the lumbar spine and making the upper knee rest on the table behind the lower leg. Illustrated by Mayank Pathak, redrawn from author's original.

inserted on the anterolateral aspects of T12, L1 and L2 up to the superior ramus of the pubic bone.

The iliac muscle is inserted proximally on the upper two-thirds of the internal surface of the iliac fossa and the internal border of the iliac crest. Distally it joins the psoas major muscle within the pelvis to form the iliopsoas muscle. Both muscle bellies become mainly tendinous on passing below the inguinal ligament and are inserted distally on the lesser trochanter of the femur.

The iliopsoas muscle is innervated by fibers from the lumbar plexus (L2 to L4), the main action of the iliopsoas muscle is anterior flexion of the hip when the spinal column is fixed. It also assists in abduction of the column.

Iliopsoas contracture may produce increased pressure in the discs of the lumbar spine, which may result in compression of the lumbar roots and the consequent nerve root pain (Insausti-Valdivia, 2006).

Symptoms

Pain primarily occurs in activities performed during load bearing and conversely is relieved in the decubitus position with the knees flexed. The patient has difficulty in rising from low places and in sitting up from the supine position.

vertebra and all the lumbar vertebrae, as well as in the anterior borders and lower surfaces of the lumbar transverse processes. Hence it is situated next to the vertebral bodies and in front of the transverse processes (Fig. 29.6).

The psoas minor muscle is anatomically inconstant and may not be found in up to half of subjects. It is located in front of the psoas major muscle and is

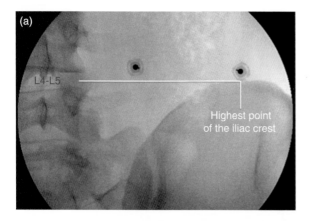

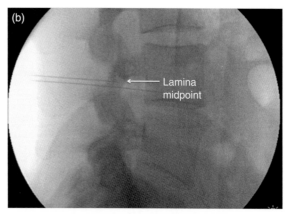

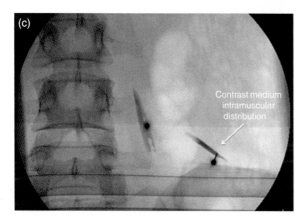

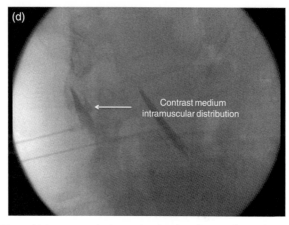

Fig. 29.4 Infiltration of the quadratus lumborum muscle under X-ray guidance. (a) Anteroposterior image showing the references for quadratus lumborum muscle puncture. The highest point of the iliac crest is located and the space between the transverse processes L4 and L5. (b) Lateral image showing the references for quadratus lumborum muscle puncture. The needle has been advanced to the point where it is in the midpoint of the lamina of the corresponding vertebra. (c) Anteroposterior view with iodine contrast, showing intramuscular distribution. (d) Lateral view with iodine contrast, showing intramuscular distribution.

Patients with a dysfunctional iliopsoas report lumbar pain distributed vertically along the spinal column and occasionally pain in the front part of the thigh and groin. When dysfunction is bilateral, the patient may report pain distributed horizontally across the entire lumbar region.

There are three main psoas trigger points:

- the front part of the thigh on the lateral border of the femoral triangle in the area of muscle insertion; compression at this level causes pain mainly radiated to the lumbar area, though also to the anteromedial aspect of the thigh and the groin
- internal aspect of the anterosuperior iliac crest where the iliopsoas muscle arises; in this case, the radiated pain is distributed over the lumbar area and sometimes to the sacroiliac joint
- area below and lateral to the navel where the muscle crosses the pelvis; this is in the trigger points of the groin and pain is primarily distributed over the lumbar area.

The patterns of radiated pain and the trigger points are illustrated in Fig. 29.7.

Examination

Patients with myofascial dysfunction of the iliopsoas muscle tend to walk with a bent-over posture, have anterior tilting of the pelvis and hyperlordosis of the lumbar spine.

251

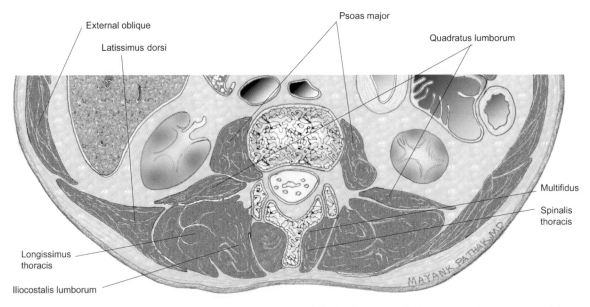

External oblique

Latissimus dorsi

Psoas major

Quadratus lumborum

Multifidus

Spinalis thoracis

Longissimus thoracis

Iliocostalis lumborum

Fig. 29.5 Anatomical section at the level of L2. When accessing the quadratus lumborum muscle, the greatest risk is penetration of the abdominal cavity or injury to the renal poles.

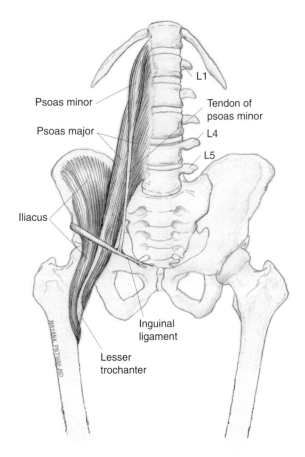

Psoas minor

Psoas major

Iliacus

Lesser trochanter

L1

Tendon of psoas minor

L4

L5

Inguinal ligament

Fig. 29.6 Insertion sites of psoas major, iliac and psoas minor muscles.

Iliopsoas muscle tension is assessed with the patient lying in a supine position on the table, checking the amplitude of the hip extension movement. The patient is placed so that the buttocks are supported on the edge of the table. The patient grasps the thigh of the contralateral leg and moves it toward the chest to stabilize the pelvis and flatten the lumbar spine. In this position, normally the leg falls below the horizontal in a normal patient; if psoas muscle contracture is present, the leg will remain above the horizontal because of shortening of the muscle (Fig. 29.8a).

Muscle force is also assessed with the patient in a sitting position, asking the patient to flex the hip without leaning forward, with and without resistance (Fig. 29.8b) (Pleguezuelos-Cobo *et al.*, 2008).

To palpate the trigger points, the patient is placed in the decubitus position. The myotendinous junction of the psoas with the iliac muscle in the femoral triangle can be compressed. To avoid compression of the femoral nerve (medial to the muscle), abducting the hip is recommended.

Using the fingers along the internal border of the iliac crest, the proximal fibers of the iliac muscle can be palpated within the iliac crest through the aponeurosis of the external oblique muscle.

The trigger points of the psoas major in its paravertebral position are difficult to access since their palpation must be done through the muscles of the

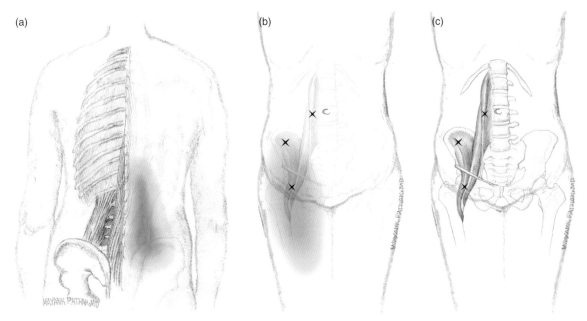

(a)　　　　　　　　　　　(b)　　　　　　　　　　　(c)

Fig. 29.7 Patterns of referred pain from the trigger points of the iliopsoas muscle: (a) ipsilateral posterior lumbar back distribution; (b) anterior groin and upper anteromedial aspect of the thigh. (c) Psoas and iliacus muscles and specific trigger points causing referred pain pattern.

abdominal wall. The patient should be asked to relax the muscles of the abdominal wall. The trigger points are usually found at the level of the navel or slightly below by attempting to sink the fingers below the anterior rectus muscle of the abdomen (Travell and Simmons, 1983).

The maneuvers for palpation of the psoas muscle are illustrated in Fig. 29.9.

Treatment

The doses of the different types of BoNT used for treatment of iliopsoas dysfunction are summarized in Table 29.2.

Although ultrasound-guided intramuscular infiltration has been used for treatment of iliopsoas myofascial syndrome, the classic and most commonly used technique to access this muscle is with fluoroscopy (Westhoff et al., 2003).

The patient is placed in a prone position, and with the X-ray unit in anteroposterior projection, the lateral processes of L4 and L5 can be located. The point of access is located at the midpoint of the line joining the external border of both spinal processes. Depending on patient size, a Quincke-type, 22-gauge, 90 mm or 140 mm spinal needle is used. After infiltration of the overlying tissues with local anesthetic, the needle is

inserted under tunnel vision about 4–5 cm or until it remains fixed. The X-ray unit is now placed in a lateral position and the needle is advanced until it reaches the midpoint of the corresponding intervertebral disc or body.

Once situated, correct positioning is checked by injection of a small amount of iodine contrast, observing the characteristic intramuscular distribution (Fig. 29.10). This is confirmed by placing the X-ray unit again in anteroposterior position. At this time, the dose of BoNT is injected in a single point, administering a volume not greater than 10 ml.

There is a risk, though very remote, of accessing the retroperitoneum. When the needle is advanced toward the muscle belly of the psoas major, it may accidentally encounter the L4 root, causing paresthesia and nerve root pain in the patient. If this occurs, the needle should be redirected upwards or downwards. Injection may cause bruising and pain in the groin area, which are normally self-limiting (Insausti-Valdivia, 2006).

Lumbar paravertebral muscles

Review of anatomy

The paravertebral muscles lie alongside the vertebral column. Located on the paravertebral canals, they are

(a)

(b)

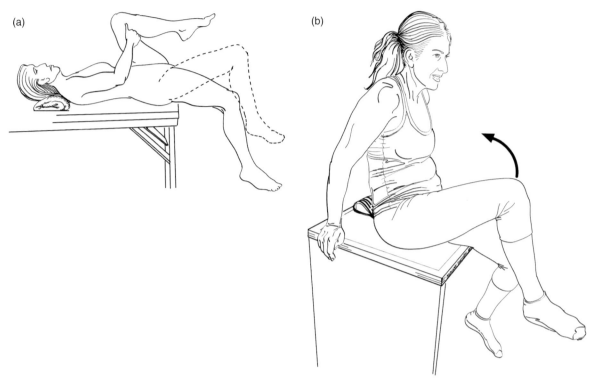

Fig. 29.8 Assessment of iliopsoas muscle contracture (a) and function (b). (a) The right lower limb shows the normal position without tension. The dotted limb shows an excessively shortened iliopsoas muscle, maintaining the hip flexed against gravity, with the leg hanging freely (normal rectus femoris muscle). (b) The patient in a sitting position is asked to make a hip flexion without leaning forward. Illustrated by Mayank Pathak, redrawn from author's original.

longitudinal muscles that play an important role in maintaining static posture of the vertebral column and also in movements of flexion, extension and rotation. For study, they can be divided into deep (also called short) muscles and superficial or long muscles.

The *deep paravertebral muscles* (Fig. 29.11a) have a more horizontal arrangement. The interspinous, intertransverse, rotators and multifidus muscles are included in this group, among others.

Of all these muscles, the ones most frequently involved in low-back pain syndromes are the multifidus muscles.

The multifidus muscles arise from the transverse processes of between two and four adjacent vertebrae and then turn upward and inward to the spinous process of the vertebra that lie immediately above the one from which the first segment arose.

Innervation is provided by divisions of the dorsal branches of the spinal nerves. These dorsal branches have a medial and a lateral division; the medial branch being responsible for innervation of the deep paraspinal muscles.

The main action of these muscles together with that of the rotators and the other deep muscles is to stabilize the spine as well as contralateral rotation of the trunk on unilateral contraction. When they contract bilaterally, they extend the vertebral column.

The *superficial paravertebral muscles* (Fig. 29.11b), known collectively as the erector spinae muscles, are arranged longitudinally and are composed of fibers of three muscles; from lateral to medial, they are the iliocostalis, the longissimus and the spinalis. Taken together, they form a thick muscular mass, easily palpated at the lumbar level. The erector spinae muscles arise from a wide and thick tendon which is inserted at the level of the sacrum (sacral thoracolumbar aponeurosis). The iliocostalis muscle inserts on posterior surfaces of the ribs and on the transverse processes of the neck region. The longissimus muscle inserts on the thoracic and lumber processes.

When they contract on both sides, the action of these muscles is to extend the vertebral column. When they contract on one side only, they produce lateral flexion of the spine to one side or the other.

(a)

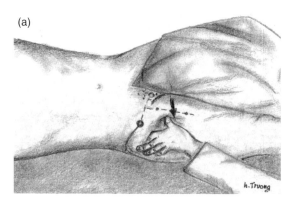

(b)

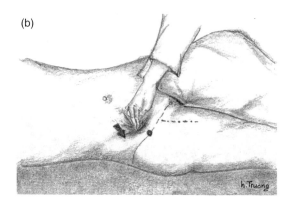

(c)

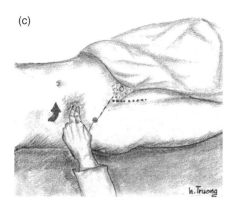

Fig. 29.9 Palpation of trigger points of the iliopsoas muscle in three locations. The iliac crest (solid line), inguinal ligament (broken line), femoral artery (dotted line), anterosuperior iliac spine (filled circle) and pubic tubercle (open circle) are marked. (a) Palpation of distal trigger points of the iliopsoas muscle in the lateral wall of the femoral triangle. (b) Palpation within the pelvic rim of the trigger points of the iliac muscle. (c) Compression of deep proximal trigger points next to the anterior rectus muscle of the abdomen. Illustrated by Dr Hiep Truong, redrawn from author's original (from Travell and Simons, 1983).

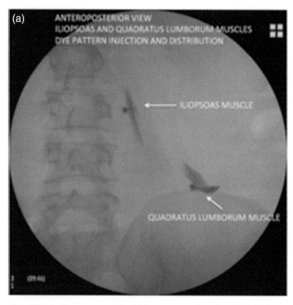

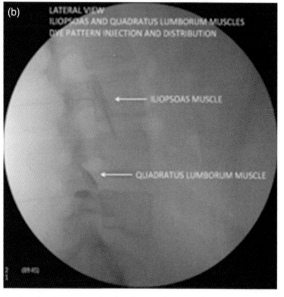

Fig. 29.10 Iliopsoas muscle. (a) Anteroposterior view with iodine contrast, showing intramuscular distribution. (b) Lateral view with iodine contrast, showing intramuscular distribution.

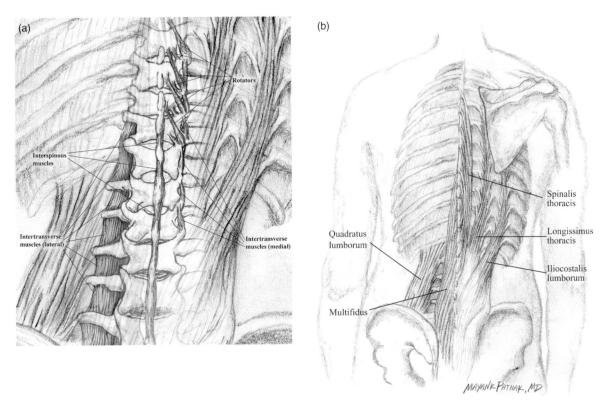

(a)

Rotators

Interspinous
muscles

Intertransverse
muscles (lateral)

Intertransverse
muscles (medial)

(b)

Spinalis
thoracis

Quadratus
lumborum

Longissimus
thoracis

Iliocostalis
lumborum

Multifidus

MAYANK PATHAK, MD

Fig. 29.11 Paravertebral muscles. (a) Deep paraspinal muscles. (b) Superficial or long paraspinal muscles.

Innervation is provided mainly from the lateral division of the dorsal branches of the thoracolumbar spinal nerves.

Symptoms

The chief complaint caused by thoracolumbar paravertebral muscle dysfunction is central pain and occasionally pain located in the buttocks and abdomen. The patterns of radiated pain are outlined in Fig. 29.12. Involvement of the deeper muscles (rotatores and multifidus) usually causes midline pain. Involvement of the multifidus muscles, particularly at the level of L2 and S1, can cause patterns of pain radiated to the abdomen.

Given the importance of these muscles in static and dynamic functions of the spinal column, bilateral disorder may cause significant disability in the patient. Bilateral dysfunction of the longissimus muscle can hinder rising from a sitting position and climbing stairs.

Examination

The best way to palpate the paravertebral muscles is with the patient in lateral position with a pillow next to the abdomen and a slight tendency toward prone. The knees are flexed toward the chest until an adequate degree of muscle tension is achieved. Dysfunction of the deep muscles can be revealed by percussion or pressure on the spinous processes. When a hypersensitive area is located, the groove between the transverse process and the longissimus muscle is palpated firmly.

Palpation of the affected muscles can cause, in addition to focal hypersensitivity to pressure, the appearance of the characteristic pain pattern (Travell and Simmons, 1983).

Treatment

Administration of BoNT in the paravertebral musculature has been shown to be effective in the treatment

(a)   (b)

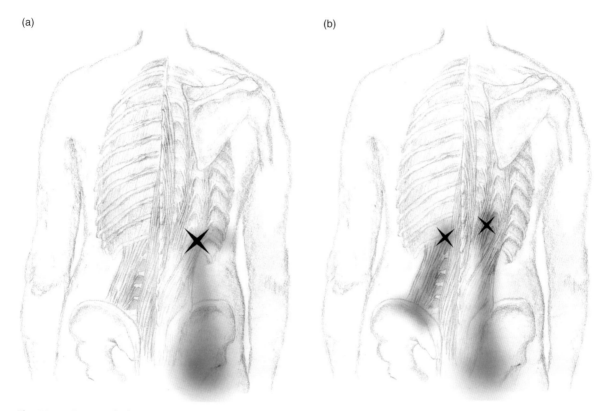

Fig. 29.12. Patterns of referred pain from the trigger points of the iliocostal muscle (a), longissimus muscle (b) and multifidus muscles in the front (c) and back (d). Illustrated by Mayank Pathak.

of low-back pain conditions (Foster *et al.*, 2001; Jabbari *et al.*, 2006; Ney *et al.*, 2006).

For treatment, the vertebral level is chosen where the patient has the greatest pain, either reported by the patient or observed by the examiner. At that level, unilaterally or bilaterally depending on the pain pattern of the patient, BoNT is administered, for example using 40–50 IU onabotulinumtoxinA. Other formulations can be used, but most experience is with this formulation. Starting from this point, successive injections are made between one and two levels above and below the point of greatest pain with the intention of covering the greatest possible length of the paraspinal musculature, taking care not to exceed 400–500 IU onabotulinumtoxinA per session.

To achieve intramuscular administration, use of electromyography is recommended, though some

authors use "blind" puncture (Jabbari *et al.*, 2006). Our group recommends the use of ultrasonography for precise intramuscular administration of the BoNT.

References

Curatolo M, Eichenberger U (2007). Ultrasound-guided blocks for the treatment of chronic pain. *Tech Reg Anesth Pain Med*, **11**, 95–102.

Foster L, Clapp L, Erickson M et al. (2001). Botulinum toxin A and chronic low back pain. *Neurology*, **56**, 1290–3.

Insausti-Valdivia J (2006). Dolor Miofascial. *Manual de exploración y tratamiento*. Majadahonda, Madrid: Ergon.

Jabbari B, Ney J, Sichani A et al. (2006). Treatment of refractory, chronic low back pain with botulinum neurotoxin A: an open-label pilot study. *Pain Med*, **7**, 260–4.

(c)

(d)

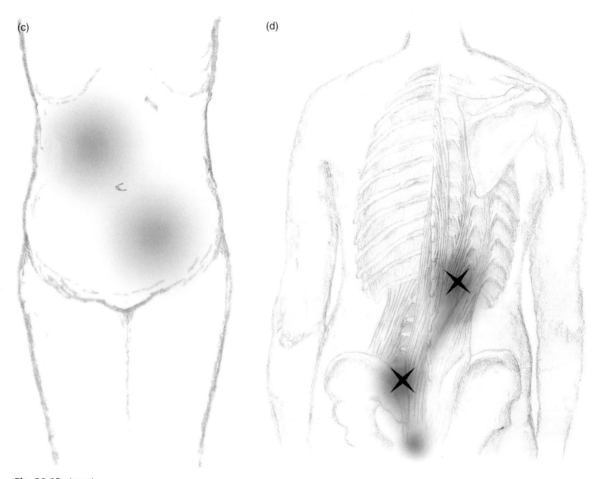

Fig. 29.12. (cont.)

Koes BW, Van Tulder MW, Thomas S (2006). Diagnosis and treatment of low back pain. *BMJ*, **332**, 1430–4.

Ney JP, Difazio M, Sichani A *et al.* (2006). Treatment of chronic low back pain with successive injections of botulinum toxin A over 6 months: a prospective trial of 60 patients. *Clin J Pain*, **22**, 363–9.

Pleguezuelos-Cobo E *et al.* (2008). *Atlas de puntos clave musculares en la práctica clínica*. Madrid: Panamericana.

Porterfield JA, DeRosa C (1998). *Mechanical Low Back Pain: Perspectives in Functional Anatomy*. Philadelphia, PA: Saunders.

Travell JG, Simmons DG (1983). *Myofascial Pain and Dysfunction: The Trigger Point Manual*. Baltimore MD: Williams & Wilkins.

Westhoff B, Seller K, Wild A, Jaeger M, Krsuspe R (2003). Ultrasound-guided botulinum toxin injection technique for the iliopsoas muscle. *Dev Med Child Neurol*, **45**, 829–32.

Use of botulinum neurotoxin in the treatment of piriformis syndrome

Loren M. Fishman and Sarah B. Schmidhofer

Introduction

Piriformis syndrome is entrapment of the sciatic nerve by the piriformis muscle, causing sciatica. One estimate puts the incidence of sciatica of non-disc origin as equal to or greater than that of herniated disc, based on comparison of the number of lumbar MRI scans versus the number of subsequent surgery for lumbar disc problems in 239 subjects in 2002 (Filler *et al.*, 2005). The same study found intensive MRI evidence that piriformis syndrome accounted for a full 67% of sciatica of non-disc origin. Regardless of exact incidence, it seems fair to say that sciatica of non-disc origin is common and that in some circumstances the diagnosis of piriformis syndrome is controversial. Some investigators (Halpin and Ganju, 2009; Miller *et al.*, 2012) find the syndrome undefined and infrequent.

In the 25-year period from 1987 to 2012, our own experience has included over 17 000 patients referred or self-referred for piriformis syndrome, approximately half of whom ultimately had the diagnosis confirmed. Since we are a referral center for the condition, our data cannot be used as a suitable sample from which to derive incidence or prevalence figures. However, the average length of time that our patients have had the pain related to piriformis syndrome has fallen from 6.5 years (Fishman *et al.*, 2002a,b) to well below 2 years, suggesting, at least, that the syndrome is being recognized and treated more quickly than in the past, and that although recognized incidence is rising, prevalence is declining.

Clinical features

Signs of piriformis syndrome are:

- sciatica
- buttock pain
- buttock tenderness.

Clinical tests for piriformis syndrome include:

- weakened abduction of the flexed thigh (Pace and Nagle, 1976)
- piriformis pain on passive adduction of flexed thigh (Solheim *et al.*, 1981).

Pathogenesis

Pathogenetic mechanisms causing piriformis syndrome are:

- compression between piriformis muscle and ischiofemoral ligament in 90%
- adhesion to ventral piriformis or dorsal obturator internis in 9%
- anatomical, gluteal arterial or, rarely, fibrous band through nerve in 1%.

There appear to be three main pathogenetic factors in the development of piriformis syndrome: anatomical variations, nerve compression and nerve adhesion. To begin with a likely misconception, it is often felt that piriformis syndrome results from any number of anatomical variations in lower extremity nerve configurations. In fact, worldwide cadaveric studies do show a 10–30% variation in the sciatic nerve's relation to the piriformis muscle (Pećina, 1979; Gotlin, 1990; Sharma *et al.*, 2010; Ogeng'o *et al.*, 2011). Perhaps surprisingly, these variations are largely –though not entirely – irrelevant to diagnosis and treatment of the syndrome.

In approximately 70–90% of patients, the anterior and posterior divisions of the L_4, L_5, S_1 and S_2 roots (the lumbosacral plexus) join to form the sciatic nerve before reaching the sciatic foramen and remain united as the sciatic nerve passes beneath the piriformis muscle, dividing into posterior tibial (anterior division) and common peroneal (posterior division) nerves in the proximal, middle or distal third of the

Manual of Botulinum Toxin Therapy, 2nd edition, ed. Daniel Truong, Mark Hallett, Christopher Zachary and Dirk Dressler.
Published by Cambridge University Press. © Cambridge University Press 2013.

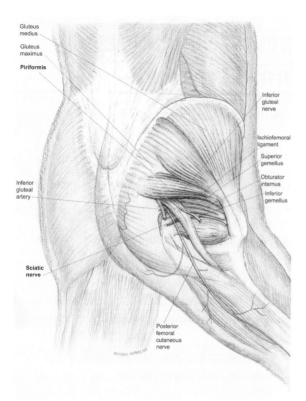

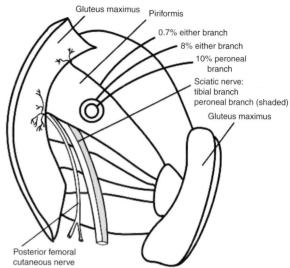

Fig. 30.2 In 10–30% of unselected cadavers, fibers of the posterior tibial and peroneal nerves never unite to form the sciatic nerve. In approximately half of these cases, one or both nerves pass through or above the piriformis muscle. (Reproduced with permission from Travell, JG and Simons, DG. *Myofascial Pain and Dysfunction: The Trigger Point Manual, Volume 2*, 2nd edn. Philadelphia, PA: Williams & Wilkins; 1998, p. 186.)

Fig. 30.1 In piriformis syndrome, the sciatic nerve is either sandwiched between the piriformis muscle and the ischiofemoral ligament or, less commonly, adherent to the ventral surface of the piriformis muscle or the dorsal aspect of the obturator internus.

thigh, in ascending order of frequency (Fig. 30.1). In the other 10–30% of patients, the anterior and posterior divisions of the lumbosacral plexus do not unite, resulting in their passage independently down the leg.

Approximately 3–4% of cases include variations involving the posterior tibial and peroneal components uniting below the piriformis muscle with or without a communicating nerve. Also included in this grouping is a variation in which the two divisions are united within the pelvis, separate at the piriformis level and reunite; effectively surrounding the muscle (Sunderland, 1868; Beaton and Anson, 1937; Sridhara and Izzo, 1985; Fishman and Zybert, 1992; Sharma *et al.*, 2010) (Fig. 30.2). In rare cases in which the muscle is divided, a small fibrous band penetrates the nerve. This can easily result in sciatic pathology at the level of the piriformis muscle.

A common opinion about the pathogenesis of piriformis syndrome is that any and all of these anomalies are responsible for it (Sharma *et al.*, 2010). However, the facts do not support this. Cadaveric studies show that anomalous passage of the sciatic nerve and the

piriformis, when it occurs, is overwhelmingly bilateral (Sunderland, 1868; Beaton and Anson, 1937; Sridhara and Izzo, 1985; Fishman and Zybert, 1992; Sharma *et al.*, 2010). Yet in our experience of 17 000 patients, the syndrome is unilateral 90% of the time it is encountered. Further, surgical reports confirm an anomalous sciatic–piriformis relationship approximately 15% of the time, the same proportion found in cadaveric studies of the general population (Fishman and Ardman, 1997). Understanding these anatomical variations is important in treating the disorder, but they do not inevitably cause it. Far from it. Tension or pressure of the muscle on the nerve causes the syndrome, but it does not appear that these anomalous nerve/muscle variations are consistently responsible for that pressure.

Anatomy books frequently picture the gemellus superior, the obturator internus and the gemellus inferior distal to the most caudal side of the piriformis muscle and adjacent to the exiting sciatic nerve (Lockhart *et al.*, 1959); in fact, there is also a sharp-edged ligament that lurks just below the muscle, the ischiofemoral ligament (Fig. 30.1). Where we *do* find this compressive pressure, and resulting piriformis syndrome, is where the sciatic nerve is held against the ischiofemoral ligament under pressure by a misbehaving piriformis muscle. Its erosive influence on the sciatic nerve, developed under pressure from the tight, shortened or scarred piriformis muscle roofing the sciatic nerve at that junction, appears to be the most common cause of piriformis syndrome. Denudation of the vaso nervorum, noted in more than 100 postsurgical reports, confirms this.

There are also cases of piriformis syndrome in which adhesions attach the nerve to the piriformis muscle or, less frequently, to the obturator internus muscle. In these cases, muscular contraction raises the risk of neuropraxia through stretching. Surgical reports and specialized scans describe both the compressive and adhesive phenomena with regularity, favoring the former considerably. For our purposes, both are important, since a botulinum neurotoxin (BoNT) injection that reduces muscle motility will be effective in either case, provided the injection is well placed.

Diagnosis of piriformis syndrome

The most common causes of piriformis syndrome are:

- sedentary occupation: financial sector, vehicle driver, secretary, clinical psychology
- athletic: track and field, rowing, hockey, football, soccer
- recreational: health club, pilates, trainer
- traumatic: rear-ended in vehicle, backward fall.

Piriformis syndrome was long considered a diagnosis of exclusion, a diagnosis to consider only when other diagnoses had been ruled out. Unfortunately, this means that piriformis syndrome is *not* considered if other diagnoses are actually present, when in fact, clinicians may often find patients with two diagnoses.

There are two methods of specifically diagnosing piriformis syndrome: electrodiagnostic testing and the MRI neural scan.

The electrophysiological method is the oldest. The diagnosis is made by measuring the delay of the H-reflex when the piriformis muscle is stretched against the sciatic nerve (Fig. 30.3). This is done by first recording an H-reflex for the posterior tibial and peroneal nerves bilaterally in the anatomical position. Then, the patient is placed in the lateral decubitus position and the affected leg is forcibly urged into flexion, adduction and internal rotation (FAIR test). The posterior tibial and peroneal H-reflexes are then re-elicited. We generally press diagonally downward on the knee in order to control hip motion while raising the ankle (Fig. 30.4). This is well tolerated by most patients. After testing 88 normal individuals in our laboratory, the mean prolongation seen in the FAIR

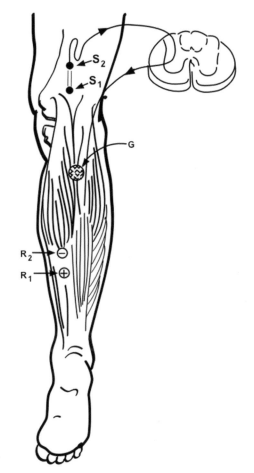

Fig. 30.3 The H-reflex is electrophysiological initiation and measurement of the monosynaptic Achilles tendon reflex. It is named after Paul Hoffmann, who discovered it in 1910. S_1 and S_2, first and second stimuli; R_1 and R_2, recording electrodes; G, ground. Illustrated by Mayank Pathak, from author's original.

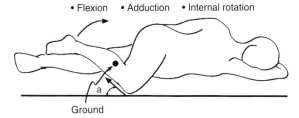

Fig. 30.4 When a patient is in 90 degrees of hip and knee flexion, forcibly adducting and internally rotating the leg to the level of the patient's or joint's tolerability (FAIR test) may compress the sciatic nerve or stretch it sufficiently to delay the H-reflex significantly (1.86 ms). Illustrated by Mayank Pathak, from author's original.

test was 0.01 milliseconds and the standard deviation (SD) was 0.62 milliseconds (Fishman *et al.*, 2002a). A delay of 3SD (1.86 milliseconds) of either branch of the sciatic nerve's H-reflex in the FAIR position is taken to denote piriformis syndrome (Figs. 30.5 and 30.6).

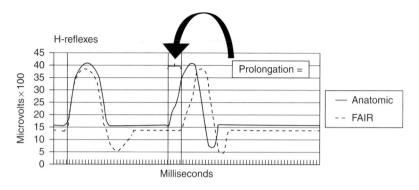

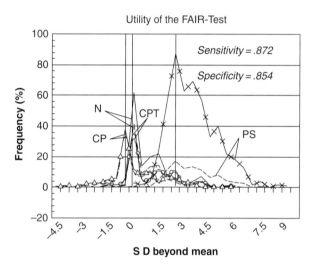

Fig. 30.5 Comparing the H-reflex in the anatomical position with one elicited in flexion, adduction and internal rotation will either confirm or refute the presence of piriformis syndrome according to whether the FAIR test generates a delay equal to or greater than 1.86 ms.

Fig. 30.6 Frequency curves for the H-reflex showing percentage with a standard deviation (SD) delay (full lines) compared with 88 normals and the percentage within each group that attained that particular prolongation of the H-reflex with FAIR positioning (dotted lines): normals (N), piriformis syndrome (PS); contralateral posterior tibial reflex (CPT), contralateral peroneal reflex (CP). Because the H-reflex crosses the piriformis muscle in both afferent and efferent limbs, the delay generated by compression is doubled, amplifying FAIR test discrepancies in patients with piriformis syndrome. Patients with piriformis syndrome can be clearly separated from normals in this FAIR test ($n = 687$) (Fishman *et al.*, 2002a).

The electrodiagnostic approach may be tempered by comparing side-to-side H-reflexes in the anatomical position with each other and with normal values, as a clue to radiculopathic involvement. It is also useful to seek additional electromyography (EMG) findings cephalad to the piriformis muscle, as well as in the muscle itself, as the S_1 and S_2 fibers that innervate the piriformis muscle do not pass under it. Unfortunately, nature has missed an opportunity for a feedback loop here, as with pronator syndrome, for if the innervation of these muscles passed below them, spasm would reduce their stimulus for further tightening, limiting compression of the sciatic and median nerves, respectively.

Findings from EMG suggestive of piriformis syndrome may be confined to one branch of the sciatic nerve with no involvement of the hamstrings, glutei, piriformis or tensor fascia latae. Further, discrepancy in the sural sensory nerve action potentials, with reduction in the amplitude on the affected side, is consistent with the clinical diagnosis of piriformis

syndrome in the context of the usual clinical criteria – sciatica, pain worsened by sitting, and tenderness in the mid-buttock. Attempts to use a 50% reduction in sural sensory nerve action potentials as a criterion for piriformis syndrome indicate that it only correlates in 30% with the FAIR test. However, placing pickups on the peroneus longus and stimulating just behind the fibular head produces a peroneal H-reflex more than 80% of the time.

The second diagnostic method is neural scanning, a technique that shims the MRI for the pelvis, does a standard MRI study and a fat-suppression study, then proceeds to digitally subtract the fat-suppression study from the standard one, leaving the myelin-rich peripheral nerves in fairly sharp relief (Filler *et al.*, 2005) (Fig. 30.7). This imaging method can detect nerve swelling proximal to and nerve attenuation distal to the site of entrapment, it may note pudendal and medial femoral cutaneous nerve involvement and can detect ischial tunnel syndrome if these are present. It may also reveal bifurcation of the piriformis muscle

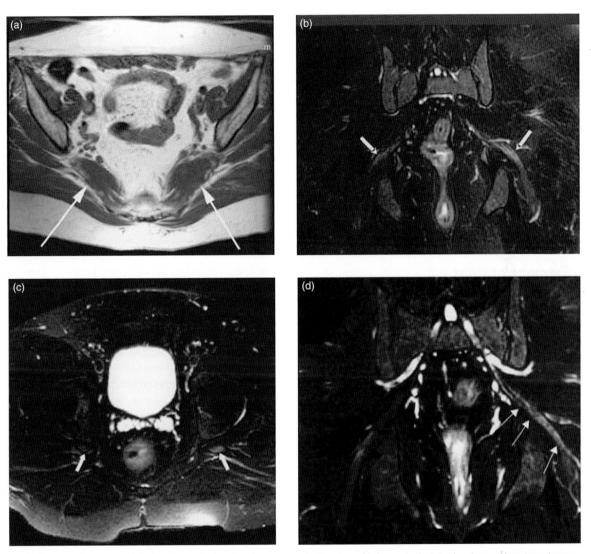

Fig. 30.7 Neural scanning. (a) Piriformis muscle showing the asymmetrically enlarged left muscle. (b,c) Axial and coronal sections. Arrows indicate sciatic nerves. (d) The curved neurographic image of hyperintense left sciatic nerve with loss of fascicular detail. Piriformis syndrome is on the reader's right in each image. (With permission from Filler *et al.*, 2005.)

and the sciatic nerve or other anomalous situations, including gluteal arterial and obturator internus complications in the course of the sciatic nerve or its components. At the time of writing there are five centers in the USA where the test is performed.

We have used neural scanning in more than 45 patients, generally in patients who had a postive FAIR test that was not straightforward or where the patient simply did not improve with treatment. Agreement of diagnosis was found in 42 of 45, the divergences being an ischial tunnel entrapment, an obturator internus adhesion and a penetration of the sciatic nerve by a

fibrous band. In each of these patients, the electro-diagnostic method has so far been unable to distinguish the actual pathology from entrapment by the piriformis muscle.

It is important here to avoid the "diagnosis of exclusion" mindset, as seen in the historical approach to piriformis syndrome diagnosis. Radiculopathy, spinal stenosis, spondylolisthesis and piriformis syndrome can coexist and even overlap in terms of pathogenesis and symptomatology. For example, any of these other conditions may cause tenderness of the sciatic nerve fibers as they descend in the buttock, mimicking piriformis syndrome. Likewise, the opposite may happen: chronic or severe piriformis compression can alter sciatic nerve conduction overall and increase the H-reflex latency in the anatomical position. In this situation, piriformis syndrome may give the electrophysiological suggestion of spinal pathology.

Imaging studies find substantial spinal abnormalities in more than 30% of never-symptomatic subjects (Jensen *et al.*, 1994). If a patient can have a herniated disc and no pain, then a patient can have a herniated disc and pain from another source. The same applies to piriformis syndrome. Diagnostic accuracy is improved with functional confirmation by the FAIR test.

Treatment options

Evidence supports that the FAIR test and the MRI neural scan can accurately identify the pain generator in the advent of non-disc sciatica. Surgery at the site of the piriformis muscle–sciatic nerve passage, be it neurolysis or partial or complete excision of the muscle, has been successful in 65–80% following accurate diagnosis of the syndrome (Freiberg, 1937; Mizuguchi, 1976; Solheim *et al.*, 1981; Sridhara and Izzo, 1985; Fishman *et al.*, 2002a; Pećina *et al.*, 2008; Martin *et al.*, 2011). There are only a few situations in which conservative treatment (injections and/or physical therapy) seems ineffective. The only patients consistently requiring surgery are those in whom the nerve surrounds or is penetrated by a fibrous or motile portion of the muscle, the gluteal vessels entwine with the sciatic nerve near the greater sciatic foramen or there are fibrous bands that surround the nerve. In our clinical experience, there have been a total of nine such patients over 25 years. In our clinical series over a 25-year period, we have sent approximately 150 patients for surgery, generally because of failure of the methods described below.

Conservative treatment with both steroid injection and physical therapy has yielded 50% or greater improvement on the visual analog scale (VAS) within 3 months of treatment for 79.56% of patients suffering for an average of 6.5 years in the 1014 leg study of Fishman *et al.* (2002b).

Botulinum neurotoxin therapy

As opposed to the steroid injections and 3 months of physical therapy required for relief in the above study, injections of BoNT serotypes A and B with the same physical therapy resulted in the same relief within 2–3 weeks of treatment for 92% of patients (Fishman *et al.*, 2004). Similarly, a recent Cochrane database study found BoNT superior to steroid injections with lidocaine and superior to acupuncture in the context of piriformis syndrome (Waseem *et al.*, 2011). The *United States Pharmacopeia* currently offers four BoNT preparations (Table 30.1).

Clinical studies indicate that when injected in four equally divided doses, each of these medications suppresses neurotransmission for 8–12 weeks (Childers *et al.*, 2002). In our experience thus far, there is no significant difference among these preparations in terms of clinical improvement.

Injection technique

We inject BoNT into four locations in the buttocks, attempting to reach as many myoneural junctions as possible. Two of these injections are given in the middle third of the muscle, where it is thickest (Sunderland, 1868; Sharma *et al.*, 2010; Ogeng'o *et al.*, 2011). A third injection is given at the muscle's lateral extreme near to the greater trochanter and a fourth injection at its medial extreme, just before the muscle disappears below the sacrum at the greater sciatic foramen.

Table 30.1 Botulinum neurotoxin preparations listed in the *United States Pharmacopeia*

Name	Commercial name	Estimated equivalents (U) in piriformis injection
OnabotulinumtoxinA	Botox	300
AbobotulinumtoxinA	Dysport	750
IncobotulinumtoxinA	Xeomin	300
RimabotulinumtoxinB	MyoBloc	12 500

Source: US Pharmacopeial Convention, 2012.

The virtual center of the piriformis muscle can be identified as the most tender point in the mid-buttock. The tenderness is partially generated by the sciatic nerve's location deeper within the buttock at that point. The muscle itself may be palpated as a gentle rise in the buttock, a beveled diagonal region of 5–7.5 cm (2–3 inches) in width that narrows to converge on the rostral tip of the greater trochanter and spreads more widely as one palpates medially and slightly rostrally.

Guidance

In the minimally landmarked region of the buttocks, injection guidance is indispensible. Different practitioners use EMG, musculoskeletal ultrasound, fluoroscopy, CT, MRI and neural scanning techniques (Hanania, 1997; Fishman *et al.*, 1998; Hanania and Kitain, 1998; Porta, 2000; Childers *et al.*, 2002; Fishman *et al.*, 2002a; Benzon *et al.*, 2003; Lang, 2004; Kirschner *et al.*, 2009; Waseem *et al.*, 2011; Masala *et al.*, 2012). We have guided BoNT injections with EMG for nearly 15 years and in doing so have improved our successful clinical outcomes (50% VAS improvement) for patients with positive FAIR tests from 60% to just above 90% (Fishman and Zybert, 1992; Fishman *et al.*, 2002b, 2004).

The patient is asked to lie in lateral decubitus with the affected side up, knees and thighs both flexed to 90 degrees (FAIR-position), facing toward the

practitioner. A 9 cm (3.5 inch) 22- or 25-gauge injectible EMG needle is inserted one-third of the distance from the greater trochanter to the point of maximum tenderness, to a depth of approximately 3.8 cm (1.5 inches). The patient is then asked to raise the ipsilateral thigh and calf vertically off of the contralateral leg. If no interference pattern appears on the EMG device, the needle is not in muscle. The needle is adjusted by 0.5 cm (0.25 inch) increments until an interference pattern appears with abduction. The interference pattern with abduction indicates that the needle is either in the piriformis or the gluteus maximus muscle. To determine which muscle the needle is in, the patient is asked to squeeze the legs together and extend the affected hip. If an interference pattern is observed at this point, the needle is in the gluteus maximus. In that case, the needle must enter the buttock 0.5 cm (0.25 inch) more deeply and the squeezed leg extension repeated until there is no interference pattern and the needle cannot be in the gluteus maximus. At this point, a further check should be made to ensure that there is an interference pattern on abducting the flexed thigh; this confirms that the needle is in the piriformis muscle. When the needle is in the piriformis muscle, an interference pattern will be seen with abduction of the leg but not with extension.

This is the time to inject one-quarter of the total dose of BoNT. The process is repeated at the other three points in the buttock (Figs. 30.8–30.10).

Although this method may seem laborious, it actually takes less than a minute at each site (Fishman *et al.*, 2004) and has the additional advantage of teaching the practitioner through feedback what the proper depth of injection is for patients of various body types. This considerably shortens the injection time after 20 injections or so.

We generally wait a minimum of 2 months before reinjection but give physical therapy at once. (The program can be seen on sciatica.org.)

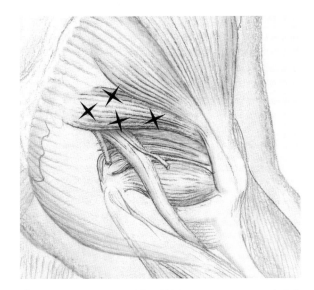

Fig. 30.8 Injection sites yielding 50% improvement or more in 2–3 weeks following botulinum neurotoxin injection and physical therapy (Fishman *et al.*, 2004).

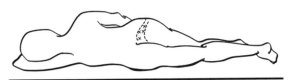

Fig. 30.9 The flexed, adducted, internally rotated (FAIR) position is used for injection, facilitating abduction and subsequent extension of the affected leg, as described in the text. Illustrated by Mayank Pathak, from author's original.

Adverse effects of botulinum neurotoxin therapy

There is no significant difference among the four BoNT preparations available in terms of efficacy. Apart from their few adverse effects, mentioned below, BoNTs have only local action. This is an important safety feature since the sciatic nerve, the superior and inferior gluteal nerves and the medial femoral cutaneous nerves all lie close to the piriformis muscle and, approximately 15% of the time, their passage is anomalous. However, because BoNTs (unlike agents such as lidocaine) have effect only on myoneural junctions, they have no paralytic or other effect on neurons or axons themselves. In this respect, BoNT injection of any kind is an extremely local treatment, chiefly affecting only the site of its injection and essentially causing discomfort or pain only at this injection site.

Serotype A has extremely benign side effect profiles. We have never seen any serious side effects with

BoNT serotype A injections into the buttock. Minor systemic side effects that have been reported with buttock injections specifically include dry mouth, fatigue, general muscle weakness and one patient with constipation lasting a week. After 1000 injections, we have seen only one instance of lower extremity weakness, lasting 8 weeks, but no generalized weakness.

Serotype B (rimabotulinumtoxinB) has a similar side effect profile, which is also probably site related, but does includes substantially more severe dry mouth, even with piriformis injection.

In a study of 57 patients receiving rimabotulinumtoxinB at 20 000–25 000 U, all but nine of whom had previous exposure to BoNT serotype A, the neurotoxin was tolerated well enough to receive additional doses in every patient. Groups of patients above and below 65 years of age have had similar adverse effect profiles (package insert for MyoBloc [rimabotulinumtoxinB]).

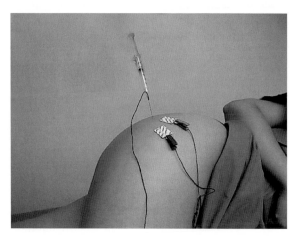

Fig. 30.10 Injection at the lateral region of the piriformis muscle.

Relapse

A considerable advantage to BoNT injection over steroid injection is the reduction in reappearance of the syndrome. In our general experience, relapse occurs in approximately 15–20% and is well reflected in serial FAIR tests (Fig. 30.11). One study with rimabotulinumtoxinB with 6-month follow-up found only 9% recurrence of sciatica or other symptoms (Fishman et al., 2004). Weakening the muscle is curative in the major group of patients in which the pathogenetic mechanism is compression and in the second largest group, in which adhesions to the muscle cause neuropraxia with forcible contraction. The longevity of the treatment is possibly a result of the coadministration of physical therapy, in which the patient

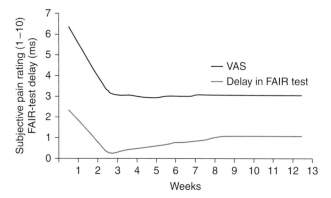

Fig. 30.11 Parallel changes of patient-reported pain on the visual analog scale (VAS) and the delay in H-reflex (SD beyond the mean in the 88 normals) seen on the FAIR test suggest that the test measures actual pathogenesis (Fishman et al., 2004).

engages the muscle in its temporarily weakened condition and is able to control its contractility 8–12 weeks later when its strength returns.

Summary

Injections of BoNT are a successful and largely innocuous treatment for piriformis syndrome. Although both serotypes A and B have similarly benign toxicity profiles, the less-potent serotype B has greater incidence of dry mouth. Using the diagnostic and injection technique described here along with physical therapy, more than 90% of patients recover 50% or more within 2–3 weeks. Relapse has been seen in less than 10% of patients following BoNT injection.

References

Beaton LE, Anson BJ (1937). Relation of sciatic nerve and subdivisions to piriformis muscle. *Anat Rec*, **70**(Suppl 1), 1–3.

Benzon HT, Katz JA, Hubert A, Benzon BA, Iqbal MS (2003). Piriformis syndrome: anatomic considerations, a new injection technique, and a review of the literature. *Anaesthesiology*, **98**, 1442–8.

Childers MK, Wilson DJ, Gnatz SM, Conway RR, Sherman AK (2002). Botulinum toxin type A use in piriformis muscle syndrome: a pilot study. *Am J Phys Med Rehabil*, **81**, 751–9.

Filler AG, Haynes J, Jordan SE *et al.* (2005). Sciatica of nondisc origin and piriformis syndrome: diagnosis by magnetic resonance neurography and interventional magnetic resonance imaging with outcome study of resulting treatment. *J Neurosurg Spine*, **2**, 99–115.

Fishman LM, Ardman CA (1997). *Back Talk, How to Diagnose and Cure Low Back Pain and Sciatica*. New York: Norton.

Fishman LM, Zybert PA (1992). Electrophysiological evidence of piriformis syndrome. *Arch Phys Med Rehabil*, **73**, 359–64.

Fishman LM, Dombi GW, Michaelsen C *et al.* (2002a). Piriformis syndrome: diagnosis, treatment and outcome- a ten year study. *Arch Phys Rehabil*, **83**, 295–302.

Fishman LM, Anderson C, Rosner B (2002b). Botox and physical therapy in the treatment of piriformis syndrome. *Am J Phys Med Rehabil*, **81**, 936–42.

Fishman LM, Konnoth C, Rozner B (2004). Botulinum neurotoxin type B and physical therapy in the treatment of piriformis syndrome: a dose-finding study. *Am J Phys Med Rehabil*, **83**, 42–50.

Fishman SM, Caneris OA, Bandman TB, Audette JF, Borsook D (1998). Injection of the piriformis muscle by fluoroscopic and electromyographic guidance. *Reg Anesth Pain Med*, **23**, 554–9.

Freiberg AH (1937). Sciatic pain and its relief by operations on muscle and fascia. *Arch Surg*, **34**, 337–50.

Gotlin R (1990). Piriformis muscle syndrome. In *Proceedings of the New York Academy of Medicine Section on Physical Medicine and Rehabilitation*, May.

Halpin RJ, Ganju A (2009). Piriformis syndrome: a real pain in the buttock? *Neurosurgery*, **65**(Suppl), A197–202.

Hanania M (1997). New technique for piriformis muscle injection using a nerve stimulator. *Reg Anesth Pain Med*, **22**, 200–2.

Hanania M, Kitain E (1998). Perisciatic injection of steroid for the treatment of sciatica due to piriformis syndrome. *Reg Anesth Pain Med*, **23**, 223–8.

Jensen MC, Brant-Zawadziki MN, Obuchowski N *et al.* (1994). Magnetic resonance imaging of the lumbar spine in people without back pain. *N Engl J Med*, **331**, 69–73.

Kirschner JS, Foye PM, Cole JL (2009). Piriformis syndrome, diagnosis and treatment. *Muscle Nerve*, **40**, 10–18.

Lang AM (2004). Botulinum toxin type B in piriformis syndrome. *Am J Phys Med Rehabil*, **83**, 198–202.

Lockhart RD, Hamilton GF, Fyfe FW (1959). *Anatomy of the Human Body*. Philadelphia, PA: Lippincott.

Martin HD, Shears SA, Johnson JC, Smathers AM, Palmer IJ (2011). The endoscopic treatment of sciatic nerve entrapment/deep gluteal syndrome. *Arthroscopy*, **27**, 172–81.

Masala S, Crusco S, Meschini A *et al.* (2012). Piriformis syndrome: long term follow-up in patients treated with percutaneous injection of anaesthetic and corticosteroid under CT guidance. *Cardiovasc Intervent Radiol*, **35**, 375–82.

Miller TA, White KP, Ross DC (2012). The diagnosis and management of Piriformis syndrome: myths and facts. *Can J Neurol Sci*, **39**, 577–83.

Mizuguchi T (1976). Division of piriformis muscle for the treatment of sciatica. *Arch Surg*, **111**, 719–22.

Ogeng'o JA, El-Busaidy H, Mwika PM, Khanbhai MM, Munguti J (2011). Variant anatomy of sciatic nerve in a black Kenyan population. *Folia Morphol*, **70**, 175–9.

Pace JB, Nagle D (1976). Piriform syndrome. *West J Med*, **124**, 435–9.

Pećina M (1979). Contribution to the etiological explanation of the piriformis syndrome. *Acta Anat (Basel)*, **105**: 181–7.

Pećina HI, Boric I, Smoljanovic T, Duvancic D, Pecina M (2008). Surgical evaluation of magnetic resonance imaging findings in piriformis muscle syndrome. *Skel Radiol*, **37**, 1019–23.

Porta M (2000). A comparative trial of botulinum toxin type A and methylprednisolone for the treatment of myofascial pain syndrome and pain from chronic muscle spasm. *Pain* **85**, 101–5.

Sharma T, Singla RK, Lalit M (2010). Bilateral eventration of sciatic nerve. *J Nepal Med Assoc*, **50**, 309–12.

Solheim LF, Siewers P, Paus B (1981). The piriformis muscle syndrome. *J Orthop Scand*, **52**, 73–5.

Sridhara CR, Izzo KL (1985). Peroneal nerve entrapment syndrome. *Arch Phys Med Rehabil*, **66**, 789–91.

Sunderland S (1868). *Nerves and Nerve Injuries*. Baltimore, MD: Williams & Wilkins.

US Pharmacopeial Convention (2012). *United States Pharmacopeia*. Rockville, MD: US Pharmacopeial Convention.

Waseem Z, Boulias C, Gordon A *et al.* (2011). Botulinum toxin injections for low-back pain and sciatica. *Cochrane Database Syst Rev*, (**1**), CD008257.

Ultrasound-guided botulinum neurotoxin injections for thoracic outlet syndrome

Katharine E. Alter

Introduction

Thoracic outlet syndrome (TOS) is a rare, often perplexing disorder caused by compression of neurovascular structures, leading to cervicogenic–brachial pain and other symptoms in neck and upper limb. Thoracic outlet syndrome is a group of disorders, not a single disorder, and patients may present with a wide variety of signs and symptoms. The wide range of symptoms and signs in TOS may confound clinicians unfamiliar with this condition (Sanders *et al.*, 2008; Ferrante, 2012; Foley *et al.*, 2012). Again, because TOS is a group of disorders, there is no "gold standard" to establish the diagnosis. This may lead to misdiagnosis or overdiagnosis of TOS in patients who present with symptoms suggesting TOS but who have other causes for their symptoms. It is, therefore, imperative that physicians be familiar with the range of symptoms and signs of TOS and testing that either supports or refutes this diagnosis. It is also critical that the diagnosis be correctly established before proceeding to invasive interventions for a presumed diagnosis of TOS, including botulinum neurotoxin (BoNT) injections.

One of the many emerging applications for BoNT therapy is for the treatment of musculoskeletal pain disorders, including TOS. While the efficacy of BoNT on decreasing pain associated with cervical dystonia and chronic migraine is established, the antinociceptive mechanism of action of BoNT is not fully understood (Mense, 2004; Aoki, 2005). Reports of reduced pain with BoNT have been reported in various musculoskeletal pain disorders, including joint pain, myofascial pain and cerebral palsy (Barwood *et al.*, 2000; Gobel *et al.*, 2006; Singh *et al.*, 2009). Although there are numerous reports in the literature citing the efficacy of BoNT for pain and other symptoms associated with TOS, additional research is needed to establish the role of BoNT in TOS and other pain disorders (Jordan *et al.*, 2007; Danielson and Odderson, 2008; Torriani *et al.*, 2010; Foley *et al.*, 2012). The proposed mechanism of action includes reduced muscle spasm leading to decreased compression of neurovascular structures (Jordan *et al.*, 2007; Tsao, 2007; Danielson and Odderson, 2008). Injection of BoNT into muscles also leads to denervation atrophy, which may reduce compression and neurogenic or vasogenic symptoms. It has also been reported that BoNT reduces the release of nociceptive neurotransmitters, which could also be a contributing factor in reduced pain in TOS.

There are also a number of reports in the literature investigating the role of anesthetic injections and BoNT as diagnostic tools to establish the diagnosis of TOS and prior to surgery to guide the surgeon's choice of procedure for TOS (Odderson *et al.*, 2009; Benzon *et al.*, 2012).

When considering BoNT therapy for TOS, accurately identifying the problematic muscle, if there is one, and then targeting this muscle for injection is often challenging. Injections in this region have an intrinsic risk associated with inserting a needle and injecting structures in a region that contains large vessels, nerves and the apex of the lung. In addition, injections of BoNT are associated with additional risks, including dysphagia and muscle weakness (Simpson *et al.*, 2008; Truong *et al.*, 2010; Hong *et al.*, 2012). Various targeting techniques have been reported to guide injection therapy for TOS, including with BoNT. Recommended techniques include electromyography (EMG) and various imaging modalities (CT, MRI, ultrasound) or imaging plus EMG (Speelman and Brans, 1995; Hong *et al.*, 2012). This chapter will briefly review TOS and the literature related to use of BoNT for TOS before giving a detailed review of

Manual of Botulinum Toxin Therapy, 2nd edition, ed. Daniel Truong, Mark Hallett, Christopher Zachary and Dirk Dressler. Published by Cambridge University Press. © Cambridge University Press 2013.

procedural techniques for ultrasound guidance in BoNT therapy for TOS.

Thoracic outlet syndrome

Thoracic outlet syndrome is a group of disorders leading to cervicobrachial pain and neurovascular symptoms and caused by compression of elements of the brachial plexus, subclavian vessels or both by musculoskeletal structures in the region of the neck known as the thoracic outlet (Sanders *et al.*, 2008; Ferrante, 2012; Foley *et al.*, 2012). While the term was coined by Peet *et al.* in 1956 and further described by Rob and Standeven in 1958, the symptoms, signs and treatment of compression of structures in this region date back to antiquity.

When the signs and symptoms of neurogenic TOS or vasogenic TOS are clear and diagnostic testing is supportive a diagnosis of true TOS is undisputed. The controversy surrounding TOS may be partly attributed to mis- or overdiagnosis of TOS in patients who have other causes for their symptoms and to diagnosis of "non-specific thoracic outlet syndrome" in patients with non-specific cervicogenic pain (Ferrante, 2012). A chapter describing a treatment technique for TOS, therefore, warrants a review of the disorder to increase the accuracy of diagnosis and to reduce unnecessary and risky interventions in patients with an alternative diagnosis.

Classification of thoracic outlet syndromes

One accepted classification system for TOS defines specific subtypes based on affected/compromised structures and/or clinical features (Sanders *et al.*, 2008; Ferrante, 2012). The defined subtypes of TOS and their symptoms include:

- *neurogenic*: compression of elements of the brachial plexus (roots, cords) leads to numbness, tingling, pain, atrophy, weakness; involvement of the lower trunk is most often described
- *arterial vasogenic*: compression of the subclavian or axillary artery leads to claudication symptoms with a cool pale extremity, decreased pulses, pain and Raynaud's symptoms
- *veno-vasogenic*: dusky discoloration of the limb with diffuse limb swelling
- *combined neurovascular*: combination of above symptoms
- *non-specific*: cervicogenic pain, numbness or parasthesiae that do not clearly fit into the above

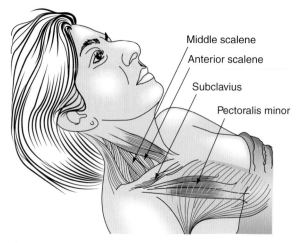

Fig. 31.1 Muscle anatomy of the thoracic outlet.

categories; non-specific TOS is a controversial diagnosis and use of this diagnosis is discouraged (Ferrante, 2012).

Anatomy of the thoracic outlet

The thoracic outlet refers to the region of body extending from the supraclavicular fossa to the axilla. From anterior to posterior, this encompasses the area located between the clavicle and first rib. The thoracic outlet is further divided into three specific regions: the interscalene triangle, the retroclavicular region and the subcoracoid region or retropectoralis minor space (Fig. 31.1).

Structures of interest contained within or traversing the region of the thoracic outlet include;

- *bone*: clavicle, first rib, C7 vertebra, cervical rib (if present), fibrous extensions from C7 (if present)
- *muscles*: anterior, middle scalenes, subclavius, pectoralis minor tendon
- *nerves*: brachial plexus including the trunks (supraclavicular), divisions (retroclavicluar) and cords (infraclavicular); axillary and musculocutaneous nerves (infraclavicular)
- *vessels*: subclavian artery and vein, axillary artery and vein.

Sites of entrapment of nerves

Reported sites of entrapment of nerves or vessels include compression between:

- *anterior and middles scalene muscles*: neurogenic symptoms in the distribution of T_1 to C_8 nerve roots. Compression is attributed to an enlarged anterior or middle scalene, muscle spasm or a fibrous band within the anterior scalene

- *anterior scalene and cervical rib or anterior scalene and a fibrous band extending from C7*: symptoms may be neurogenic or arterial/vasogenic, including decreased pulse, cool, pale extremity or Raynaud's symptoms
- *clavicle and first rib*: largely post-traumatic (most often at the level of the cords of the brachial plexus or axillary vessels) following a mid-shaft clavicle fracture with robust callus formation; the callus may compress neurovascular elements and patients most often present with combined neurovascular TOS symptoms
- *beneath the pectoralis minor muscle or tendon*: compression may be neurogenic (medial or lateral cord), arterial (axillary) or venous (axillary).

Epidemiology

Thoracic outlet syndrome is a rare disorder. The reported incidence of true neurogenic TOS approaches 1 in a million. Given that neurogenic TOS is diagnosed in 95% of those with TOS, the vasogenic causes will be exceedingly rare (Torriani *et al.*, 2010). Given the vague symptoms and lack of anatomical correlates, there can be no good information about non-specific TOS.

Work up and differential diagnosis

Neurogenic, arterial/vasogenic and veno-vasogenic TOS have objective criteria and can be evaluated with clinical, electrophysiological and vascular studies. When a patient presents with pain in the arm with or without numbness, the first thought should be cervical spine disease even if anatomical findings are not obvious. It is when anatomical findings are not obvious that the diagnosis of non-specific TOS is often considered (Ferrante, 2012; Foley *et al.*, 2012). This diagnosis should be made only rarely, hopefully when at least some objective evidence is documented.

Clearly establishing a diagnosis should be the first step when evaluating a patient with suspected TOS. Given the various presentations and perplexing symptoms associated with TOS, this often requires extensive diagnostic testing including imaging, electrodiagnostic testing and/or vascular studies. A full discussion of this topic is beyond the scope of this chapter and the reader is referred to several reviews (Urschel and Kourlis, 2007; Ferrante, 2012; Foley *et al.*, 2012).

Diagnostic testing is directed by the patient's history, symptoms. Electrodiagnostic testing including nerve conduction and EMG should be considered in patients presenting with neurogenic TOS symptoms, and such testing should be definitive. While a normal electrodiagnostic test result does not exclude other forms of TOS, the test may also reveal an alternative cause of the patient's symptoms such as other peripheral nerve entrapments, peripheral neuropathy, plexopathy, radiculopathy or focal anterior horn cell loss (Tsao, 2007; Urschel and Kourlis, 2007; Ferrante, 2012). Abnormal results for the median, ulnar or medial antebrachial cutaneous sensory nerve action potentials have been reported in TOS, and abnormality of the ulnar potentials from the fifth finger is almost mandatory for diagnosis of neurogenic TOS. Denervation in those muscles innervated by C_8–T_1 is also characteristic, and atrophy in these muscles may also be seen in long-standing neurogenic TOS (Ferrante, 2012; Foley *et al.*, 2012).

Diagnostic imaging in patients with TOS generally includes plain radiographs to evaluate for a cervical rib, clavicular callus, other bony abnormalities or mass effect. Fibrous bands will not be visible on plain films but are detected by MRI. Imaging with MRI or CT may also be useful when an apical lung mass, tumor or malignancy is suspected (Ferrante, 2012).

When venovascular symptoms predominate, venography is the gold standard. For patients with suspected arterial vasogenic TOS, MRI, CT angiography or duplex ultrasonography should be considered (Stapleton *et al.*, 2009). High-frequency ultrasound is useful for both procedural guidance and as a diagnostic tool for arterial vasogenic TOS and has the advantage of portability, lower cost and no exposure to ionizing radiation. Ultrasound in B-mode can also provide a dynamic assessment of vascular flow and can be used during provocative clinical maneuvers to assess the effect of a maneuver or neck/limb position on flow within a vessel (Jordan *et al.*, 2007; Danielson and Odderson, 2008; Odderson *et al.*, 2009; Torriani *et al.*, 2010). It is important to recognize that arterial or venous compression with various maneuvers is also seen in asymptomatic individuals, so thoughtful clinical correlation is needed.

Treatment

Various treatments for TOS have been proposed including postural or physical therapy, manipulation, acupuncture, BoNT injections and various surgical procedures. The focus of this text is on BoNT therapy for diagnostic or therapeutic intervention for TOS. There are several excellent reviews that contain a full discussion of the various proposed treatments for TOS (Jordan *et al.*, 2007; Ferrante, 2012; Foley *et al.*, 2012). Only certain therapies make sense for certain conditions. For example, if the brachial plexus is compressed by a first rib, there is no way in which BoNT can help and surgery would be necessary. The utility of BoNT is currently supported only by anecdotal case reports, and there is certainly no logic in using BoNT therapy if entrapment by a muscle is not the issue.

Botulinum neurotoxin therapy under ultrasound guidance

As noted above, BoNT therapy for TOS is associated with risks related to the needle insertion/injection procedure itself as well as the risks inherent with BoNT. It is incumbent on the clinician to establish both a diagnosis of true TOS and the correct site of compression and the involved structures prior to proceeding with BoNT therapy. Clearly, BoNT has no place in treatment of TOS caused by callus formation from a clavicle fracture or compression from a true cervical rib. Additionally, BoNT has no place in treatment of non-specific TOS where no objective compression can be identified. However, BoNT may be useful for patients with compression of neurovascular structures caused by the effects of muscle hypertrophy or muscle action on bones (anterior scalene on first rib), leading to TOS.

Since the mid 2000s, several reviews of ultrasound-guided BoNT therapy have been published (Jordan *et al.*, 2007; Danielson and Odderson, 2008; Le *et al.*, 2010; Torriani *et al.*, 2010; Foley *et al.*, 2012).

Techniques

Ultrasound guidance for TOS has been described for BoNT injections in the anterior and middle scalene, pectoralis minor and subclavius muscles. Accurately localizing any of these muscles may be challenging without imaging-based guidance, such as ultrasound or fluoroscopy.

A general review of ultrasound and ultrasound guidance techniques useful for BoNT injections is provided elsewhere in this text (e.g. Chapter 7). For a more detailed review of ultrasound guidance and procedural techniques, see Smith and Finnoff (2009), Alter (2010) and Alter *et al.* (2012).

Both the in-plane and out-of-plane injection techniques are useful when performing ultrasound-guided

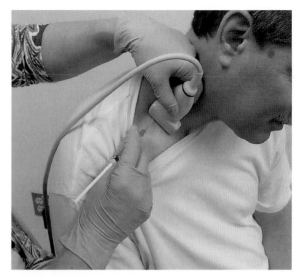

Fig. 31.2 Needle/transducer orientation for transverse ultrasound out-of-plane injection of the scalene muscles.

BoNT injections for TOS. Clinicians should be at ease with both techniques and familiar with the advantages and disadvantages of both. Therefore, a brief discussion, specific to the topic of these techniques for TOS is provided below (Smith and Finnoff, 2009; Alter, 2010). Because of anatomical variations, patient-related issues with positioning and other factors, one specific technique may be required for a given procedure.

In an out-of-plane injection technique, the needle is inserted across the short axis of the transducer (Fig. 31.2). Using this technique, a cross-sectional view of the needle is obtained and the needle is viewed as a bright (i.e. hyperechoic) dot (Fig. 31.3). The out-of-plane technique may provide a more direct path to the target. However, the entire length of the needle and its path is not visualized. During needle insertion, care must be used to keep the tip of the needle within the ultrasound beam. If the tip is inserted beyond the ultrasound transducer, it may be in an untargeted structure. When using the out-of-plane technique to track the path of the needle to the target, a walk-down technique is recommended. In this approach, the needle is vibrated or jiggled during insertion. Jiggling the needle creates movement in the tissue through which the needle is passing. The clinician tracks the position of the needle by observing movement of tissue as the needle passes from superficial through deeper structures. When the needle tip reaches the target, a small quantity of the injectate is injected, confirming the correct location.

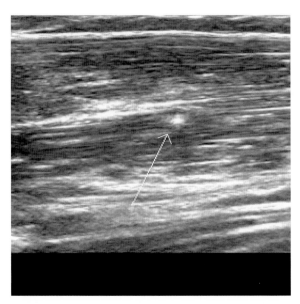

Fig. 31.3 Ultrasound (B-mode) view of the needle using the out-of-plane technique. The needle is visualized as a bright (hyperechoic) dot (arrow).

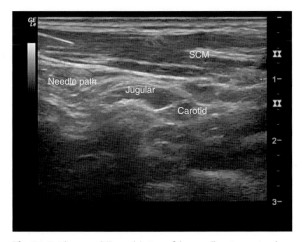

Fig. 31.5 Ultrasound (B-mode) view of the needle using an in-plane injection technique. Needle is viewed as a thin, bright or hyperechoic line. SCM, sternocleidomastoid muscle.

Many clinicians prefer the in-plane technique when performing ultrasound-guided BoNT injections. When using this technique, the needle is inserted along the length of the transducer (Fig. 31.4). The advantage of an in-plane approach is that this provides a long axis view of the needle and, therefore, the entire length of the needle and its path to the target is visualized (Fig. 31.5). This technique may be challenging to perform and often requires an indirect path of the needle to the target (to keep it in the ultrasound beam). This may be difficult in the anterior neck where an indirect

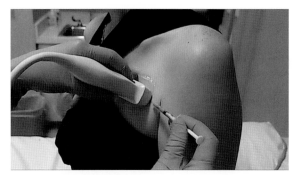

Fig. 31.4 Needle/transducer orientation for the in-plane injection technique, transverse view, for pectoralis minor muscle.

path may traverse regions with various large vessels and nerves.

Anterior scalene injections

The anterior scalene is the most frequently targeted muscle for BoNT injections for TOS, although some clinicians target both the anterior and middle scalenes. Spasm or hypertrophy of the muscle may cause direct compression of neurovascular structures in the supraclavicular fossa, specifically within the interscalene triangle. Spasm or overactivity of the anterior scalene may also elevate the first rib, leading to compression of neurovascular structures (Jordan *et al.*, 2007; Torriani *et al.*, 2010).

The scalene muscles run from their origin on the transverse processes of C3–C6 to their insertion on the first rib (anterior scalene). After exiting their respective neural foramina, the trunks of the brachial plexus descend into the interscalene triangle, running between the anterior and middle scalene muscles. The transverse cervical artery also transverses this space (Fig. 31.1).

The scalene muscles are best viewed in the transverse plane (Jordan *et al.*, 2007; Torriani *et al.*, 2010; Alter *et al.*, 2012). The transverse imaging plane provides a more distinct view of the fascial planes between the sternocleidomastoid, anterior scalene, middle scalene and the adjacent neurovascular structures (brachial plexus, carotid, jugular, subclavian artery/vein, transverse cervical artery) (Fig. 31.6).

In most non-obese patients the scalene muscles are relatively superficial; therefore, a relatively high-frequency linear transducer (10 or 12 MHz to 5 MHz) is selected for imaging the cervical region including the TOS. Because ultrasound transducers

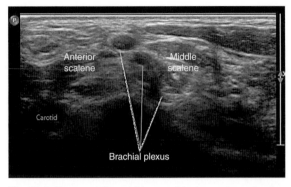

Fig. 31.6 Ultrasound (B-mode) image of the interscalene triangle, with transverse view of the scalene muscles and brachial plexus.

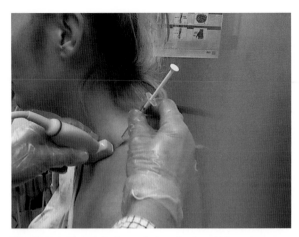

Fig. 31.7 In-plane injection technique for the middle scalene. Transducer is positioned for cross sectional (i.e. transverse) view of the scalenes and brachial plexus.

create a narrow beam of ultrasound (thickness of a credit card), only a thin image slice is created. This mandates that the sonographer slides or moves the transducer back and forth over a structure of interest to image it in its entirety.

For ultrasound-guided scalene injections, the transducer is placed over the interscalene triangle in a plane perpendicular to the underlying scalene muscles (i.e. transverse view of scalene muscles; Fig. 31.6). The transducer is then moved, rocked or toggled to image the anterior scalene, middle scalene, brachial plexus and adjacent vessels (Smith and Finnoff, 2009; Alter, 2010; Alter et al., 2012).

To localized the scalene muscles, a useful technique, particularly for a less experienced sonographer, is to first scan the anterior neck in the transverse plane and locate the sternocleidomastoid muscle and carotid and jugular vessels. These structures serve as easily identifiable landmarks or reference structures to help to localize the anterior and middle scalene. The sternocleidomastoid muscle and carotid and jugular vessels are located anterior and superficial to the scalene muscles.

As noted above, either an in-plane or an out-of-plane technique can be used for ultrasound-guided scalene injections. Many authors prefer an in-plane technique, where the needle is inserted from lateral to medial and advanced into the anterior or middle scalene (Fig. 31.7) (Jordan et al., 2007; Torriani et al., 2010). However, for scalene injections, the out-of-plane technique often provides a more direct path to the muscle while avoiding the adjacent plexus and vessels. The in-plane technique may be challenging to perform in some patients because of the close proximity of the carotid, jugular, transverse cervical artery and trunks of the brachial plexus. Physicians should

use the technique that provides the best view of the muscle, needle and adjacent structures.

For scalene injections, the dose range reported in the literature for onabotulinumtoxinA is from 12 to 20 U in the anterior scalene and 20 U in the middle scalene (Jordan et al., 2007; Danielson and Odderson, 2008; Le et al., 2010; Torriani et al., 2010). Saline dilution volume was not reported by all authors but was reported at 2 ml preservative-free saline per 100 U onabotulinumtoxinA by Torriani et al. (2010). Other BoNT products could be used, but there is most experience with onabotulinumtoxinA.

Pectoralis minor injections

The pectoralis minor lies deep to the overlying pectoralis major. The origin is on ribs 3–5 and insertion is on the coracoid process of the scapula. The pectoralis major forms a bridge from the thorax to the coracoid process/upper limb beneath which the brachial plexus and vascular structures travel into the arm. The actions of the pectoralis minor are to depress the shoulder and draw the scapula inferior and forward towards the chest wall and the posterior angle away from the chest wall. The cords of the brachial plexus may be compressed under the muscle fibers or the tendon of the pectoralis minor.

For ultrasound-guided BoNT injections, the pectoralis minor is visualized at its insertion on the coracoid process (Figs. 31.4, 31.8, 31.9 and 31.10). The muscle is imaged either in an oblique longitudinal or a longitudinal plane (Torriani et al., 2010). The coracoid process is used as a landmark and the transducer

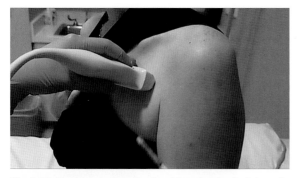

Fig. 31.8 Transducer orientation for oblique longitudinal view of pectoralis minor.

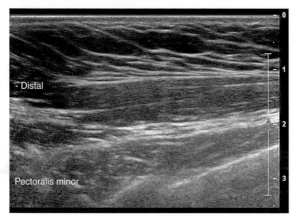

Fig. 31.10 Ultrasound (B-mode) view of pectoralis major (superficial) and minor (deep).

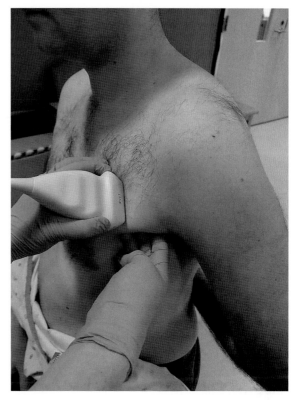

Fig. 31.9 Transducer position/orientation for oblique transverse view of pectoralis minor.

is moved inferior and medially to visualize the pectoralis muscle. The position of the axillary vessels and nerve are observed. An in-plane injection approach from lateral to medial is used, inserting the needle parallel to the chest wall superficial to the ribs to avoid entry into the intercostal space and underlying lung tissue. Reported doses of onabotulinumtoxinA for the pectoralis minor muscle range from 15 U (Torriani *et al.*, 2010) to 35 U (Jordan *et al.*, 2007). Reported dilution of 2 ml preservative-free saline per 100 U onabotulinumtoxinA was reported by Torriani *et al.* (2010).

Subclavius muscle injections

The origin of the subclavius muscle is at the junction of the costal cartilage and first rib. The muscle runs from its origin to its insertion on the underside of the middle one-third of the clavicle. It has several actions including drawing the shoulder medial, raising the first rib or depressing the clavicle. Because the subclavius narrows the space between the first rib and

clavicle, structures traversing this region may be compressed by a hypertrophied or overactive muscle or poor shoulder posture.

A hypertrophied or aberrant subclavius is reported to be one potential source of neurovascular compression in TOS. Ultrasound-guided injections are reported by several authors (Ozçakar *et al.*, 2010; Jordan *et al.*, 2007; Torriani *et al.*, 2010); however, the precise techniques for ultrasound-guided injection of this muscle is not described in any of the published articles.

Ultrasound guidance for subclavius injections requires the transducer to be placed inferior and parallel to the clavicle. The transducer is then rocked or toggled to steer the ultrasound beam under the clavicle to visualize the muscle. The smaller foot print of a hockey stick transducer is useful when scanning the subclavius. The needle is then inserted using an in-plane approach from medial to lateral directing the needle between the clavicle and first rib (Fig. 31.11). Care must be taken to keep the needle parallel and superficial to the underlying chest wall to avoid

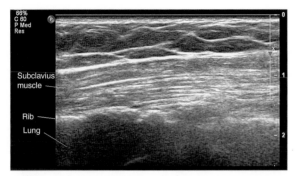

Fig. 31.11 Longitudinal view of the subclavius muscle.

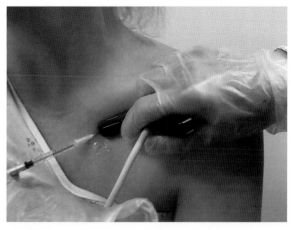

Fig. 31.12 Transducer/needle orientation demonstrating a longitudinal scan/injection of the subclavius muscle using an in-plane needle insertion technique.

penetration of the intercostal muscles and lung (Fig. 31.12). Doses reported for onabotulinumtoxinA injections in the subclavius range from 12 U (Torriani *et al.*, 2010) to 35 U (Jordan *et al.*, 2007). Torriani *et al.* (2010) reported a dilution of 2 ml preservative-free saline per 100 U onabotulinumtoxinA.

Summary

While some studies report that BoNT provides long-lasting symptomatic relief for some patients with TOS, others have reported only a short duration of, or limited degree of, benefit. Possible factors in this variation include patient selection, proper diagnosis, dose of BoNT, injection targeting technique and post-injection therapy or intervention. Injections of BoNT are clearly less invasive than surgical intervention and may provide some patients with long-lasting symptomatic improvement. In other patients in whom BoNT injections provide inadequate or short-lived improvement, this intervention may help to guide surgical procedures.

Because of the risks associated with muscle injections in the region affected in TOS, clinicians performing BoNT injections for TOS should consider ultrasound or other imaging-based guidance (fluoroscopy or CT). The addition of EMG to ultrasound guidance provides information about muscle activity, which may be useful when selecting muscles for injection. The muscles targeted for TOS injections are adjacent to many important neurovascular structures and other organs; consequently, ultrasound guidance provides an additional level of safety for these high-risk procedures. Additional research is necessary to clarify the role of BoNT therapy for TOS, including whether specific subtypes of TOS or patient populations may benefit from BoNT intervention. Additional research is

also needed related to treatment – dosage and injection technique – to establish the role of BoNT.

References

Alter KE (2010). High-frequency ultrasound guidance for neurotoxin injections. *Phys Med Rehabil Clin N Am*, **21**, 607–30.

Alter KE, Hallett M, Karp B (eds.) (2012). *Ultrasound Guided Chemodenervation Procedures. Text and Atlas.* New York: Demos Medical, pp. 108–23.

Aoki KR (2005). Review of proposed mechanism for the antinoceptive action of botulism toxin type A. *Neurotoxicology*, **6**, 785–93.

Barwood S, Baillieu C, Boyd R *et al.* (2000). Analgesic effects of botulinum toxin A: a randomized, placebo-controlled clinical trial. *Dev Med Child Neurol*, **42**, 116–21.

Benzon HT, Rodes ME, Chekka K *et al.* (2012). Scalene muscle injections for neurogenic thoracic outlet syndrome: case series. *Pain Pract*, **12**, 66–70.

Danielson K, Odderson IR (2008). Botulinum toxin type A improves blood flow in vascular thoracic outlet syndrome. *Am J Phys Med Rehabil*, **87**, 956–9.

Ferrante MA (2012). The thoracic outlet syndromes. *Muscle Nerve*, **45**, 780–95.

Foley JM, Finlayson H, Travlos A (2012). A review of thoracic outlet syndrome and the possible role of botulinum toxin in the treatment of thoracic outlet syndrome. *Toxins*, **4**, 1223–35.

Gobel H, Heinze A, Reichel G (2006). Efficacy and safety of a single botulinum type A toxin complex treatment for the relief of upper back myofascial pain syndrome: results from a randomized double-blind placebo controlled multicentre study. *Pain*, **125**, 82–8.

Hong JS, Sathe GG, Niyonkuru C *et al.* (2012). Elimination of dysphagia using ultrasound guidance for botulinum toxin injections in cervical dystonia. *Muscle Nerve*, **46**, 535–9.

Jordan SE, Ahn SS, Gelabert HA, Danielson K, Odderson IR (2007). Combining ultrasonography and electromyography for botulinum chemodenervation treatment of thoracic outlet syndrome: comparison with fluoroscopy and electromyography guidance. *Pain Physician*, **10**, 541–6.

Le EN, Freischlag JA, Christo PJ *et al.* (2010). Thoracic outlet syndrome secondary to localized scleroderma treated with botulinum toxin injection. *Arthritis Care Res*, **62**, 430–3.

Mense S (2004). Neurobiological basis for the use of botulinum toxin in pain therapy. *Neurology*, **251**, 11–17.

Odderson IR, Chun ES, Kolokythas O, Zierler RE (2009). Use of sonography in thoracic outlet syndrome due to a dystonic pectoralis minor. *J Ultrasound Med*, **28**, 1235–8.

Ozçakar L, Güney MS, Ozdağ F *et al.* (2010). A sledgehammer on the brachial plexus: thoracic outlet syndrome, subclavius posticus muscle, and traction in aggregate. *Arch Phys Med Rehabil*, **91**, 656–8.

Peet RM, Henriksen JD, Anderson TP, Martin GM (1956). Thoracic-outlet syndrome: evaluation of a therapeutic exercise program. *Proc Staff Meet Mayo Clin*, **31**, 281–7.

Rob CG, Standeven A (1958). Arterial occlusion complicating thoracic outlet compression syndrome. *BMJ*, **20**, 709–12.

Sanders RJ, Hammond SL, Rao NM (2008). Thoracic outlet syndrome: A review. *Neurologist*, **14**, 365–73.

Simpson DM, Blitzer A, Brashear A *et al.* (2008). Assessment: botulinum neurotoxin for the treatment of movement disorders (an evidence-based review). Report of the Therapeutics and Technology Assessment Subcommittee of the American Academy of Neurology. *Neurology*, **70**, 1699–706.

Singh JA, Mahowald ML, Noorbaloochi S (2009). Intraarticular botulinum toxin type A for refractory shoulder pain A randomized, double-blinded, placebo-controlled trial. *Transl Res*, **153**, 205–16.

Smith J, Finnoff JT (2009). Diagnostic and interventional musculoskeletal ultrasound: part 1. Fundamentals. *PM R*, **1**, 64–75.

Speelman JD, Brans JW (1995). Cervical dystonia and botulinum treatment: is electromyographic guidance necessary? *Mov Disord*, **10**, 802.

Stapleton C, Herrington L, George K (2009). Sonographic evaluation of the subclavian artery during thoracic outlet syndrome shoulder manoeuvres. *Man Ther*, **14**, 19–27.

Torriani M, Gupta R, Donahue DM (2010). Botulinum toxin injection in neurogenic thoracic outlet syndrome: results and experience using a ultrasound-guided approach. *Skel Radiol*, **39**, 973–80.

Truong D, Brodsky M, Lew M *et al.* (2010). Long-term efficacy and safety of botulinum toxin type A (Dysport) in cervical dystonia. *Parkinsonism Relat Disord*, **16**, 316–23.

Tsao B (2007). True neurogenic thoracic outlet syndrome. Case report 18, *AANEM*, **7**, 1–7.

Urschel HC, Kourlis H (2007). Thoracic outlet syndrome: a 50-year experience at Baylor University Medical Center. *Proc Bayl Uni Med Cent*, **20**, 125–35.

Chapter 32

Botulinum neurotoxin in the gastrointestinal tract

Vito Annese and Daniele Gui

Cricopharyngeal dysphagia

The cricopharyngeal muscle, or upper esophageal sphincter (UES), corresponds to the most inferior portion of the inferior constrictor muscle. It creates a sphincter separating the hypopharynx from the esophagus, preventing the inlet of air into the esophagus during inspiration and esophageal reflux into the pharynx. It is myoelectrically silent at rest and active during swallowing.

Cricopharyngeal dysphagia arises from dysfunction of the cricopharyngeal muscle, which can be primary or secondary to a number of pathological conditions, including cerebrovascular accidents, amyotrophic lateral sclerosis, oculopharyngeal muscular dystrophy and skull basal lesion. Oropharyngeal dysphagia is the clinical presentation and possibly correlates with aspiration or penetration of liquid or food into the upper airways. During manometry, incomplete relaxation of the UES or an increase in intrabolus pressure may be demonstrated (Fig. 32.1).

Cricopharyngeal muscle dysfunction has been traditionally treated with surgical myotomy, mechanical dilatation or plexus neurectomy. Localized injections of botulinum neurotoxin (BoNT) into the dorsomedial or ventrolateral parts of the muscle have also been successfully performed endoscopically, percutaneously (Fig. 32.1a) and eventually under CT or fluoroscopic control, with or without electromyographic (EMG) guidance (Fulmer *et al.*, 2011). Unfortunately, there are no standards or guidelines and the administered dose reported ranges widely between 10 and 120 U onabotulinumtoxinA, usually selected on the basis of symptom severity.

Currently, there is no head-to-head comparison or dose-equivalance study in this setting with different BoNTs. It is generally believed, however, that 100 U onabotulinumtoxinA has a similar efficacy to 250 U abobotulinumtoxinA and 100 U incobotulinumtoxinA in this setting.

Local injections are relatively simple, safe (complication rate about 7%) and effective, although the effect wanes after 4–6 months (Fulmer *et al.*, 2011). Injection in the horizontal part of the muscle and an adequate (i.e. high enough) starting dose are predictors of greater efficacy. The BoNT can be used as part of the diagnostic evaluation to ascertain the role of cricopharyngeal spasm in a patient's symptoms; moreover, it may help to identify those patients who are more likely to benefit from surgical myotomy.

Paradoxically, BoNT can cause transient oropharyngeal dysphagia as a complication of local injections for cervical and oromandibular dystonia.

Achalasia

Achalasia is a rare neuromuscular disorder of the esophagus characterized by loss of peristalsis and failure of the lower esophageal sphincter (LES) to relax normally. This results in functional obstruction with retention of food and saliva in the lumen, and subsequent risk of aspiration, malnutrition and weight loss. The etiology is unknown but the early pathological changes consist of a myenteric plexus inflammation with subsequent loss of ganglion cells and fibrosis. Degenerative changes of the vagal nerves and dorsal vagal nuclei have also been described. The impairment of LES relaxation and peristaltic propagation of contractions is caused by selective loss of inhibitory nerve endings releasing the neurotransmitters nitric oxide and vasoactive intestinal polypeptide. Conversely, the excitatory cholinergic pathway is preserved and may lead to increased resting LES pressure.

Current therapies are aimed to mechanically reduce LES tone through pneumatic dilatation or surgical myotomy. Both procedures, although effective in the

Manual of Botulinum Toxin Therapy, 2nd edition, ed. Daniel Truong, Mark Hallett, Christopher Zachary and Dirk Dressler. Published by Cambridge University Press. © Cambridge University Press 2013.

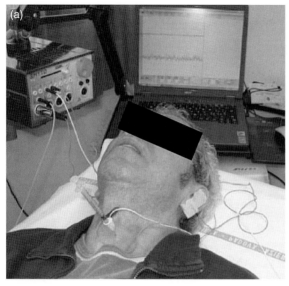

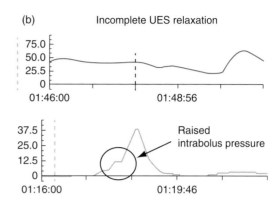

Fig. 32.1 Electromyography of the upper esophageal sphincter (UES). (a) Portable computer-assisted equipment. A 26-gauge concentric needle electrode of 50 mm length is inserted at the inferolateral aspect of the cricoid cartilage and rotated medially after insertion to record the cricopharyngeal muscle electrical activity. Subsequently, the electrode can be connected to a insulin syringe for injection of 4–10 U onabotulinumtoxinA. (b) Example of manometry demonstrating incomplete relaxation of the UES and raised intrabolus pressure at the pharyngeal level. Manometry should be combined with videofluoroscopy in the careful evaluation of UES dysfunction. (With permission from Zaninotto *et al.*, 2004).

large majority of patients (65 to 90%), carry a significant risk of complications: a 2% rate of perforation and reduced efficacy over time (about 50%) for dilatation and a 10–30% risk of gastroesophageal reflux after myotomy (Pehlivanov and Pasricha, 2006). The functional results, particularly for myotomy, are largely influenced by the surgeon's experience.

These limitations prompted Pasricha and colleagues in 1994 to assess, for the first time, the usefulness of intrasphincteric injection of BoNT. The rationale behind this was that the selective loss of the inhibitory nerves in achalasia upset the excitatory (cholinergic) influences on the LES. By blocking acetylcholine release, locally injected BoNT might reduce LES pressure and improve esophageal emptying. The efficacy of this treatment modality has been evaluated in a number of uncontrolled and controlled trials, also comparing its cost–effectiveness with dilatation and surgical myotomy (Annese and Bassotti, 2006; Leyden *et al.*, 2006). The BoNT is injected through a standard sclerotherapy needle during upper gastrointestinal endoscopy under conscious sedation with 80–100 U onabotulinumtoxinA/incobotulinumtoxinA (or 250 U abobotulinumtoxinA) (Annese *et al.*, 1999) injected in each quadrant of the LES at four or eight (preferred) sites in 1 or 0.5 ml portions (Fig. 32.2). Injections of BoNT via endoscopic

fundic retroversion or endoscopic ultrasonography do not enhance efficacy.

Although BoNT injection is remarkably safe, (about 10% of patients report a mild chest pain) and effective in the short term (70–90%) (Annese and Bassotti, 2006; Leyden *et al.*, 2006), there are a number of limitations: (1) the mean duration of efficacy is 1 year or less, although single patients with prolonged benefit (3–4 years) have been reported; (2) after repeated injections, a decline of efficacy (antibody formation?) has been reported; and (3) repeated BoNT injections may increase the difficulty of a subsequent surgical myotomy, although functional results seem similar (Leyden *et al.*, 2006). The use of BoNT is currently recommended in poor candidates for surgery, old and very old patients or as temporizing measure (Pehlivanov and Pasricha, 2006). A potential benefit of BoNT prior to pneumatic dilatation has been suggested but not adequately proven.

Spastic esophageal disorders

Diffuse esophageal spasm is a rare esophageal motility disorder characterized by a severe reduction of esophageal peristalsis, often accompanied by prolonged and high-amplitude esophageal contractions and impaired LES relaxation. Isolated LES hypertension is another

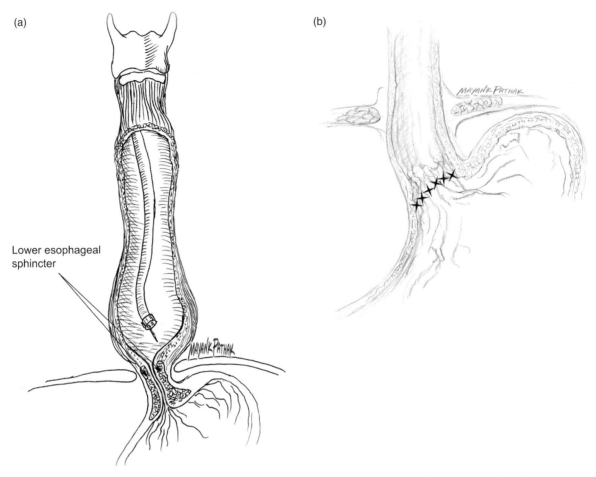

(a)

Lower esophageal
sphincter

(b)

Fig. 32.2 Esophageal achalasia. (a) Botulinum neurotoxin is injected during a standard endoscopy with conscious sedation, through a sclerotherapy needle (23-gauge); 100 U onabotulinumtoxinA or 250 U abobotulinumtoxinA diluted in 4 ml is delivered in four or (preferably) eight radial sites starting at the Z-line and 1 cm above. (b) Following the injection, the pressure of lower esophageal sphincter is reduced and the esophagus empties by gravity. In the early stages of disease, this also allows reduction of esophageal diameter.

infrequent motility disorder, usually characterized by normal esophageal peristalsis and LES relaxation. The etiology for both disorders is unknown but deranged function of the myenteric plexus is suspected. The major symptom for both disorders is chest pain, with or without concurrent dysphagia. No satisfactory pharmacologic therapy is available, and rarely a surgical myotomy is required. Moreover, pneumatic dilatation is usually poorly effective for the chest pain. A therapeutic role of BoNT has been reported in the literature, although in limited case series and uncontrolled observations (Bashashati *et al.*, 2010). For LES hypertension, the treatment technique used for achalasia has been employed, while in patients with diffuse esophageal spasm, multiple injections along the esophageal wall are suggested, beginning at the LES region and moving

proximally at 1–2 cm intervals into endoscopically visible contraction rings (Fig. 32.3) (Bashashati *et al.*, 2010).

Sphincter of Oddi dysfunction

Recurrent upper abdominal pain is a common clinical problem affecting 10% or more patients undergoing cholecystectomy. Sphincter of Oddi dysfunction has been implicated in the etiology of 10–20% of these patients. Although rare, sphincter of Oddi dysfunction can cause recurrent pancreatitis. Unfortunately, this disorder is difficult to diagnose with non-invasive techniques; sphincter of Oddi manometry is useful in diagnosis but carries a potential risk of pancreatitis and cholangitis. Moreover, it shows a great technical complexity, with a considerable rate of false positives

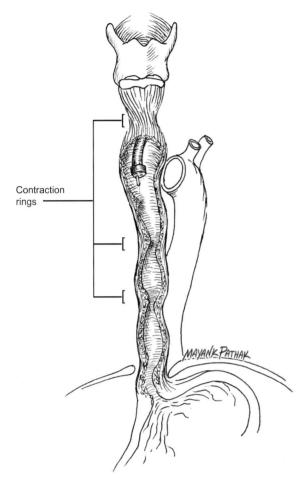

Contraction rings —

Fig. 32.3 In patients with diffuse esophageal spasm, the same amount of neurotoxin is delivered half at the level of the lower esophageal sphincter and half 5 cm proximally to reduce the strength of esophageal contractions.

and negatives. High pressure at the sphincter is relieved by endoscopic sphincterotomy, which is considered as the treatment of choice for sphincter of Oddi dysfunction; however, in many patients this procedure does not relieve symptoms and might carry a risk of pancreatitis, bleeding and perforation.

Preliminary studies on animals demonstrated that locally injected BoNT significantly reduces the sphincter wave amplitudes and phasic contractile activity, probably through selective inhibition of cholinergic influences. In this setting, two potential uses of BoNT could be hypothesized: first, intrasphincteric injection may serve as a simple test to identify patients whose pain is really caused by sphincter of Oddi dysfunction. Second, once efficacy is established, BoNT may prove to be an effective and safer therapeutic modality than

sphincterotomy (Murray, 2011). The technique is rather simple, consisting of a single injection into the major papilla of 100 U BoNT with a sclerotherapy needle (Fig. 32.4). However, controlled and prospective studies are lacking.

Obesity

Genetic, social, psychological and behavioral factors make it difficult either to prevent or to treat obesity. High caloric intake in obese patients is difficult to control and the achievement of early satiety is an important goal in reducing intake. In the stomach, rings of contraction originate in the antrum and sweep distally; the strongest ones occlude the gastric lumen entirely, propelling chyme through the pylorus, into the duodenum (Fig. 32.5). Even though several neuromediators are present in the gastrointestinal tract, and the complex gastric activity is influenced by endocrine and paracrine mediators, motility is mostly dependent on acetylcholine. This suggests a possible effect of BoNT injections into the antral muscles, weakening the propulsive contractions and interfering with gastric emptying.

Rats treated with BoNT gastric injections have a parallel reduction of body weight and food intake (Gui *et al.*, 2000), probably related to a significant delay of gastric emptying (Coskun *et al.*, 2005).

Currently, BoNT intraparietogastric injections in obese patients are still in early development (Foschi *et al.*, 2006; Gui *et al.*, 2006). Injections of BoNT (100–500 U type A) were made under endoscopic control, using a sclerotherapy injector needle, in 8, 16, 20 or 24 sites around the gastric antral circumferences, starting at a distance of 3 cm from the pyloric ring. In other studies, the fundus and the angulus were also injected (Fig. 32.6) (Gui *et al.*, 2006). The procedure was safe, without side effects. Early satiety was consistently reported as the most frequent subjective effect of the treatment. Body weight variations differed greatly; in one randomized study the difference between treated and control patients reached statistical significance (11 ± 1.09 kg versus 5.7 ± 1.1 kg; $p < 0.001$) (Foschi *et al.*, 2006). In another randomized controlled trial, a significant decrease of body weight and body mass index, together with a decrease of ghrelin and peptide YY levels was demonstrated (Li *et al.*, 2012). Botulinum neurotoxin may act by increasing the solid gastric emptying time and reducing the solid eating capacity of the stomach (Foschi *et al.*, 2008).

In conclusion, BoNT intraparietogastric injections seem to play a role in the manipulation of appetite, but

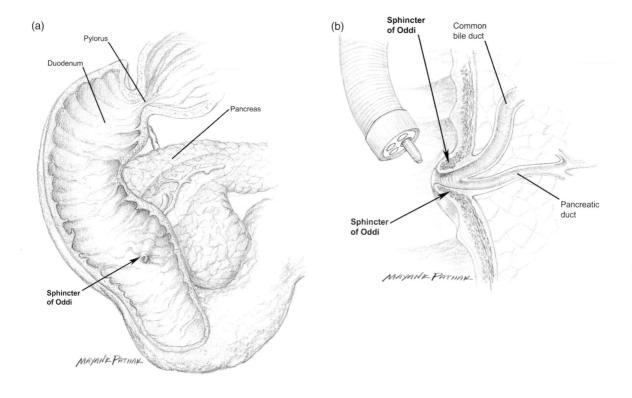

Fig. 32.4 Sphincter of Oddi dysfunction (demonstrated by biliary manometry and/or colangio-magnetic nuclear resonance imaging plus secretin stimulation). (a) The position of the sphincter of Oddi. (b) Toxin is delivered with a side view endoscope through a sclerotherapy needle at the papilla.

further studies are required to explore optimal modalities and possibilities of this new application.

Gastroparesis

Gastroparesis is an uncommon gastric motility disorder, mostly idiopathic or related to diabetes, that results in delayed gastric emptying, early satiety, postprandial fullness, bloating, epigastric pain, nausea, vomiting and weight loss. Motility-increasing drugs such as metoclopramide, erythromycin and domperidone (and the recently introduced tegaserod), have been extensively used, unfortunately, with poor results and prominent side effects.

Injection of BoNT into the pyloric ring, aimed at relaxing the sphincter, can reduce pyloric resistance and accelerate gastric emptying, as shown in several small series where 80–200 U onabotulinumtoxinA was administered in four or five sites circumferentially, using an endoscope (Fig. 32.7). The reported reduction in symptoms lasted for 1–3 months in the majority of patients.

Recently a systematic review evaluating 15 studies; almost all non-randomized controlled trials, reported significant improvement in subjective symptoms and gastric emptying. However, two randomized controlled trials did not confirm the efficacy of BoNT injection (Bai *et al.*, 2010).

OnabotulinumtoxinA has been administered to resolve pyloric spasm after the Whipple procedure (duodeno-cephalo-pancreatectomy) with pylorus preservation, but the results were inconsistent (Gui *et al.*, 2003). Occasionally, BoNT has been used for pyloric obstruction syndrome (after pyloroplasty for ulcer, pancreas transplantation, total esophagectomy) and in infants with hypertrophic pyloric stenosis, but results were unsatisfactory.

Chronic anal fissure

Anal fissure is a frequent, highly painful condition affecting both sexes in the young, otherwise healthy, population. The principal symptom is intense, long-lasting, postdefecatory pain. The first lesion is a mucosal tear,

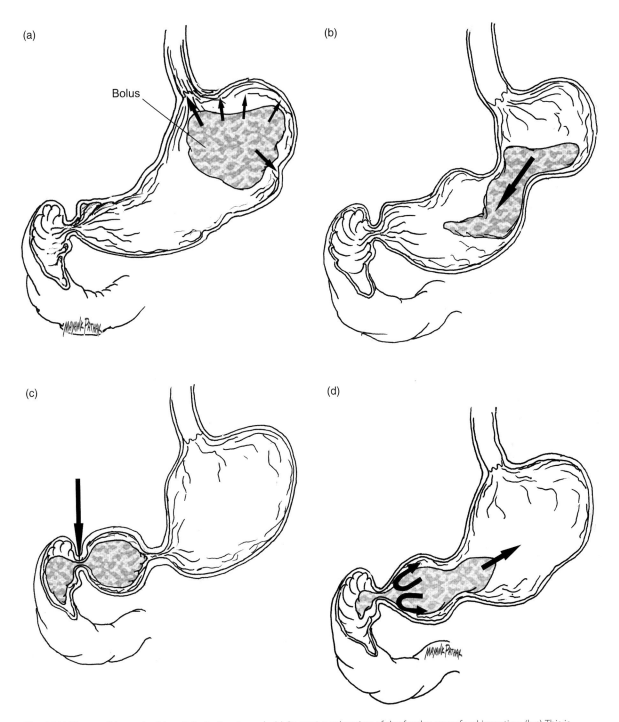

Fig. 32.5 Phases of the peristaltic activity in the stomach. (a) Receptive relaxation of the fundus upon food ingestion. (b,c) This is followed by the peristaltic movements, causing the food to advance towards the antrum and pylorus. (d) Based on antral pump strength and pylorus contraction strength, food may partly go through the duodenum or be totally repelled towards the gastric body and remixed.

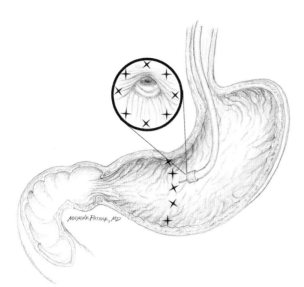

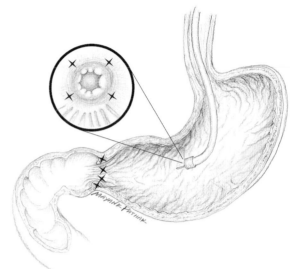

Fig. 32.6 Endoscopic injection of the stomach for obese patients in order to reduce antral propulsive peristalsis. A gastroscope is inserted into the stomach. A sclerotherapy needle advances inside the endoscope and is inserted in the gastric wall to inject the neurotoxin (not shown). The eight sites (X), frontal and lateral, where the neurotoxin was injected.

Fig. 32.7 Endoscopic injection of the stomach. A gastroscope is inserted into the stomach. A sclerotherapy needle advances inside the endoscope and is inserted in the gastric wall to inject the neurotoxin (not shown). The sites (X), frontal and lateral, on the pylorus quadrants where the neurotoxin is injected.

usually in the posterior anal commissure (Fig. 32.8). Even though constipation is frequently associated, the pathogenesis has not been completely elucidated and hypertonus of the internal anal sphincter (IAS) is deemed to play a critical role. The mucosal lesion causes intense pain and the reflex action to the pain seems to cause spastic contraction of the IAS, leading to compression of the small arterial vessels running through the muscular fibers of the sphincter. Blood shortage in the mucosa impairs the healing of the lesion – a vicious circle. If the lesion lasts over 3 months, it is considered "chronic" as it does not tend to heal spontaneously.

Current therapies for chronic anal fissure aim to reduce IAS tone, interrupting the sequence of pain and spasm. Surgical treatment (lateral internal sphincterotomy, anal dilatation) achieves this mechanically, reducing the strength of the muscle. Anal dilatation techniques have been progressively abandoned because of poor results and frequent side effects; lateral sphincterotomy is the most frequent surgical technique applied today, with a high success rate (97%), although incontinence of flatus or feces, up to 35% and 5.3%, respectively, has been reported (Khubchandani and Reed, 1989).

Medical spasmolitic therapies (i.e. topically applied nitroglycerin, isosorbide dinitrate or nifedipine) are effective to a limited extent but are often unpractical

and may be associated with tedious general side effects such as headache.

"Chemical sphincterotomy" with a single injection of onabotulinumtoxinA into the IAS was introduced in 1994 (Gui *et al.*, 1994). It has the advantage of a long-term effect (up to 4 months), reversibility of action, minimal invasiveness and a healing rate slightly short of results offered by surgery. The very rare side effects include short-term incontinence of flatus or feces, anal hematomas, acute inflammation of hemorrhoids and hemorrhoidal prolapse. Botulinum treatment is performed in the outpatient setting. No sedation or local analgesia is required.

In most cases, the IAS is easily identified by the surgeon's finger and the BoNT is injected in the muscle using a syringe with a 27-gauge needle (Fig. 32.8). Although the optimal dose of BoNT has not yet been established, usually a total of 10–50 U onabotulinumtoxinA is administered, preferentially in both sides of the anterior commissure (Gui *et al.*, 2003). The efficacy of BoNT was found equivalent to that of topical nitroglycerin and calcium channel blockers (Nelson *et al.*, 2012).

Puborectalis syndrome

Outlet obstruction related to pelvic floor dyssynergia is not an infrequent cause of constipation in the elderly and

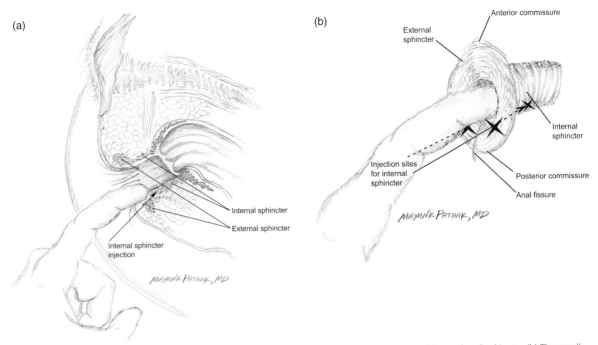

Fig. 32.8 Chronic anal fissure injection. (a) The surgeon's finger tip is used to identify the contracted internal anal sphincter. (b) The needle is inserted into the sphincter and the neurotoxin is injected.

middle-aged woman. It is characterized by a failure of the puborectalis muscle to relax during evacuation efforts or by its paradoxical contraction, with reduction of the ano-rectal angle, thus impeding the expulsion of feces from the rectum. Biofeedback training and relaxation exercises are beneficial in many patients; however, they are time consuming and lose effectiveness over time. Surgical division of the puborectalis muscle has been proposed, but it is associated with a high rate of incontinence.

Injection of BoNT into the muscle is a reversible and less invasive approach that can relax the spasm and increase the ano-rectal angle during straining, thus allowing for evacuation. A few studies have been reported in the literature (Gui *et al.*, 2003). Injections are administered without sedation, in the outpatient setting, under ultrasound or EMG control or other-wise guided by the surgeon's finger. With the patient in the lithotomy position, the needle is inserted into the perianal skin, 2–2.5 cm laterally of the anal orifice (Fig. 32.9) (Maria *et al.*, 2006).

Although the treatment remains an experimental procedure and optimal dose or standard technique have yet to be determined, BoNT injections seem to be an effective approach in outlet obstruction syndrome related to pelvic floor dyssynergia, particularly in patients with Parkinson's disease (Cadeddu *et al.*, 2005).

However, a study comparing the efficacy of BoNT injections with partial division of the puborectalis muscle demonstrated reduced efficacy with BoNT (86% and 100%, respectively) and shorter duration of the efficacy (40% and 66%, respectively, at 1 year)(Farid *et al.*, 2009).

Proctalgia fugax

Proctalgia fugax is defined as a sudden and severe pain in the anal region, mostly occurring at night and lasting for several seconds or minutes, then completely disap-pearing. The pathophysiology of this rare condition remains unclear, but it has been suggested that spasm of the IAS might be the cause. Data concerning the treatment of this disorder are very scarce. Diltiazem, clonidine, salbutamol and nitroglycerin ointments have been applied with some beneficial results (Bharucha *et al.*, 2006).

A few cases of BoNT injections into the IAS have been reported in literature. The injection technique is quite similar to the one used in anal fissure (Fig. 32.8), but in proctalgia the four quadrants of the IAS are injected. Results are described as promising; however, only a small proportion of patients benefit in the long term (Hollingshead *et al.*, 2011).

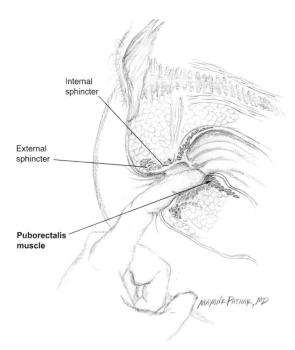

Internal
sphincter

External
sphincter

Puborectalis
muscle

MAYANK PATHAK, MD

Fig. 32.9 Puborectalis muscle injection. The procedure is basically the same as that for the internal anal sphincter (Fig. 32.8). The surgeon inserts his finger more deeply into the anal canal in order to perceive the bulging muscle, which encompasses the rectum in a semicircular way. This procedure may also be performed under transanal ultrasonographic guidance.

References

Annese V, Bassotti G (2006). Non-surgical treatment of esophageal achalasia. *World J Gastroenterol*, **12**, 5763–6.

Annese V Bassotti G, Coccia G et al. (1999). Comparison of two different formulations of botulinum toxin A for the treatment of oesophageal achalasia. The Gismad Achalasia Study Group. *Aliment Pharmacol Ther*, **13**, 1347–50.

Bai Y, Xu MJ, Yang X et al. (2010). A systematic review on intrapyloric botulinum toxin injection for gastroparesis. *Digestion*, **81**, 27–34.

Bashashati M, Andrews C, Ghosh S, Storr M (2010). Botulinum toxin in the treatment of diffuse esophageal spasm. *Dis Esophagus*, **23**, 554–60.

Bharucha AE, Wald A, Enck P, Rao S (2006). Functional anorectal disorders. *Gastroenterology*, **130**, 1510–18.

Cadeddu F, Bentivoglio AR, Brandara F et al. (2005). Outlet type constipation in Parkinson's disease: results of botulinum toxin treatment. *Aliment Pharmacol Ther*, **22**, 997–1003.

Coskun H, Duran Y, Dilege E et al. (2005). Effect on gastric emptying and weight reduction of botulinum toxin-A injection into the gastric antral layer: an experimental study in the obese rat model. *Obes Surg*, **15**, 1137–43.

Farid M, Youssef T, Mahdy T et al. (2009). Comparative study between botulinum toxin injection and partial division of puborectalis for treating anismus. *Int J Colorectal Dis*, **24**, 327–34.

Foschi D, Corsi F, Lazzaroni M et al. (2006). Treatment of morbid obesity by intraparietogastric administration of botulinum toxin: a randomized, double-blind, controlled study. *Int J Obes*, **31**, 707–12.

Foschi D, Lazzaroni M, Sangaletti O et al. (2008). Effects of intramural administration of botulinum toxin A on gastric emptying and eating capacity in obese patients. *Dig Liver Dis*, **40**, 667–72.

Fulmer SL, Merati AL, Blumin JH (2011). Efficacy of laryngeal botulinum toxin injection: comparison of two techniques. *Laryngoscope* **121**, 1924–8.

Gui D, Cassetta E, Anastasio G et al. (1994). Botulinum toxin for chronic anal fissure. *Lancet*, **344**, 1127–8.

Gui D, De Gaetano A, Spada PL et al. (2000). Botulinum toxin injected in the gastric wall reduces body weight and food intake in rats. *Aliment Pharmacol Ther*, **14**, 829–34.

Gui D, Rossi S, Runfola M, Magalini SC (2003). Review: botulinum toxin in the therapy of gastrointestinal motility disorders. *Aliment Pharmacol Ther*, **18**, 1–16.

Gui D, Mingrone G, Valenza V et al. (2006). Effect of botulinum toxin antral injection on gastric emptying and weight reduction in obese patients: a pilot study. *Aliment Pharmacol Ther*, **23**, 675–80.

Hollingshead JR, Maeda Y, Brown TJ, Warusavitarne J, Vaizey CJ (2011). Long-term outcome of the use of botulinum toxin injection for functional anal pain. *Colorectal Dis*, **13**, 293–6.

Khubchandani IT, Reed JF (1989). Sequelae of internal sphincterotomy for chronic fissure in ano. *Br J Surg*, **76**, 431–4.

Leyden JE, Moss AC, MacMathuna P (2006). Endoscopic pneumatic dilation versus botulinum toxin injection in the management of primary achalasia. *Cochrane Database Syst Rev*, (4), CD005046.

Li L, Liu QS, Liu WH et al. (2012). Treatment of obesity by endoscopic gastric intramural injection of botulinum toxin A: a randomized clinical trial. *Hepatogastroenterology*, **59**, 2003–7

Maria G, Cadeddu F, Brandara F, Marniga G, Brisinda G (2006). Experience with type A botulinum toxin for treatment of outlet-type constipation. *Am J Gastroenterol*, **101**, 2570–5.

Murray WR (2011). Botulinum toxin-induced relaxation of the sphincter of Oddi may select patients with acalculous biliary pain who will benefit from cholecystectomy. *Surg Endosc* **25**, 813–16.

Nelson RL, Thomas K, Morgan J, Jones A (2012). Non surgical therapy for anal fissure. *Cochrane Database Syst Rev*, (**2**), CD003431.

Pasricha PJ, Ravich WJ, Hendrix TR *et al.* (1994). Treatment of achalasia with intrasphincteric injection of botulinum toxin. A pilot trial. *Ann Intern Med*, **121**, 590–1.

Pehlivanov N, Pasricha PJ (2006). Achalasia: botox, dilatation or laparoscopic surgery in 2006. *Neurogastroenterol Motil*, **18**, 799–804.

Zaninotto G, Marchese Ragona R, Briani C *et al.* (2004). The role of botulinum toxin injection and upper esophageal sphincter myotomy in treating oropharyngeal dysphagia. *J Gastrointest Surg*, **8**, 997–1006.

Chapter 33

Botulinum neurotoxin applications in urological disorders

Brigitte Schurch and Stefano Carda

Introduction

Botulinum neurotoxin (BoNT) is licensed for the treatment of a number of conditions characterized by striated muscle spasticity. However, in recent years, their unlicensed use in the treatment of lower urinary tract conditions has been described (Smith *et al.*, 2004). Chief amongst these are conditions characterized by detrusor overactivity. Treatment of vulvodynia and chronic pelvic pain, benign prostate hyperplasia (BPH) and detrusor sphincter dyssynergia (DSD) are other emerging indications with promising positive results.

Overactive bladder

The International Continence Society (ICS) report of 2002 defined overactive bladder syndrome as urgency, with or without urge incontinence, usually with frequency and nocturia, and in the absence of local pathological or hormonal factors (Abrams *et al.*, 2002). The prevalence in Europe and USA was estimated to be 3% among men 40–44 years of age, 9% among women 40–44 years of age, 42% among men 75 years of age or older and 31% among women 75 years of age or older (Tubaro, 2004). The symptoms of overactive bladder have many potential causes and contributing factors. Urination involves the cerebral cortex, the pons, the spinal cord, the peripheral autonomic, somatic and sensory afferent innervation of the lower urinary tract and the anatomical components of the lower urinary tract itself. Disorders of any of these structures may contribute to the symptoms of overactive bladder (Fig. 33.1).

A variety of efferent and afferent neural pathways, reflexes and central and peripheral neurotransmitters are involved in urine storage and bladder emptying. Acetylcholine, which interacts with muscarinic receptors on the detrusor muscle, is the predominant peripheral neurotransmitter responsible for bladder contraction. The muscarinic receptor subtype M_3 appears to be the most clinically relevant in the human bladder. Acetylcholine interacts with the M_3 receptor, initiating a cascade of events that result in contraction of the detrusor muscle. The M_2 receptor may also facilitate bladder contraction by reducing intracellular levels of cyclic AMP. Pathological states can alter sensitivity to muscarinic stimulation. For example, bladder outflow obstruction appears to enhance responsiveness to

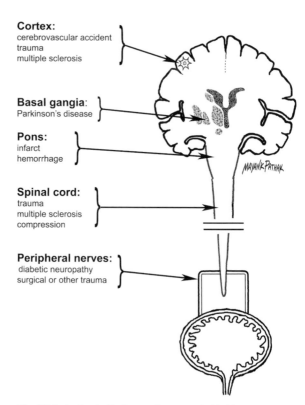

Cortex:
cerebrovascular accident
trauma
multiple sclerosis

Basal ganglia:
Parkinson's disease

Pons:
infarct
hemorrhage

Spinal cord:
trauma
multiple sclerosis
compression

Peripheral nerves:
diabetic neuropathy
surgical or other trauma

MAYANK PATHAK

Fig. 33.1 Anatomical lesions and neurogenic bladder.

Manual of Botulinum Toxin Therapy, 2nd edition, ed. Daniel Truong, Mark Hallett, Christopher Zachary and Dirk Dressler. Published by Cambridge University Press. © Cambridge University Press 2013.

acetylcholine, a phenomenon similar to denervation supersensitivity.

Many classes of drug, particularly anticholinergics, have been studied or proposed for the treatment of symptoms of overactive bladder. All anticholinergic drugs can have bothersome side effects. Although dry mouth is the most common, constipation, gastroesophageal reflux, blurry vision, urinary retention and cognitive side effects can also occur. Since various forms of dementia are routinely treated with cholinesterase inhibitors, the potential for adverse cognitive effects and delirium with antimuscarinic drugs is a particular concern in the older population. Direct injection of BoNT into the detrusor muscle (which inhibits acetylcholine at the presynaptic cholinergic junction but may also have an important role on the afferent pathways of the lower urinary tract [Ikeda et al., 2012]) appears to ameliorate detrusor hyperreflexia in patients with spinal cord injury (Cruz et al., 2011; Herschorn et al., 2011; Ginsberg et al., 2012). It also has therapeutic value in selected patients with severe refractory overactive bladder (Duthie et al., 2011). Injection technique consists of injecting mainly the detrusor and sparing the trigone (Fig. 33.2) using a rigid or a flexible cystoscope. However, a recent randomized study comparing trigone-sparing with trigone-including injections showed better results in the latter group (Manecksha et al., 2012).

Patients have either mild conscious sedation or general anesthesia. Injection doses reported in the literature have varied between 100 and 300 U (mouse units) onabotulinumtoxinA and 500 and 1000 U abobotulinumtoxinA for neurogenic detrusor overactivity. Injection doses have varied between 100 and 300 U onabotulinumtoxinA (diluted from 10 to 30 ml with 0.9% saline) and 300 to 1000 U abobotulinumtoxinA (dilution from 100 UI/ml to 25 UI/ml) for idiopathic detrusor overactivity. Injection sites have varied between 20 and 30 for neurogenic detrusor overactivity and 10 to 30 for idiopathic detrusor overactivity. For each treatment, the recommended dose for abobotulinumtoxinA seems to be 500–750 U and for onabotulinumtoxinA from 100 to 300 U.

Mean duration of improvement has varied between 6 and 9 months with onabotulinumtoxinA and between 5 and 10 months with abobotulinumtoxinA. The continence improvement rate is 86.5% with onabotulinumtoxinA and 86% with abobotulinumtoxinA. No side effects related to the injection itself

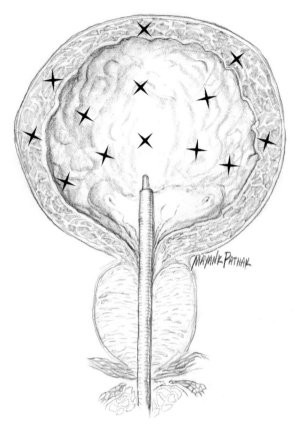

Fig. 33.2 Botulinum neurotoxin A injection into the bladder: detrusor mapping.

have been reported with the exception of a risk of urinary tract infections of 7.1–24%; for this reason, some authors recommend the use of antibiotic prophylaxis with a short course of trimethoprim or quinolones. There are occasional reports of general weakness using onabotulinumtoxinA (2 of the 340 treated patients [0.6%]), whereas general weakness has been described in 2.5–5% with abobotulinumtoxinA (255 treated patients). RimabotulinumtoxinB is efficient in treating idiopathic detrusor overactivity, but because of its short duration of effect, it is better used as a secondary treatment in patients who become resistant to BoNT type A products.

Conclusions

Injection with BoNT for overactive bladder appears to be a treatment with high efficacy that meets evidence-based medicine level I criteria (i.e. prospective, randomized controlled clinical trial with masked outcome assessment, in a representative population), with an acceptable safety profile. Repeated injections appear as effective as the first one (Giannantoni *et al.*, 2009; Sahai *et al.*, 2010; Dowson *et al.*, 2012). Additional controlled, double-blind studies are needed and particularly studies in idiopathic detrusor overactivity to further explore this treatment option.

Vulvodynia and chronic pelvic pain

Vulvodynia

Vulvodynia is a chronic disorder in women defined as vulvar discomfort, most often described as burning pain, occurring in the absence of relevant findings or a specific clinically identifiable neurological disorder (Moyal-Barracco and Lynch, 2003) and characterized by provoked or unprovoked vulvar pain of varying intensity without obvious concomitant clinical pathology. Two subtypes of vulvodynia are recognized: generalized and localized. The latter is currently referred to as vestibulodynia or vestibulitis.

In addition to vulvar pain, there is typically burning and, less often, itching. Onset is usually abrupt and the typical patient is between 20 and 45 years of age. Vulvodynia has been shown to affect 15–20% of the female population in the USA (Bachmann and Rosen, 2006). There is a limited number of studies on the use of BoNT for the treatment of vulvodynia (Brin and Vapnek, 1997; Shafik and El-Sibai, 2000; Gunter *et al.*, 2004; Dykstra and Presthus, 2006; Bertolasi *et al.*, 2009; Pelletier *et al.*, 2011). Initial studies targeted overactive muscle sites in the vagina and pelvic floor with the intention of decreasing muscle spasm and, therefore, pain. Because recent research has suggested that BoNT may affect peripheral and central sensitization, researchers have targeted overactive muscle and painful tissue areas with the intention of relaxing muscle and inhibiting the release of neurotransmitters that can cause pain and inflammation (substance P and calcitonin gene-related peptide) (Dykstra and Presthus, 2006).

Injection techniques with BoNT for vulvodynia range from 10 U to 50 U onabotulinumtoxinA and 150 U to 400 U abobotulinumtoxinA. Dilutions of BoNT have ranged from 0.5 ml to 1.0 ml. Injection sites have included the anterior vaginal wall muscles, the puborectalis, pubococcygeus, perineal body, bulbocavernosus and bulbospongiosus muscle (Figs. 33.3 and 33.4). The number of injection sites in each muscle has varied from one to three. Needle size

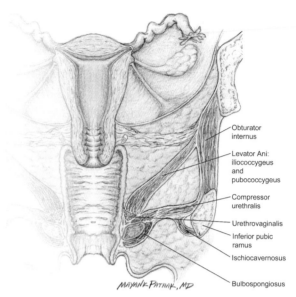

Fig. 33.3 Vaginal and pelvic floor muscles.

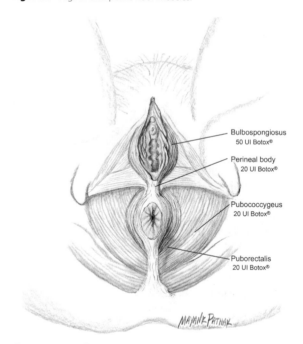

Fig. 33.4 Pelvic floor muscles.

has been between 23- and 30-gauge. Patients had either no sedation or mild conscious sedation. Electromyography has been used in a few studies to locate the muscle being injected. Studies have been mainly single or multiple case series with single or multiple follow-up injections. One study was controlled (Shafik and El-Sibai, 2000), whereas all others were prospective cohort studies or case reports. All studies showed improvement in most patients regarding pain, muscle spasm, quality of life and sexual activity. Duration of effects lasted from 4 weeks to 2 years. A small number of patients were cured. No significant adverse effects were noted in any study. Therapy with BoNT is suggested for women with hyperactive pelvic floor at physical examination, or for those who respond poorly to oral drugs and/or surgical procedures. It should be noted that the actual level of evidence for use of BoNT in vulvodynia is low, and it is not currently recommended as a first-line treatment by current guidelines (Nunns *et al.*, 2010).

Chronic pelvic pain

Non-malignant pain may be perceived in structures related to the pelvis of both males and females. Pain must have been continuous or recurrent for at least 6 months. If non-acute and central sensitization pain mechanisms are well documented, the pain may be regarded as chronic, irrespective of the time period. In all cases, there are often associated negative cognitive, behavioral, sexual and emotional consequences (Fall *et al.*, 2010).

Approximately 15–20% of women aged 18–50 years have chronic pelvic pain of greater than 1 year in duration (an estimated number greater than for migraine, asthma and back pain) (Howard, 2003). Chronic pelvic pain may result from psychological disorders or neurological diseases, both central and peripheral. Sufficient evidence strongly suggests that several of the most common disorders in women, such as endometriosis, interstitial cystitis, irritable bowel syndrome and pelvic inflammatory disease, are causes of chronic pelvic pain. In men, chronic pelvic pain syndrome is an enigmatic medical condition that has been classified as category III chronic pelvic pain syndrome or non-bacterial chronic prostatitis, and, more recently, as prostate pain syndromes (Fall *et al.*, 2010).

Patients with chronic pelvic pain may have generalized or localized pelvic pain, pain with intercourse, pain with ejaculation, pain exacerbation after sexual intercourse, pain exacerbated both premenstrually and menstrually and complaints of voiding symptoms of frequency, urgency and nicturia (Howard 2003).

There are a few studies on the use of BoNT for the treatment of chronic pelvic pain (Jarvis *et al.*, 2004; Thomson *et al.*, 2005; Abbot *et al.*, 2006; Meredeth *et al.*, 2006; Gottsch *et al.*, 2011). These studies have included both male and female patients. Injection techniques with BoNT for chronic pelvic pain have ranged from 40 to 200 U onabotulinumtoxinA. Dilutions have ranged from 2 to 4 ml. Injection sites have included the puborectalis (20 to 50 U onabotulinumtoxinA), pubococcygeus (25 U onabotulinumtoxinA), the bulbospongiosus (25 U onabotulinumtoxinA), the perineal body (25 U onabotulinumtoxinA) and the external urethral sphincter muscles (Fig. 33.4). The number of injections into each muscle has ranged from three to five sites, and a 22-gauge needle is usually used. Patients have had either no sedation or only mild conscious sedation. Electromyography was used in two studies to improve muscle localization. Two studies were randomized and placebo controlled (Abbott *et al.*, 2006; Gottsch *et al.*, 2011), while the others were prospective cohort studies or case series. All studies showed improvement in most patients regarding pain, spasm, quality of life and sexual activity. Duration of effect was 3 to 18 months. No adverse effects were noted. There was a reduction in dyspareunia and non-menstrual pelvic pain, associated with a significant reduction in pelvic floor pressure, in the BoNT-treated group (Abbott *et al.*, 2006) and a modest but significant reduction of the Global Response Assessment and of the pain subdomain of the Chronic Prostatitis Symptom Index in the BoNT group compared with placebo group (Gottsch *et al.*, 2011).

Conclusions

The use of BoNT for the treatment of vulvodynia and chronic pelvic pain may be a viable option for patients. Adequately powered, controlled, double-blind studies are needed to further explore this treatment option.

Benign prostatic hyperplasia

Non-malignant enlargement of the prostate (BPH) is regarded as a major cause of bladder outlet obstruction. Because surgical denervation was known to produce profound atrophy in the rat prostate, onabotulinumtoxinA was used to show selective chemical denervation and subsequent atrophy in the rat prostate. The pathophysiology of BPH may involve a dynamic component that reflects the smooth muscle tone within the gland and a static component that is related to the mass effect of the enlarged prostate. Botulinum neurotoxin may have an effect on both components by relaxing smooth muscle and causing atrophy of the glandular tissue.

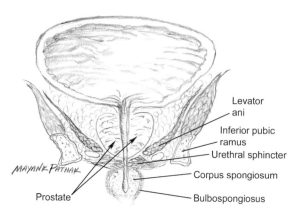

Fig. 33.5 Male genetalia and prostate.

There have been a few studies on the use of BoNT in humans. Injections of 100–300 U onabotulinumtoxinA have been made at two to ten sites, with a 4–20 ml dilution factor. The injections were made into the transition zone at the lateral lobes and median lobes of the prostate or into both lateral lobes of the prostate (Fig. 33.5). Needle size was 21-, 22- or 23-gauge and injections were guided by rectal utrasound, transrectal ultrasound or cystoscope. The procedure was carried out without sedation or anesthesia, under light intravenous sedation or under general anesthesia. No meaningful difference was observed between using 100 or 300 U onabotulinumtoxinA (Crawford *et al.*, 2011). Most studies were case series, while one was a double-blind, placebo-controlled randomized study (Maria *et al.*, 2003).

In all studies, patients showed improvement in mean prostate volumes, symptom scores, quality-of-life measurements, postvoid residual volumes, peak flow rates and serum prostate-specific antigen concentration (Maria *et al.*, 2003; Silva *et al.*, 2008, 2009; Brisinda *et al.*, 2009; Crawford *et al.*, 2011). Onset of effects was within 1 week of injection and duration was from 3 to 9 months.

Conclusions

The use of onabotulinumtoxinA for treatment of BPH may be a viable option for selected patients. Controlled, double-blind studies are needed to further explore this treatment option.

Detrusor sphincter dyssynergia

Detrusor sphincter dyssynergia (DSD) is an involuntary contraction of the external urethral sphincter (Figs. 33.6 and 33.7) during detrusor contraction.

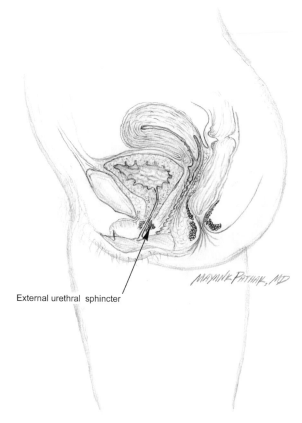

Fig. 33.6 External urethral sphincter injection using EMG in a woman. The arrowhead indicates approximate injection site.

Patients with spinal cord injuries are particulary vulnerable to this problem. It causes voiding dysfunction and can lead to high intravesical pressure, autonomic hyperreflexia, hydroureteronephrosis, infection and renal failure.

There are a limited number of studies on the use of BoNT for the treatment of DSD. Doses have ranged from 40 to 100 U onabotulinumtoxinA and 150 to 250 U abobotulinumtoxinA. Injections have been performed either transperineally or endoscopically with 21- to 23-gauge needles using both EMG (Figs. 33.6 and 33.7) (Chen *et al.*, 2008, 2011) and non-EMG techniques. Early techniques used frequent injections (weekly or monthly) because initial findings suggested that more frequent injections lasted longer. Because of immunogenic concerns, however, injections are now limited to at least 3-month intervals. Currently, injections into the external sphincter are performed using one to four injection sites with a volume of 1–4 ml (Figs. 33.6 and 33.7).

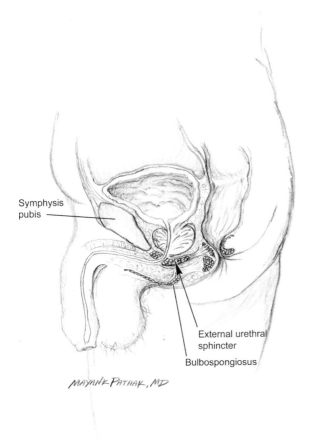

Symphysis
pubis

External urethral
sphincter

Bulbospongiosus

MAYANK PATHAK, MD

Fig. 33.7 External urethral sphincter injection using EMG in a man. The arrowhead indicates approximate injection site.

Autonomic dysreflexia is monitored during the injections.

Results in patients with spinal cord injury and DSD show improvement in urodynamic parameters such as postvoid residual volume, detrusor pressure on voiding and urethral pressure profiles. Duration of effects lasts from 2 to 9 months. However, patients with multiple sclerosis and DSD who were injected with a single dose of 100 U onabotulinumtoxinA did not show similarly favorable results (Gallien *et al.*, 2005). We recommend a dilution of 50 to 100 UI/ml for onabotulinumtoxinA.

Conclusions

The use of BoNT for patients with spinal cord injury and DSD appears to be a viable treatment option. Its use in patients with multiple sclerosis and DSD does not appear helpful. Further controlled studies are needed to clarify dose, technique, response and ideal patient population.

References

Abbott JA, Jarvis SK, Lyons SD, Thomson A, Vancaille TG (2006). Botulinum toxin type A for chronic pain and pelvic floor spasm in women: a randomized controlled trial. *Obstet Gynecol*, **108**, 915–23.

Abrams P, Cardozo L, Fall M *et al.* (2002). The standardisation of terminology of lower urinary tract function: report from the Standardisation Subcommittee of the International Continence Society. *Neurourol Urodyn*, **21**, 167–78.

Bachmann GA, Rosen R (2006). Vulvodynia: a state-of-the-art consensus on definitions, diagnosis and management. *J Reprod Med*, **51**, 447–56.

Bertolasi L, Frasson E, Cappelletti JY *et al.* (2009). Botulinum neurotoxin type A injections for vaginismus secondary to vulvar vestibulitis syndrome. *Obstet Gynecol*, **114**, 1008–16.

Brin MF, Vapnek JM (1997). Treatment of vaginismus with botulinum toxin injections. *Lancet*, **349**, 252–3.

Brisinda G, Cadeddu F. Vanella S *et al.* (2009). Relief by botulinum toxin of lower urinary tract symptoms owing to benign prostatic hyperplasia: early and long-term results. *Urology*, **73**, 90–4.

Chen SL, Bih LI, Huang YH *et al.* (2008). Effect of single botulinum toxin A injection to the external urethral sphincter for treating detrusor external sphincter dyssynergia in spinal cord injury. *J Rehabil Med*, **40**, 744–8.

Chen SL, Bih LI, Chen GD, Huang YH, You YH (2011). Comparing a transrectal ultrasound-guided with a cystoscopy-guided botulinum toxin A injection in treating detrusor external sphincter dyssynergia in spinal cord injury. *Am J Phys Med Rehabil*, **90**, 723–30.

Crawford ED, Hirst K, Kusek JW *et al.* (2011). Effects of 100 and 300 units of onabotulinum toxin A on lower urinary tract symptoms of benign prostatic hyperplasia: a phase II randomized clinical trial. *J Urol*, **186**, 965–70.

Cruz F, Herschorn S, Aliotta P *et al.* (2011). Efficacy and safety of onabotulinumtoxinA in patients with urinary incontinence due to neurogenic detrusor overactivity: a randomised, double-blind, placebo-controlled trial. *Eur Urol*, **60**, 742–50.

Dowson C, Watkins J, Khan MS, Dasgupta P, Sahai A (2012). Repeated botulinum toxin type A injections for refractory overactive bladder: medium-term outcomes, safety profile, and discontinuation rates. *Eur Urol*, **61**, 834–9.

Duthie JB, Vincent M, Herbison GP, Wilson DI, Wilson D (2011). Botulinum toxin injections for adults with overactive bladder syndrome. *Cochrane Database Syst Rev*, **(12)**, CD005493.

Dykstra DD, Presthus J (2006). Botulinum toxin type A for the treatment of provoked vestibulodynia: an open-label, pilot study. *J Reprod Med*, **51**, 467–70.

Fall M, Baranowski AP, Elneil S *et al.* (2010). EAU guidelines on chronic pelvic pain. *Eur Urol*, **57**, 35–48.

Gallien P, Reymann JM, Amarenco G *et al.* (2005). Placebo controlled, randomised, double blind study of the effects of botulinum A toxin on detrusor sphincter dyssynergia in multiple sclerosis patients. *J Neurol Neurosurg Psychiatry*, **76**, 1670–6.

Giannantoni A, Mearini E, Del Zingaro M, Porena M (2009). Six-year follow-up of botulinum toxin a intradetrusorial injections in patients with refractory neurogenic detrusor overactivity: clinical and urodynamic results. *Eur Urol*, **55**, 705–12.

Ginsberg D, Gousse A, Keppenne V *et al.* (2012). Phase 3 efficacy and tolerability study of onabotulinumtoxinA for urinary incontinence from neurogenic detrusor overactivity. *J Urol*, **187**, 2131–9.

Gottsch HP, Yang CC, Berger RE (2011). A pilot study of botulinum toxin A for male chronic pelvic pain syndrome. *Scand J Urol Nephrol*, **45**, 72–6.

Gunter J, Brewer A, Tawfik O (2004). Botulinum toxin a for vulvodynia: a case report. *J Pain*, **5**, 238–40.

Herschorn S, Gajewski J, Ethans K *et al.* (2011). Efficacy of botulinum toxin A injection for neurogenic detrusor overactivity and urinary incontinence: a randomized, double-blind trial. *J Urol*, **185**, 2229–35.

Howard FM (2003). Chronic pelvic pain. *Obstet Gynecol*, **101**, 594–611.

Ikeda Y, Zabbarova IV, Birder LA *et al.* (2012). Botulinum neurotoxin serotype A suppresses neurotransmitter release from afferent as well as efferent nerves in the urinary bladder. *Eur Urol*, **62**, 1157–64.

Jarvis SK, Abbott JA, Lenart MB, Steensma A, Vancaillie TG (2004). Pilot study of botulinum toxin type A in the treatment of chronic pelvic pain associated with spasm of the levator ani muscles. *Aust N Z J Obstet Gynaecol*, **44**, 46–50.

Manecksha RP, Cullen IM, Ahmad S *et al.* (2012). Prospective randomised controlled trial comparing trigone-sparing versus trigone-including intradestrusor injection of abobotulinumtoxinA for refractory idiopathic detrusor overactivity. *Eur Urol*, **61**, 928–35.

Maria G, Brisinda G, Civello IM *et al.* (2003). Relief by botulinum toxin of voiding dysfunction due to benign prostatic hyperplasia: results of a randomized, placebo-controlled study. *Urology*, **62**, 259–64.

Meredeth M, Karp B, Bartrum D, Zimmer C, Stratton P (2006). Botulinum toxin in the treatment of chronic pain and endometriosis. *J Soc Gynecol Invest*, **13**, 276A.

Moyal-Barracco M, Lynch PJ (2004). 2003 ISSVD terminology and classification of vulvodynia: a historical perspective. *J Reprod Med*, **49**, 772–7.

Nunns D, Mandal D, Byrne M for the British Society for the Study of Vulvar Disease Guideline Group (2010). Guidelines for the management of vulvodynia. *Br J Dermatol*, **162**, 1180–5.

Pelletier F, Parratte B, Penz S *et al.* (2011). Efficacy of high doses of botulinum toxin A for treating provoked vestibulodynia. *Br J Dermatol*, **164**, 617–22.

Sahai A, Dowson C, Khan MS, Dasgupta P (2010). Repeated injections of botulinum toxin-A for idiopathic detrusor overactivity. *Urology*, **75**, 552–8.

Shafik A, El-Sibai O (2000). Vaginismus: results of treatment with botulin toxin. *J Obstet Gynaecol*, **20**, 300–2.

Silva J, Silva C, Saraiva L *et al.* (2008). Intraprostatic botulinum toxin type A injection in patients unfit for surgery presenting with refractory urinary retention and benign prostatic enlargement. Effect on prostate volume and micturition resumption. *Eur Urol*, **53**, 153–9.

Silva J, Pinto R, Carvalho T *et al.* (2009). Intraprostatic botulinum toxin type A injection in patients with benign prostatic enlargement: duration of the effect of a single treatment. *BMC Urol*, **9**, 9.

Smith CP, Somogyi GT, Boone TB (2004). Botulinum toxin in urology: evaluation using an evidence-based medicine approach. *Nat Clin Pract Urol*, **1**, 31–7.

Thomson AJ, Jarvis SK, Lenart M, Abbott JA, Vancaillie TG (2005). The use of botulinum toxin type A (BOTOX) as treatment for intractable chronic pelvic pain associated with spasm of the levator ani muscles. *BJOG*, **112**, 247–9.

Tubaro A (2004). Defining overactive bladder: epidemiology and burden of disease. *Urology*, **64**, 2–6.

Index

Note: page numbers in *italics* refer to figures and tables; those in **bold** refer to boxes.